The Mind-Brain Continuum

The Mind-Brain Continuum

Sensory Processes

edited by
Rodolfo Llinás and Patricia S. Churchland

A Bradford Book
The MIT Press
Cambridge, Massachusetts
London, England

This book was set in Palatino by Asco Trade Typesetting Ltd., Hong Kong and was printed and bound in the United States of America.

Library of Congress Cataloging-in-Publication Data

The mind-brain continuum : sensory processes / edited by Rodolfo
   Llinás and Patricia S. Churchland.
      p.   cm.
   "A Bradford book."
   Proceedings of a meeting held in Madrid in 1995.
   Includes bibliographical references and index.
   ISBN 0-262-12198-0
   1. Perception—Congresses. 2. Neuropsychology—Congresses.
3. Senses and sensation—Congresses. I. Llinás, Rodolfo R.
(Rodolfo Riascos), 1934–   . II. Churchland, Patricia Smith.
QP441.M56   1996
612.8—dc20   95-46160
                                                           CIP

Contents

Foreword

The idea of generating a set of encounters between members of the different fields of neuroscience, to include neurophilosophy, in order to propose global views concerning the so-called mind-body problem was conceived in a discussion between ourselves and Rodolfo Llinás. Having concluded that such could be an intellectually attractive possibility, the three of us sat down in Madrid at the Instituto Marañon to discuss the possibilities of organizing such an encounter to be housed in Spain and to consider possible sponsors. After a long deliberation it became clear that such a meeting would be extraordinarily useful and that probably the very distinguished BBV Foundation (Banco de Bilbao y Viscaya) could defer the cost of such a meeting. A year or so later the meeting took place in Madrid, where Spanish intellectuals and a set of international scientists and philosophers gathered to have one of the most enlightening four days that we have seen on this topic. The book that you now read was put together by the invitees to the symposium and, while it may not represent a point of view relating to the "mind" that the BBV Foundation necessarily endorses, it is, in our view, an outstanding compilation of present-day ideas concerning what the authors have chosen to call the "mind-brain continuum." As instigators of the initial idea, we therefore choose to write this prologue to thank the BBV Foundation for their support and in the hopes that the Foundation will support other meetings in this realm in years to come. Indeed, in our first discussion, we were expecting to generate a set of consecutive encounters that would initially cover the sensory domain and then proceed to the motor, emotional, mnestic, and cognitivity aspects of this mind-brain continuum.

Finally, we are very happy to see that this vision of four years ago has come to fruition in this very elegant and thought-provoking book.

Antonio Fernandez de Molina
Pedro Lain Entralgo

Introduction

Mental activity, it appears, *is* brain activity. After the empirical rough and tumble of the last hundred years, that is by far the most parsimonious and productive hypothesis left on the table. The traditional Cartesian posit of a radical discontinuity between the mental and the neural has weathered poorly as biology in general, and neuroscience in particular, inched forward. Our phrase "mind-brain continuum" conveys the absence of any discontinuity. In addition, it commands a more succinct and forward-looking profile than the doubly negated, heavily freighted rendition, the mind and brain are not discontinuous in the Cartesian sense.

Recognizing that the notion of a continuum has its roots in mathematics, we are taking the liberty of using the word in a modified fashion to suit the neurobiological context. The nub of what we mean to convey is quite straightforward: first, that perceiving, thinking, introspecting, and so forth, are activities of the brain. Second, the expression connotes the smooth integration of functional properties at all levels of organization, from cells, networks, and systems, to behavior, which in turn connotes the likelihood of their ultimate explanatory unification in a large-scale, top-to-bottom theory. Finally, it reflects the profoundly important fact that humans brains evolved from the brains of preceding animals, sharing much with them structurally and functionally as well as cognitively. However remarkable the human brain is, it is a product of Darwinian evolution, with all the constraints that such a history implies.

True to the scientist's old saw, God is in the details. Assuming mental activities are brain activities, it is in the factual details—the details of anatomy, physiology, neurochemistry, developmental neuroscience, and psychophysics—that the truth is to be found. None of us can really be satisfied until we understand how brains do what they do—exactly how it is that the mind-brain is a continuum. Needless to say, the details do not just arrange themselves into an explanatory framework. To wrest an explanatory understanding of how the brain makes a mind, a necessary continuing task is to integrate facts into a common theoretical framework. What are especially needed are the invention of new ideas together with an airing of meaningful patterns, pregnant possibilities, and newly discerned puzzles.

Given the extraordinary complexity of nervous systems, the vast reach of the neurobiological enterprise, and the technological difficulties confronting research, powerful centrifugal forces send individual research off into distant data-rich hinterlands. Since explanation is our goal, these exploratory forces must be counterbalanced by forces pulling the discoveries back into a common, integrative framework. Only then do we get the real—explanatory— pay-off. It is not surprising that there are different but mutually supporting strategies for achieving coherence. One common strategy is to go narrow, deep, and exhaustive, pulling together, for example, research on a particular type of neuronal property such as synaptic plasticity in hippocampal neurons or the properties of pyramidal cells in visual area V1 of the macaque. A different kind of utility derives from taking a broad sweep and exposing to critical discussion seminal, if yet-to-be confirmed, ideas. An uneasy tension exists in the current (largely) pretheoretical state of neuroscience, between the need to be finer and finer grained, and the need to keep the general contours of the problem in view. The dangers of fact-poor, smitten-by-grand-theory-ism are complemented by the dangers of hypothesis-poor, isolated-fact infatuation.

Our particular strategy in this volume aims for the benefits of the broad sweep format, narrowed for manageability to a subset of brain functions, namely, the sensory capacities, where each topic is firmly tethered by hard data. In this design we were guided by the conviction that a specific integrative purpose is served by counterpoising different sensory modalities (not just vision), different brain structures (not just the cortex), different species (not just the macaque), different stages of development (not just adults), ranging across human lesion studies, single-cell physiology, to behavioral manipulations in ecologically normal as well as highly abnormal conditions that push the limits of a sensory capacity. Our hope is that this format will midwife the birth of empirically healthy, if sometimes rambunctious, theoretical ideas.

While the concept of the mind-brain continuum is the major backdrop for this work, the second framework feature looming out the empirical data is what one might call, for want of a better word, "endogenesis." The crux here is that sensory experience is not created by incoming signals from the world, but by intrinsic, continuing processes of the brain. The essential functions of incoming signals on this view are to trellis, shape, and otherwise sculpt the intrinsic activity to yield a survival-facilitating, me-in-the-world representational scheme.

How then does the brain's internal activity actually represent the external world? How do we know reality? In simplest terms, the answer would be that biological evolution has provided the basic intrinsic wherewithal, and learning in its many forms tunes up the wherewithal. Remarkably, nervous systems are both highly constrained in their overall structural and functional properties by genetic and dynamic considerations, and yet within those constraints they are also astonishingly plastic. To consider but one example, amputees typically have an enduring experience of a phantom limb, yet specific somatosensory feelings in the phantom can be generated by touching existing body parts in the the corresponding region. They can even be produced by the right visual interactions. Receptive field properties of single cells are clearly not fixed and final even in the adult, but shift within certain yet-to-be quantified limits. This suggests, therefore, that it is also *because* of the nature of general genetic constraints, whatever precisely they really are, that nervous systems display the specific dimensions of plasticity that they do. Part of the brain's business is to make it possible for us to learn, but learning seems to be more a matter of reconfiguring or returning or recalibrating what is there than building from scratch. Which means that it is part of the genes' business to make brains that can appropriately tune their internal worlds to permit successful, causally propitious interactions with the external world. In highly complex organisms such as humans, these interactions can even involve deployment of representational schemata that have emerged from the broadly scientific enterprise, representations such as "atom" and "voltage." The reality we know is, inevitably, reality as portrayed by the brain. Nevertheless, given our evolutionary bequest, including our capacity to devise theories, tools, and instruments, the brain's portrait of reality can become ever more harmonious with what's really out there.

P. S. Churchland and R. Llinás

The Mind-Brain Continuum

1 The Brain as a Closed System Modulated by the Senses

R. Llinás and D. Paré

In reviewing the progress of neuroscience during the last decades, it is clear that truly fundamental discoveries relating to the structure and function of the nervous system—ranging from the molecular to the cellular and systems levels—have surfaced. It is also evident that many properties germane to the global functioning of the system still elude our analysis and, often, our attention.

Present-day science has been characterized by a trend toward analysis rather than synthesis. The study of neuroscience is no exception; our research has often failed to extend beyond the description of the properties of neurons and of the networks they weave. Fortunately, this trend is less prevalent in sensory physiology, where it is accepted that the geometric and refractive properties of the eye, by transforming light wavefronts into images, provide the context for the organization of the visual system at all levels of evolution. Thus, a continuum in levels of analysis from the molecular to the psychophysical has been implemented.[8] Similarly, the spatial arrangement of the semicircular canals or the resonant properties of the basilar membrane in the organ of Corti provide the necessary coordinate systems that allow neuronal activity to represent angular acceleration and sound, respectively.[1] However, context-dependent analysis becomes difficult, and therefore uncommon, when moving away from the peripheral sensory systems. In this paper we intend to outline a possible path toward cognition on the basis of cellular neuroscience.

COMPUTATION IN THE BRAIN AND THE ESTABLISHMENT OF CATEGORIES

If we follow the flow of activity into the nervous system away from the peripheral sensory apparatus or the output effector organs (i.e., muscles and glands), we observe that the geometrical transformations that allow the functional communication between sensory and motor frames of reference become more abstract.[4,57] In addressing these remote transformations and in referring to the complexity or "distance" that the process under study has in relation to the peripheral metric, neuroscientists often use the term "higher computational levels." Since computation is an accepted term in neuroscience, it is essential to clarify its meaning: *what is actually being computed when nerve cells fire? or, how is the activity of networks computational?*

One view concerning computation is typified by the attempt to equate the activation of given neurons with macroscopic motor, sensory, or cognitive events. This isomorphic tendency is reflected in the literature by the use of terms such as face cell and memory cell (for a critical discussion of face cells, see 14). This grandmother cell approach[29] expresses the belief that nerve cells may be capable of selectivity based on a type of computational (algorithmic-like) circuit property reaching *categorical* interpretations of universals such that they may form the substrate for labeled lines (i.e., each action potential from a given cell has a preestablished meaning within the function of the brain). However, recently accumulated evidence suggests that in the visual[14] and motor[11,40] domains, representation is achieved by the pattern of activity in a population of cells, and not by the electrical activity of single cells. For instance, even though the selectivity of inferior temporal cells for faces or hands may appear striking, it is still true that these neurons respond weakly to a variety of dissimilar visual stimuli.[7,15] Furthermore, in simian experiments it has thus far been impossible to find inferior temporal neurons with selective responses to a variety of equally important stimuli, such as apples or bananas. More fundamentally, however, the number of sensory percepts that could potentially be distinguished by an individual is probably much higher than the number of available neurons.

THE FUNCTIONING OF CELL ASSEMBLIES AND NEURONAL SILENCE

The functional properties of entire cellular assemblies (not single neurons) are the important variable if we assume that computation in the Von Neuman[73] algorithmic sense is probably not present in central nervous system (CNS) function.[45] Indeed, what people generally mean by computation is the presence of large functional states that approximate, more or less faithfully (a homomorphism), certain aspects of the external world. Thus the term computation is actually used to mean internal representation; for example, the retina does not compute, it transforms functional states from one coordinate system to another.[56]

This latter point is quite significant. If we assume that the patterns of activity in distributed populations of neurons are involved in creating a consistent representation of external reality, it follows that, at any given time, the silence of some neurons is as important as the firing of others. In this sense, as in the case of music, timing and duration are as essential during sound emission as during silence. Thus, to generate the necessary patterns, nervous system function requires that some cells fire and others remain quiescent, and as in the case of vectorial spaces, null-value vector components are as important in determining the computational space as vector components having a value.[56]

Neuronal silence is difficult to address, however, as present technology has been developed toward analyzing neuronal activity but cannot as easily grasp the functional meaning of the absence of neuronal activity, especially when single-electrode recording techniques are used.

Another relevant question that eludes our understanding relates to whether the patterns of neuronal activity within a given region of the brain are necessary and sufficient for perception, or whether some other parts of the brain have a "reading function" that interprets such patterns. In other words; *if inactive cells could be transiently removed from a neuronal circuit during its function, would the outcome of the reduced network be modified by this deletion?* The answer, clearly, is yes. The reason for such an emphatic statement is that, as indicated above, neuronal silence is not necessarily lack of participation; rather, it constitutes the counterpart that ultimately generates the patterns that exist only in a relational sense.

What about neuronal activity distant from the functional state under study? Clearly, the importance of remotely situated cells to intervene, modulate, or "remember" specific patterns of neuronal activity may be minimal, but, as in the case of inertia, they may exert an effect, if only by limiting the system in terms of generating boundaries.

In the latter case, no ultimate reader would be required for such patterns in neuronal assemblies, as their activity would be the necessary and sufficient functional state that characterizes nervous system function. This concept is being crystallized slowly as we understand more about the properties of cellular ensembles.

As we approach conclusions relating to patterns of activity in neuronal assemblies more or less asymptotically, questions about the mechanism that generates such states and their modulation by the intrinsic electrical characteristics of individual neurons are of the essence. Let us assume that brain function embeds a type of reality emulation that evolved to specify internally the salient aspects of the surrounding world.[36] This reality emulator acts primarily as the prerequisite for coordinated, directed movement (motricity), as it creates a predictive image of an event (i.e., causes one to react if one sees a dangerous object moving toward one). Along the lines of this preface, certain corollaries may be considered.

The nervous system may implement the transformation of activity patterns obtained by sensory inputs into coherent images. Such an image is considered here to be a premotor template that would serve as a planning platform for behavior, the prerequisite to purposeful action and even to human consciousness.

A second corollary may be proposed. Since the brain did not appear suddenly, but rather was subjected to the vicissitudes of evolution, it may possess at birth as much of an a priori order to its organization as does the rest of our body. All the muscles, bones, and joints, and most of what they

The Brain as a Closed System Modulated by the Senses

are capable of doing, are in principle inscribed in the geometry of the system at birth.[57] We possess the ability to adapt to the parameters of the universe we live in. This capacity is expressed as plasticity—the ability to change those parameters that have been predesigned to be malleable. For example, we hone our ability to recognize human phonemes by discarding those we do not hear during our developing years,[72] thereby enhancing our ability to acquire one human language as opposed to another. Plasticity is possible only within very well-defined constraints. For example, regardless of training we will not be able to move much faster than 10 Hz.[41] Also, although our muscle mass can greatly increase with exercise, we cannot change the number of cells in each muscle, only their individual volume. Thus, we arrive at an important conclusion: the order of the organization of nervous systems can be enriched by plasticity and learning, but only up to a point.

The question then arises, if such perceptual properties are not learned, where do they originate? The answer is, through evolution. These aspects of nervous system function are clearly demonstrable in the visual system where, from the first time that light hits the retina, the ability to assign meaning to visual images is present in many animals, including primates.[74] This concept of a neurological a priori toward which we now gravitate[34] has long been the concern of philosophers beginning with Kant,[27] but as a epistemological rather than a developmental term, in the sense of phylogeny.

THE CNS AS A CLOSED SYSTEM

From the above discussion, it is evident that we regard as fundamental the issue of whether the functional organization of the CNS is to be considered to have a closed or an open architecture. An open system is one that accepts inputs from the environment, processes them, and returns them to the external world as a reflex regardless of their complexity. This view, supported by William James,[23] suggests a tabula rasa organization of the CNS at birth. The interactions between the CNS and its surroundings propose the mechanism for acquisition of cognition: a learning machine. This view, which is still pervasive, explains nothing about the function of the CNS or the invariance of its function among individuals. Indeed, neurobiology and neuroscience in general assume a basic similarity among phenotypes and even among species as related to neuronal function, and thus assume a degree of genetic determinism far from the tabula rasa view.

Some of us consider the CNS to be a fundamentally closed system with its basic organization geared toward the generation of intrinsic images (thoughts or predictions), where inputs *specify* internal states[34] rather than *inform* "homuncular vernacles."

If we opt for the closed-system intrinsic hypothesis,[34] it follows that the nervous system is primarily self-activating and capable of generating a cognitive representation of the external environment even in the absence of sensory input, for example in dreams, as we will discuss later. From this we may draw a further conclusion. This intrinsic order represents the core activity of the brain, which may then be modified through sensory experience and through the effects of motor activity, the latter in response to the external world or to internally created images and concepts. Emotions are examples of internally generated intrinsic events that are clearly premotor templates in primitive forms. They are also evident in higher vertebrates if the motor suppression that often constrains their behavioral manifestations of emotion (e.g., basal ganglia activity) is also considered part of the motor realm.

If we assume that a closed system uses analyzers to define the external world and that these analyzers are placed into context relative to each other to coordinate cognition, one of the central dilemmas of brain function arises: how is unity of cognition created, given the fractured nature of sensory input and motor output? It is clear that we experience consciousness as a single continuous process and that a voluntary movement is thought to represent the execution of only one motor directive at any time. When we move, we think in terms of our goal-oriented movement, not about combining the myriad of motor elements required to create a whole movement.[21] So is the case when one speaks: one is not concerned with controlling intracostal, diaphragm, larynx, tongue, and cheek muscles during phonation, but rather, with what one is saying.

We face the same problem in the sensory domain. Available data indicate that within each modality, sensory inputs are processed by activity in a constellation of cortical regions that analyze specific aspects of the stimuli (i.e., color, orientation) in a limited portion of the receptive surface. Nevertheless, the sensory percepts appear as unitary events.

As a closed system, the CNS must have developed over evolutionary time as a neuronal network that initially mediated simple reflex relations between sensory-motor connectivity. As the system evolved, the constraints generated by the coordinate systems that characterize the body were embedded into functional space and genetically determined.[57] Thus, a neurological a priori was developed over the very protracted period of vertebrate and invertebrate phylogenesis.

From this perspective, cognition as a functional state may be considered as an a priori property of the brain; that is, one that does not have to be learned. Only the particular content of cognition, as it relates to the particulars of the world around us, must be learned. Not so, for instance, is the ability to hear in the most general of terms, or the ability to see colors, or even the ability to acquire a human language.[3] It is also obvious that perceptions are, of necessity, stand-ins for external reality. On the other hand, the concept that many percepts such as colors and sounds do not exist in the external world, but are adaptive inventions of the CNS, is not universally accepted. Of interest, the correspondence between this internal representation and external reality is ultimately inconsequential as long as it permits adequate transactions with the environment.

The premotor nature of this perceptual world (i.e., the necessity for a sensory template that allows predictive behavioral interaction with the environment) is illustrated in the experience of individuals who wear inverting lenses for extended periods of time.[5] Initially, the visual world seems to be inverted to these subjects as they receive contradictory information through visual, vestibular, and proprioceptive modalities. After a period of practice, however, the environment appears upright and consistent with sensory inputs transmitted through other modalities.[28] However, subjects exposed to the same sensory stimuli, but who experience them passively (e.g., in a chair on wheels), never adapt to inverted lenses.[18] This implies that the perception of reality (a "reality emulator") has evolved to allow predictive interactions with the environment, and that such interaction is modifiable by experience and practice, but clearly not by experience alone.

As the CNS has only an indirect relationship with external reality, perceptive states may be generated by two distinct mechanisms: through the process of dreaming, or in response to sensory input during wakefulness. In fact, dreaming and wakefulness are so similar from electrophysiological and neurological points of view that wakefulness may be described as a dreamlike state modulated by sensory input.[36]

COGNITION: AN INTRINSIC PROPERTY OF THE CNS

Cognition may then be considered an intrinsic property of the CNS. From a connectivity viewpoint, CNS function requires a series of parallel, distributed, and interactive networks whose activities covary with external inputs. Such covariant activities must be related to each other with sufficient speed and precision to implement an effective interaction with the environment. The thalamocortical system,[26,67] which comprises a collection of specific thalamic nuclei and a set of cortical counterparts that can create resonant functional states, is a plausible candidate for such a cognitive role.[36]

The cerebral cortex receives information from, and projects back to, the specific and nonspecific thalamic nuclei. Coordination of activities in these distinct sensory channels is achieved at several levels. First, there is the reticular thalamic nucleus, a sheet of interconnected γ-aminobutyric acid (GABA)-ergic neurons at the interface of the thalamus and neocortex.[6,16] This nucleus, which surrounds the dorsal thalamus, receives collaterals of corticothalamic and thalamocortical axons and projects to the dorsal thalamus.[25,69] Second, in parallel with the specific thalamocortical sensory channels is a nonspecific system comprising the intralaminar thalamic nuclei and posterior thalamic group, which are reciprocally connected with widespread cortical territories.[67] Finally, one of the main targets of reticular thalamic neurons is the intralaminar thalamic complex.[69]

The distinct anatomical and functional organization of the specific and intralaminar thalamic channels is reflected in the effects of lesions circumscribed to these systems. The effects of lesions placed in one of the specific thalamic nuclei are a function of the sensory inputs that they relay to layers III and IV of the cerebral cortex. For instance, lesioning the nucleus transmitting visual inputs (the dorsal lateral geniculate nucleus) causes blindness, not deafness.

In contrast, something quite different follows damage to the intralaminar or nonspecific nuclei. Patients are not aware of the inputs conveyed to the cortex by the intact specific thalamocortical circuit. Although inputs from the specific thalamus are received, the injured individual cannot perceive or respond to them.[17] In essence, the individual no longer exists, from a cognitive point of view, and although specific sensory inputs to the cortex remain intact, they are completely ignored.

These results suggest that the nonspecific system is required to achieve binding; that is, to place the representation of specific sensory images into the context of ongoing computational activities.[39] Thus, two entirely different events occur in the CNS: the receipt of specific information, and the contextual integration of that input relative to ongoing activity.

MAGNETIC RECORDING IN HUMANS

The question now is one of how to apply the data and insights obtained from the analysis of single-cell electrophysiology to further our understanding of the nature of cognition and of the essential responses that characterize human nervous system function.

During the last decades, several noninvasive technologies were developed that allow a partial window into human brain function. They will have much to offer in years to come. Such techniques as positron emission tomography (PET) and magnetic resonance imaging (MRI) are quite powerful in visualizing localized activity in certain areas of the brain during particular functional states. These images of activity may be correlated to visual inputs, voluntary movements, and even premotor potentials, and can be accurately localized, at least at the macroscopic level with an accuracy of 1–3 mm.

These imaging methods are quite limited in the time domain, however. Only recently has it been possible, with the use of magnetoencephalography (MEG), to measure human brain function with a temporal resolution comparable to that of the CNS itself. The frequency response of the MEG instruments —1 kHz—ensures that the electrical events coexisting with cognition may be measured in real time. Moreover, this instrument allows us to localize activity with accuracy on the order of a few millimeters.

With this technique, we have been able to localize phenomena such as the sensory representation of visual, auditory, or somatosensory activity.[50,62,70] In particular, MEG allowed us to demonstrate directly, for the first time, plasticity in the human adult CNS (figure 1.1).[47–49] In these experiments, adults with syndactyly were able to reorganize their somatosensory cortex within weeks after surgical separation of the congenitally fused fingers.[47]

The Brain as a Closed System Modulated by the Senses

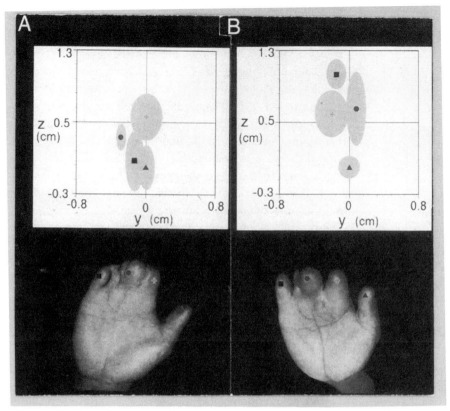

Figure 1.1 Surgical correction of syndactyle of digits two through five, coronal sections. (A) Preoperative map of dipole source locations for the thumb, index, middle, and little fingers of the hand. Data are shown normalized to the thumb in the yz (coronal) place. Note the abnormal, nonsomatotopic organization of the hand area (thumb-little-middle-index). The distance between the representation of the thumb and little finger was significantly ($p < 0.05$) smaller than normal. (B) Twenty-six days after surgical separation of the digits. The organization of the hand is now somatotopic. The distance between the representation of the thumb and little finger has increased to 1.06 cm. (Modified from reference 48.)

The issue of plasticity in the somatosensory cortex is of interest, as it may be viewed as contrary to the concept of the brain as a closed system. In this particular case, the fact that the sensory map was modified by the organizational arrangement of the peripheral sensory system could be taken to suggest that the system is, in fact, deeply modifiable. On the other hand, looking at the new hand map in the patient with syndactyly, it is clear that this spatial representation resembles the normal map. In this case, the somatosensory system must be considered as plastic, even in the adult human brain.

TIME COHERENCE AND NEURONAL OSCILLATIONS

The mechanisms responsible for the integration of specific sensory occurrences into single percepts, which clearly depend on large functional brain states, remain to be understood. Thus, (a) the fragmented representations of individual stimulus properties observed in primary sensory areas must be

R. Llinás and D. Paré

linked to obtain a complete pattern, and (b) the reconstituted patterns produced by the conjunction of different sensory modalities must be linked to the prevailing context of that functional state. One possible solution to this conjunctional problem is to superimpose a temporal dimension to the spatially segregated, but anatomically connected, functional events in the thalamocortical system. The addition of a temporal component to the topographic representations of the sensory areas could sustain an indefinitely large number of representations. According to this scheme, the activity of cells coding for different aspects of a given object would form a coherent, synchronized group, leading to the transient formation of functional cell assemblies.

Electrophysiological studies of neurons in vivo and in vitro indicate that the propensity of the nervous system to engage in coherent oscillatory activities is inscribed in the intrinsic membrane properties of constituent elements. Indeed, CNS neurons have been shown to generate both action potentials and subthreshold oscillations[33] that cyclically modulate their synaptic responsiveness.[32] Such membrane properties are present in a large variety of interconnected neurons of the thalamus[22,45,53,59,64,66,68] and cerebral cortex,[42,54] thus promoting network resonance[34] and the emergence of attractor states.[20] The fact that all frequencies are not equally probable determines that certain resonant frequencies will be observed preferentially.

40-HZ COHERENCE AND COGNITIVE BINDING

In addition to demonstrating the distribution of sensory maps and their plasticity, other experiments using MEG demonstrated that the issue of coherence and oscillations at 40 Hz may be centrally related to cognition. In alert subjects, continuous 40-Hz oscillations can be recorded over large areas of the surface of the head.[35,38,39] However, these oscillations are not in phase, but exhibited a 12- to 13-msec phase shift between the rostral and caudal parts of the brain that appeared as a continuous phenomena in space when recordings from adjacent sites were compared. On presentation of sensory stimuli, the oscillations show phase locking,[35,38,39] which is proposed to be related to cognitive processing[37,71] and to the temporal binding of sensory stimuli.[38]

Neuropsychological and psychophysical observations indicate that the auditory system is capable of discriminating the tonality of two stimuli that are separated by only 1 to 2 msec,[46] whereas 15 to 20 msec are required for the perceptual separation of two stimuli.[19] This was taken as an appropriate paradigm to test the above hypothesis.

To investigate the role of coherent 40-Hz oscillations in sensory segmentation and binding, MEG recordings were made from the auditory cortex while subjects were presented with six sets of two clicks at interstimulus intervals from 3 to 30 msec. At the end of each trial, the subjects reported whether the auditory stimuli could be identified as consisting of one or two clicks. In each set, a lower threshold was defined as the last interval reported as one click

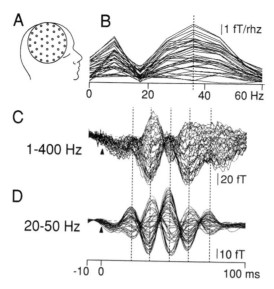

Figure 1.2 Average magnetic responses recorded from a representative subject and power spectrum (1000 epochs) after binaural auditory stimulation [10 kHz, 60-decibel (sound pressure level) click]. (A) Schematic diagram of the sensor distribution over the right hemisphere. (B) Superposition of the power spectra and responses recorded from the 37 positions. Individual traces show a clear activation near 40 Hz. (C) Band-pass filtering from 1 to 400 Hz. The 40-Hz activity is visible in addition to a small low-frequency activation (arrowhead indicates stimulus onset). (D) Twenty- to 50-Hz filtering isolates only the 40-Hz events. Broken lines indicate peak latencies. For this subject the mean latencies were 20.8, 34.2, 47.6, 64.4, and 75.6 msec (SD 0.63 msec, $n = 5$) as measured in a replicate experiment. (Modified from reference 25.)

while going through the set of intervals from 3 to 30 msec. The upper threshold was defined as the first interval reported as two clicks while going from 30 to 3 msec.

A power spectral analysis of the raw data revealed a significant component near 40 Hz (figure 1.2), indicating the presence of a synchronized 40-Hz event.[10,55,61] The data were filtered at 20 to 50 Hz for further analysis to remove a 10-Hz component in that particular channel. The high-frequency rhythm near 40 Hz in the raw data was well correlated with the 40-Hz response in the filtered data. Based on these findings, we define the 40-Hz response produced by a single stimulus as a 2.5-oscillation cycle, demonstrating two and a half oscillations at 40 Hz.

Magnetic recordings demonstrated a single 40-Hz response after the presentation of two auditory stimuli at interstimulus intervals less than 12 msec. The response was identical to that after a single stimulus (figure 1.3). When the stimuli were presented at longer intervals, a second response abruptly appeared. This second response overlapped with that elicited by the first stimulus.

Modeling of the possible origin for the second 40-Hz wave[24] indicates that at interstimulus intervals of 14.2 msec or less, only the first stimulus induced its own 40-Hz activity. The abruptness of the response probably

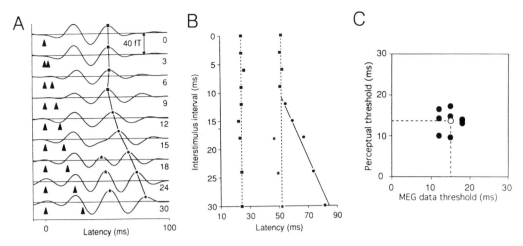

Figure 1.3 Effect of increasing the interstimulus interval on MEG activity. (A) The largest of the 37 responses, obtained by the single-click experiment and filtered at 20 to 50 Hz, was selected, and that same channel recording is the one illustrated in each block. Arrowheads indicate the onset of the clicks, and the number to the right gives the interstimulus interval in milliseconds. (B) The peak latencies of the responses shown on the left are plotted as a function of interstimulus interval. Broken lines indicate the peak latencies for the response to the single click. Note that the response latencies for intervals below 12 msec are similar to those for a single stimulus. As the interval increased, a second 40-Hz response was observed (solid line). Asterisks indicate the interaction between the second peak of the first response and the first peak of the second response. (C) Relationship between the perceptual and MEG thresholds for identifying two clicks (minimum interstimulus interval). The graph plots the thresholds for each of the nine subjects (●) and the mean across all subjects (o). (Modified from reference 25.)

relates to nonlinear single-cell oscillatory properties as observed in vitro and in vivo.[42,66]

Comparing perceptual thresholds with the responses observed by the 40-Hz reset indicated that stimuli presented at an interstimulus interval longer than 13.7 msec could be identified as two clicks. The minimum interstimulation interval required to elicit a second MEG response and that required for the recognition of a second auditory stimulus as a distinct event were not statistically different. No significant regression between the two variables was found, indicating a clusterlike correlation near 12 to 15 msec.

These findings were viewed as correlating well with neuropsychological and psychophysical observations. The ability to judge the temporal order of a sequence of sounds was reported to depend on whether the task required actual identification of the individual global patterns.[51] Whereas the finest acuity for discrimination tasks is on the order of 1 to 2 msec,[48] the identification of individual elements is on the order of 15 to 20 msec.[19] These results coincide closely with the classic interstimulus interval required to identify individual stimuli.[20]

Equally significant was the finding that delivering double stimuli at intervals less than 12 to 15 msec changes the tonality of the perceived sound. This indicates that stimuli coming within one perceptual quantum (12–15 msec) are actually bound into one cognitive event rather than perceived as separate entities. Other observations concluded that sensory information is processed in discrete time segments[43,60] as low as 12 msec.[31]

These findings suggest that 40-Hz oscillatory activity is not only involved in primary sensory processing per se, but forms part of a time conjunction or binding property that amalgamates sensory events occurring in perceptual time quanta into a single experience.[38] Indeed, 40-Hz oscillatory activity is prevalent in the mammalian CNS,[9,52] as seen at both single-cell[42,66] and multicellular[2,10,55,61] levels. This oscillatory activity, which also may be studied using electrical recording,[63,71] has been viewed as a possible mechanism for the conjunction of spatially distributed visual sensory activity[4] or multiregional cortical binding.[37,52] Other findings suggest that binding could occur in steps or quanta of 12 to 15 msec and further support our hypothesis that 40-Hz oscillatory activity could serve a broad cognitive binding function.[38]

Whereas the 12.5-msec time for the alleged quantum of cognition has been determined psychophysically, it is interesting that another very distinct measurement of the phase shift of 40-Hz oscillatory activity over the human cortex has a 12.5-msec duration as well. These two measurements, which were obtained totally independent of each other, tie the issue of sensory binding with 40-Hz activity recorded by MEG.

COINCIDENCE DETECTION, THE BINDING, AND SPECIFIC AND NONSPECIFIC 40-HZ RESONANT CONJUNCTIONS: THE ISSUE OF CONTENT AND CONTEXT IN BRAIN FUNCTION

The results reported above and other recent findings indicate that 40-Hz oscillations are present at many levels in the CNS, including the retina,[12] olfactory bulb,[3] specific and nonspecific[65] thalamic nuclei, reticular thalamic nucleus,[59] and neocortex.[42] Some of the 40-Hz activity recorded in the visual cortex is correlated with 40-Hz activity in the retina.[12] A scheme through which the correlation of thalamic and cortical 40-Hz oscillation may subserve temporal binding is presented in the left side of figure 1.4. The neuronal oscillation in specific thalamic nuclei[67] establish cortical resonance through direct activation of pyramidal cells and feed-forward inhibition through activation of 40-Hz inhibitory interneurons in layer III–IV.[69] These oscillations reenter the thalamus by way of layer VI pyramidal cell axon collaterals,[67] producing thalamic feedback inhibition by way of the reticular nucleus.[69] This view differs from the binding hypothesis proposed by Crick and Koch[4] in which cortical binding is attributed to the activation of cortical V4, pulvinar, or claustrum.

A second system is illustrated on the right side of figure 1.4. Here, the intralaminar nonspecific thalamic nuclei projection to cortical layers I and V and to the reticular nucleus[58] is illustrated. Layer V pyramidal cells return

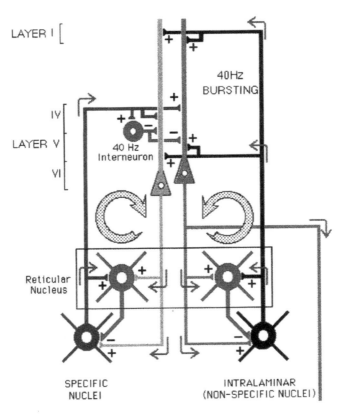

Figure 1.4 Thalamocortical circuits proposed to subserve temporal binding. Diagram of two thalamocortical systems. (Left) Specific sensory or motor nuclei project to layer III–IV of the cortex, producing cortical oscillation by direct activation and feed-forward inhibition by way of 40-Hz inhibitory interneurons. Collaterals of these projections produce thalamic feed-back inhibition by way of the reticular nucleus. The return pathway (circular arrow on the right) re-enters this oscillation to specific and reticular thalamic nuclei by way of layer VI pyramidal cells. (Right) The second loop shows nonspecific intralaminar nuclei projecting to the most superficial layer of the cortex and giving collaterals to the reticular nucleus. Layer V pyramidal cells return oscillation to the reticular and the nonspecific thalamic nuclei, establishing a second resonant loop. The conjunction of the specific and nonspecific loops is proposed to generate temporal binding. (Modified from reference 39.)

oscillations to the reticular nucleus and intralaminar nuclei. The cells in this complex have been shown to oscillate in 40-Hz bursts[65] and to be organized macroscopically as a toroidal mass input having the possibility of recursive activation.[30] This could result in the recurrent activity ultimately responsible for the rostrocaudal cortical activation found in the present MEG recordings.

It is also evident from the literature that neither of these two circuits alone can generate cognition. As stated above, damage to the nonspecific thalamus produces deep disturbances of consciousness, whereas damage to specific systems produces loss of the particular modality. This suggests a hypothesis regarding the overall organization of brain function that rests on two tenets. First, the specific thalamocortical system is viewed as encoding specific sensory and motor information through the resonant thalamocortical system specialized to receive such inputs (e.g., lateral geniculate and visual cortex). The specific system is understood to comprise those nuclei, whether sensorimotor or associative, that project mainly, if not exclusively, to layers III to IV in the cortex. Second, after optimum activation, any such thalamocortical loop would tend to oscillate near 40 Hz, and activity in the specific thalamocortical system could be easily recognized over the cortex by this oscillatory characteristic.

In this scheme, areas of cortical sites peaking at 40 Hz would represent the different components of the cognitive world that have reached optimum activity at that time. The problem now is the conjunction of such a fractured description into a single cognitive event. We propose that this could come about by the concurrent summation of specific and nonspecific 40-Hz activity along the radial dendritic axis of given cortical elements; that is, by the superposition of spatial and temporal mapping (coincidence detection).

In short, the system would function by inciting central neurons to optimum firing patterns through integrations based on passive and active dendritic conduction along the apical dendritic core conductors. In this way, the time-coherent activity of the specific and nonspecific oscillatory inputs, by summing distal and proximal activity in given dendritic elements, would enhance de facto 40-Hz cortical coherence by their multimodal character, and in this way would provide one mechanism for global binding. The specific system would thus provide the *content* that relates to the external world and the nonspecific system would give rise to the temporal conjunction, or the *context* (on the basis of a more interoceptive context concerned with alertness) that would together generate a single cognitive experience.

CONCLUSION

Although demonstration of causal relations cannot be ascribed from electrophysiological measurements alone, the types of results described here strongly suggest that integration of sensory events into the larger computational state that underlies cognition is a function of its temporal relation to ongoing oscillatory activities.

Similar hypotheses were proposed for the visual cortex experimentally by Gray and Singer[13] and theoretically by Crick and Koch[4] in important papers. At this time, however, the study of neuronal-coherence oscillation and its relation to cognition seems to be coming of age. We suggest that perception at a given moment is represented by a small percentage of coherently oscillating cellular elements over the whole thalamocortical system. The rest of the thalamocortical system, being silent to such coherence, may in fact represent the necessary counterpart to the temporal pattern of neuronal activity that we recognize individually as cognition.

ACKNOWLEDGMENT

This research was made possible by a grant from the National Institutes of Health and National Institutes of Neurological Disorders and Strokes (NIH-NINDS) (NS13742) to RL and a fellowship from the Canadian Medical Research Council (MIT-11562) to DP.

REFERENCES

1. Aitkin LM. (1990). Coding for auditory space. In: *Information processing in the mammalian auditory and tactile system*. MJ Rowe, LM Aitkin eds. Alan R. Liss, New York, 169–178.

2. Bressler SL, Freeman WJ. (1980). Frequency analysis of olfactory system EEG in cat, rabbit and rat. *Electroencephalogr Clin Neurophysiol* 50:19–24.

3. Chomsky N. (1986). *Knowledge of language: Its nature, origin and use*. Praeger Publishers, Westport, CT.

4. Crick F, Koch C. (1990). Some reflections on visual awareness. *Cold Spring Harbor Symposium Quant Biol* 55:953–962.

5. Delorme A. (1982). *Psychologie de la perception*. Editions Etudes Vivantes, Montreal.

6. Deschênes M, Madariaga DA, Steriade M. (1985). Dendrodendritic synapses in the cat reticularis thalami nucleus: A structural basis for thalamic spindle synchronization. *Brain Res* 334:165–168.

7. Desimone R, Albright TD, Gross CG, Bruce C. (1984). Stimulus-selective properties of inferior temporal neurons in the macaque. *J Neurosci* 4:2051–2062.

8. Dowling J. (1992). *Neurons and networks—An introduction to neuroscience*. Harvard University Press, Cambridge.

9. Eckhorn R, Bauer R, Jordan W, Brosch M, Kruse W, Munk M, Reitboeck HJ. (1988). Coherent oscillations: A mechanism of feature linking in the visual cortex? *Biol Cybernet* 60:121–130.

10. Galambos R, Makeig S, Talmachoff PJ. (1981). A 40-Hz auditory potential recorded from the human scalp. *Proc Natl Acad Sci USA* 78:2643–2647.

11. Georgopoulos AP, Taira M, Lukashin A. (1993). Cognitive neurophysiology of the motor cortex. *Science* 260:47–52.

12. Ghose GM, Freeman RD. (1992). Oscillatory discharge in the visual system: Does it have a functional role? *J Neurophysiol* 68:1558–1574.

13. Gray CM, Singer W. (1989). Stimulus-specific neuronal oscillations in orientation columns of cat visual cortex. *Proc Natl Acad Sci USA* 86:1698–1702.

14. Gross CG. (1992). Representation of visual stimuli in inferior temporal cortex. *Philos Trans R Soc Lond (Biol)* 335:3–10.

15. Gross CG, Rocha-Miranda CE, Bender DB. (1972). Visual properties of neurons in inferotemporal cortex of the macaque. *J Neurophysiol* 35:96–111.

16. Hauser CR, Vaughn JE, Barber RP, Roberts E. (1980). GABA neurons are the major cell type of the nucleus reticularis thalami. *Brain Res* 200:341–354.

17. Heilman KM, Valenstein E (eds). (1993). *Clin Neuropsychol* (3rd ed). Oxford University Press, New York, Oxford.

18. Held R. (1965). Plasticity in sensory-motor systems. *Sci Am* 212:84–94.

19. Hirsh IJ. (1959). Auditory perception of temporal order. *J Acoust Soc Am* 31:759–767.

20. Hopfield JJ, Tank DW. (1986). Neural architecture and biophysics for sequence recognition. In: *Neural models of plasticity—Theoretical and empirical approaches*. J Byrne, WO Berry, eds. Academic Press, New York.

21. Jackson JH. (1931). *Selected writings of John Hughlings Jackson*. Hodder & Stoughton, London.

22. Jahnsen H, Llinás R. (1984). Electrophysiological properties of guinea-pig thalamic neurons: An in vitro study. *J Physiol (Lond)* 349:202–226.

23. James W. (1890). *The principles of psychology*. Henry Holt, London.

24. Joliot M, Ribary U, Llinás R. (1994). Human oscillatory brain activity near 40 Hz coexists with cognitive temporal binding. *Proc Natl Acad Sci USA* 91:11748–11751.

25. Jones EG. (1975). Some aspects of the organization of the thalamic reticular complex. *J Comp Neurol* 162:285–308.

26. Jones EG. (1985). *The thalamus*. Plenum Press, New York.

27. Kant I. (1781). *Critique of pure reason*. Doubleday, Garden City, NY.

28. Kohler I. (1964). Experiments with Goggles. *Sci Am* 205:62–72.

29. Konorski J. (1967). *Integrative activity of the brain*. University of Chicago Press, Chicago.

30. Krieg WJS. (1966). *Functional neuroanatomy*. Brain Books, Pantagraph Printing, Bloomington, Ill.

31. Kristofferson AB. (1984). Quantal and deterministic timing in human duration discrimination. *Ann NY Acad Sci* 423:3–15.

32. Lampl I, Yarom Y. (1993). Subthreshold oscillations of the membrane potential: A functional synchronizing and timing device. *J Neurophysiol* 70:2181–2186.

33. Llinás R. (1988). The intrinsic electrophysiological properties of mammalian neurons: Insights into central nervous system function. *Science* 242:1654–1664.

34. Llinás R. (1987). "Mindness" as a functional state of the brain. In: *Mind Waves*. C Blakemore, SA Greenfield, eds. Basil Blackwell, Oxford, 339–358.

35. Llinás R. (1991). Depolarization release coupling: An overview. *Ann NY Acad Sci* 635:3–17.

36. Llinás R, Paré D. (1991). Of dreaming and wakefulness. *Neuroscience* 44:521–535.

37. Llinás R, Ribary U. (1992). Rostrocaudal scan in human brain: A global characteristic of the 40-Hz response during sensory input. In: *Induced rhythms in the brain*. E Basar, T Bullock, eds. Birkhauser, Boston, 147–154.

38. Llinás R, Ribary U. (1993). Coherent 40-Hz oscillation characterizes dream state in humans. *Proc Natl Acad Sci USA* 90:2078–2081.

39. Llinás R, Ribary U, Joliot M, Wang X-J. (1994). Content and context in temporal thalamo-cortical binding. In: *Temporal coding in the brain*. G Buzsáki, R Llinás, W Singer, A Berthoz, Y Christen, eds. Springer-Verlag, Berlin, Heidelberg, 251–272.

40. Llinás R, Welsh J. (1994). On the cerebellum and motor learning. *Curr Opin Neurobiol* 3:958–965.

41. Llinás R. (1991). The noncontinuous nature of movement execution. In: *Motor control: concepts and issues*. DR Humphrey, HJ Freund, eds. John Wiley & Sons, New York, 223–242.

42. Llinás R, Grace AA, Yarom Y. (1991). In vitro neurons in mammalian cortical layer 4 exhibit intrinsic oscillatory activity in the 10-Hz to 50-Hz frequency range. *Proc Natl Acad Sci USA* 88:897–901.

43. Madler C, Keller I, Schwender D, Poppel E. (1991). Sensory information processing during general anaesthesia: Effect of isoflurane on auditory evoked neuronal oscillations. *Br J Anaesth* 66:81–87.

44. McClelland JL, Rumelhart DE. (1986). *Parallel distributed processing*. MIT Press, Cambridge.

45. McCormick DA, Pape HC. (1990). Properties of a hyperpolarization-activated cation current and its role in rhythmic oscillation in thalamic relay neurones. *J Physiol (Lond)* 431:291–318.

46. Miller GA, Taylor WG. (1948). The perception of repeated bursts of noise. *J Acoust Soc Am* 20:171–182.

47. Mogilner A, Grossman JA, Ribary U, Joliot M, Volkmann J, Rapaport D, Beasley RW, Llinás R. (1993). Somatosensory cortical plasticity in adult humans revealed by magnetoencephalography. *Proc Natl Acad Sci USA* 90:3593–3597.

48. Mogilner A, Grossman JA, Ribary U, Lado F, Volkmann J, Joliot M, Llinás R. (1992). Abnormal somatosensory cortical organization and cortical plasticity in humans revealed by magnetoencephalography. *Soc Neurosci Abstr* 18:748.

49. Mogilner A, López L, Ribary U, Lado F, Grossman JA, Llinás R. (1991). Neuromagnetic assessment of somatosensory cortical organization following peripheral nerve injury and reconstruction. *Soc Neurosci Abstr* 17:1126.

50. Mogilner A, Ribary U, Nomura M, Lado F, Lopez L, Llinás R. (1991). Neuromagnetic mapping of the somatosensory homunculus onto three-dimensional MRI reconstructions. *Third International Brain Research Organization (IBRO) World Congress of Neuroscience*, Montreal, Canada, pp. 320, P48.20.

51. Moore BCJ. (1993). Temporal analysis in normal and impaired hearing. *Ann NY Acad Sci* 682:119–136.

52. Murthy VN, Fetz EE. (1992). Coherent 25- to 35-Hz oscillations in the sensorimotor cortex of awake behaving monkeys. *Proc Natl Acad Sci USA* 89:5670–5674.

53. Nuñez A, Amzica F, Steriade M. (1992). Intrinsic and synaptically generated delta (1–4 Hz) rhythms in dorsal lateral geniculate neurons and their modulation by light-induced fast (30- to 70-Hz) events. *Neuroscience* 51:269–284.

54. Nuñez A, Amzica F, Steriade M. (1992). Voltage-dependent fast (20–40 Hz) oscillations in long-axoned neocortical neurons. *Neuroscience* 51:7–10.

55. Pantev C, Makeig S, Hoke M, Galambos R, Hampson S, Gallen C. (1991). Human auditory evoked gamma-band magnetic fields. *Proc Natl Acad Sci USA* 88:8996–9000.

56. Pellionisz A, Llinás R. (1980). Tensorial approach to the geometry of brain function cerebellar coordination via a metric tensor. *Neuroscience* 5:1125–1136.

57. Pellionisz A, Llinás R. (1982). Space time representation in the brain. The cerebellum as a predictive space time metric tensor. *Neuroscience* 7:2949–2970.

58. Penfield W, Rasmussen T. (1950). *The cerebral cortex of man*. Macmillan, New York.

59. Pinault D, Deschênes M. (1992). Voltage-dependent 40-Hz oscillations in rat reticular thalamic neurons in vivo. *Neuroscience* 51:245–258.

60. Poppel E. (1970). Excitability cycles in central intermittency. *Psychol Forsch* 34:1–9.

61. Ribary U, Ioannides AA, Singh KD, Hasson R, Bolton JPR, Lado F, Mogilner A, Llinás R. (1991). Magnetic field tomography of coherent thalamocortical 40-Hz oscillations in humans. *Proc Natl Acad Sci USA* 88:11037–11041.

62. Ribary U, Llinás R, Lado F, Mogilner A, Jagow R, Nomura N, Lopez L. (1991). The spatial and temporal organization of the 40-Hz response during auditory processing as analyzed by MEG on the human brain, *Third International Brain Research Organization (IBRO) World Congress on Neuroscience*, Montreal, Canada, pp. 320, P48.22.

63. Sheer DE. (1989). Sensory and cognitive 40-Hz event related potentials: Behavioral correlates, brain function and clinical application. In: *Brain dynamics*. E Basar, T Bullock, eds. Springer-Verlag, Berlin, 339–374.

64. Steriade M. (1993). Central core modulation of spontaneous oscillations and sensory transmission in thalamocortical systems. *Curr Opin Neurobiol* 3:619–625.

65. Steriade M, CurroDossi DR, Contreras D. (1993). Electrophysiological properties of intralaminar thalamocortical cells discharging rhythmic (approximately 40-Hz) spike-bursts at approximately 1000-Hz during waking and rapid eye movement sleep. *Neuroscience* 56:1–9.

66. Steriade M, CurroDossi RC, Pare D, Oakson, G. (1991). Fast oscillations (20 to 40 Hz) in thalamocortical systems and their potentiation by mesopontine cholinergic nuclei in the cat. *Proc Natl Acad Sci USA* 88:4396–4400.

67. Steriade M, Jones EG, Llinás R. (1990). *Thalamic oscillations and signaling*. John Wiley & Sons, Somerset, NJ.

68. Steriade M, McCormick DA, Sejnowski TJ. (1993). Thalamocortical oscillations in the sleeping and aroused brain. *Science* 262:679–685.

69. Steriade M, Parent A, Hada J. (1984). Thalamic projections of nucleus reticularis thalami of cat: A study using retrograde transport of horseradish peroxidase and fluorescent tracers. *J Comp Neurol* 229:531–547.

70. Suk J, Ribary U, Cappell J, Yamamoto T, Llinás R. (1991). Anatomical localization revealed by MEG recordings of the human somatosensory system. *Electroencephalogr Clin Neurophysiol* 78:185–196.

71. Tiitinen H, Sinkkonen J, Rainikainen K, Alho K, Lavikainen J, Näätänen R. (1993). Selective attention enhances the auditory 40-Hz transient response in humans. *Nature* 364:59–60.

72. Trevarthen C. (1983). Cerebral mechanisms for language: Prenatal and postnatal development. In: *Neuropsychology of language, reading and spelling*. U Kirk, ed. Academic Press, New York, 45–80.

73. Von Neuman J. (1951). The general and logical theory of automata. In: *Cerebral mechanisms in behavior: The Hixon symposium*. Jeffress LA, ed. John Wiley & Sons, New York.

74. Wiesel TN, Hubel DH. (1974). Ordered arrangement of orientation columns in monkeys lacking visual experience. *J Comp Neurol* 158:307–318.

2 Making Images and Creating Subjectivity

A. R. Damasio and H. Damasio

The comments in this chapter concern consciousness and its possible neural basis. They are based on the general assumption that consciousness can be approached neurobiologically, and on the idea that for progress to occur in this area, neurobiology must first address two critical questions: how do brains create images in our minds? and how do images acquire the property of subjectivity; in other words, what makes those images our own? We realize that the neurobiological solution to both questions would not provide a comprehensive explanation of the neural basis of consciousness, but we believe it might constitute a useful beginning.

MAKING IMAGES

How do brains create images in our minds? Where in neuroanatomical terms are those images occurring? When neuroimaging studies reveal regions of activation in a sensory cortex, how do such patterns relate, if at all, to the experience of an image? These are some of the problems posed by the neurobiology of making images. We will begin by making some qualifications on our use of the word "images." First, we refer to images based on any sensory modality—sound images, images of movement in space—rather than to visual images only. Images describe both the world external to the organism as well as the world within the organism, such as visceral states, musculoskeletal structure, body movement, and so forth; and convey both nonverbal and verbal entities. That is, word forms or sign denotations in auditory or visual modes are images too.

Second, we use images to refer both to patterns generated in perception as well as to patterns generated from memory, during recall. Finally, the capacity to generate images probably evolved and endured because images allowed organisms to optimize responses; that is, to perfect existing repertoires of movement and plan even more successful ones.

We believe that a substantial part of image making depends on early cortices. In this brief chapter, we cannot discuss all the reasons why, but here are the principal ones. We know that partial destruction of early visual cortices precludes both the perception and the recall of certain aspects of vision.

After damage in cortical areas V2 and V4, for instance, color is neither perceivable nor recallable in imagination. No consciousness of color is possible even if other aspects of vision can be appreciated and even if one can note the absence of the color experience. The fact that perception and recall are compromised by damage at the same site, and the fact that no other known site of damage produces such a defect, suggest that early sensory cortices are the critical base for processes of image making. Another relevant finding is that damage to higher-order association cortices, which are located outside of the early sensory region, does not preclude the making of images (Damasio and Damasio, 1993, 1994; H. Damasio et al., 1993a,b; Kosslyn, 1994).

Relying on results of lesion studies in humans, on results of neurophysiological studies in nonhuman primates, and on known patterns of neuroanatomical connectivity, we have hypothesized that the early sensory cortices of each modality construct, with the assistance of structures in the thalamus and the colliculi, neural representations that are the basis for images. The process seems to require the cooperative action of several, massively interconnected early cortical regions. Although the precise mechanisms underlying this process are not known, it appears that the temporally coordinated activity of those varied early cortices and of the subcortical stations with which they are interconnected yields the essence of what we call an image (Churchland, Sejnowski, and Ramachandran, 1994; Crick, 1994; Tononi, Sporns, and Edelman, 1992; Zeki, 1993).

An important characteristic of images is that they have spatially and temporally organized patterns, and in the case of visual, somatosensory, and auditory images, those patterns are topographically organized. The correspondence between the structure of the neural activity pattern in early sensory cortices and the structure of the stimulus that evoked the pattern can be quite striking (Tootell et al, 1988; see also comment on this issue in A. Damasio, 1994). We proposed that topographic representations can be committed to memory in the form of nontopographically organized dispositional representations, and can be stored in dormant form in both cortical regions or subcortical nuclei. The subsequent reactivation of those dormant dispositional representations, followed by signaling from their storage sites back to early sensory cortices, can regenerate topographically organized representations. Artificial neural nets provide a conceptual framework for understanding how this might be done (P. M. Churchland, 1995). Whether the brain avails itself of similar techniques is not yet determined. The retroactivation process uses the rich connectional patterns of feed-forward and feedback that characterize the architecture of cortical regions and subcortical nuclei. In short, topographic representations can arise in turn as a result of signals external to the brain in the perceptual process, or in the process of recall, from signals inside the brain, coming from memory records held in dispositional representation form.

A. R. Damasio and H. Damasio

Most of our experiences are based on images of several sensory modalities occurring within the same window of time. Since the early sensory cortices for each modality are not contiguous and are not directly interconnected, it follows that our polymodal experiences must result from concurrent activity in several separate brain regions rather than in a single one. In other words, the making of images is a spatially parcellated process. But since our experiences appear integrated to our mind rather than parcellated, we must consider how integration occurs. Our idea is that timing, that is, synchronization of separate activities, plays an essential role in integration. We suspect that the neural mechanism behind synchronization requires signaling from both cortical and subcortical neuron ensembles, capable of simultaneous firing toward many separate neuron populations. Such ensembles do seem to exist and we call them convergence zones (Damasio, 1989a,b). They receive convergent signals and originate divergent signals toward the sites from which convergent signals came. In a manner of speaking, convergence zones contain a storehouse of knowledge in the form of dispositional representations, ready to be activated. They are located throughout the association cortices and subcortical nuclei. Knowledge and timing properties help convergence zones to generate images in recall and they also assist perceived images by enhancing their coherence.

The idea that timing plays a role in the making of images within a modality has been presented by several other theorists (von der Malsburg, 1986; Singer et al., 1990; Edelman, 1987). The idea that timing may be essential for polymodal integration is present in our work and in that of Llinás (1993, this volume) among others.

Are the temporally and topographically organized sensory patterns discussed here sufficient to generate the experience of an image? Our answer is a definite no. Although we believe that recall or perception of a human face cannot occur without the concerted activity of early visual cortices, lateral geniculate, and superior colliculi, we do not believe that activity in such cortices is sufficient to sustain the experience of an image. Other structures, cortical and otherwise, and other processes are required for consciousness to occur. This also means that the attractive images of sensory activation that modern neuroimaging techniques permit us to obtain are not the counterparts of visual experiences, although they probably index a subset of the neural activity required to make images.

SUBJECTIVITY

We turn now to the issue of subjectivity, the critical ingredient in the notion of consciousness as we see it, and inevitably, to the issue of self. Assuming our brain-mind is capable of generating states of subjectivity, it seems reasonable to presume that the self is a key agent in the process. First let us define the word self. What we mean when we talk about self, and what we would like to understand in neurobiological terms, is the antecedent and foundation for a process Jerome Kagan (1989) described as "the universal emergence" of a sense "that one can have an effect on people and objects, together with a consciousness of one's feelings and competences." We see the self as the neural structure and neurobiological states that help us know, without the help of inferences based on language, that the images we perceive are our own rather than somebody else's. This general idea of self—the core structures and operations necessary but not sufficient for subjectivity to emerge—does not include meanings such as self-esteem and social self, although it is likely that the processes to which those terms refer are rooted in the same structures and states.

Postulating a cognitive sense of self, as well as neurobiological structures and operations that support it, does not mean we believe that all images and image manipulations that take place in a brain are controlled by a single and central knower and master, and even less that such a knower-master would be in a single brain place sitting in judgment as the audience in a theater. Our view is in line with the criticisms that have been aimed at "the single brain region view" of consciousness (A. R. Damasio, 1989a,b; Dennett, 1991; Churchland and Sejnowski, 1992; P. M. Churchland, 1984; P. S. Churchland, 1995). We simply mean that our experiences have a consistent point of view, that of the individual person. That point of view is diminished or suspended only in pathological brain states such as extreme forms of anosognosia, some types of seizures, multiple personality disorder, and schizophrenia.

Our idea of self is not anchored in the pronouns I and me. In fact, it is hard to imagine how language-making devices would have been selected and evolved had animals not possessed prelanguage selves. Nonlanguaged creatures probably have a self in the sense described above, although its complexity is greater in higher primates and greatest in humans. Language enriches the human self even if it does not serve as its source.

The usual solution to the problem of the self is the homunculus. It consists of postulating a spatially defined creature to whom images are referred within the brain, and assuming that the creature is equipped with the knowledge necessary to interpret the images. But this solution would work only if the thinking homunculus had its own brain and its own knowledge so that, in turn, its images would be interpretable. Since this is not the case, the spatial homunculus solution is not acceptable. It simply removes the problem by one step, whereupon the problem starts again ad infinitum. The homunculus pitfall is now well recognized, but because the self has traditionally been conceptualized in homuncular terms, the attempt to avoid homuncular thinking has entailed a rejection of the notion of self and, by extension, of subjectivity.

This poses yet another problem. Rejecting the idea of a homunculus in our brains does not alter the fact that most images in our minds are processed from a consistent perspective. To say that our brains just form images and that we are aware of those images is not a satisfactory solution. The nature of

A. R. Damasio and H. Damasio

the neural entity that is aware of those images remains unclear. What is needed, as we see it, is a plausible and testable hypothesis for a neural structure underlying the self such that the problems of the spatial homunculus can be avoided.

A Nonhomuncular Self

The solution we proposed elsewhere (Damasio and Damasio, 1994; A. R. Damasio, 1994) includes the following features and components.

We conceptualize the self as a collection of images about the most invariant aspects of our organism and its interactions. This includes certain aspects of body structure, and certain aspects of body operation, including a repertoire of motions possible with the whole body and its varied parts. It includes also identity-defining traits (kinships to certain persons, activities, places; typical motor and sensory patterns of response) These images have a high probability of being evoked repeatedly and continuously by direct signaling, as happens in body states, or by signals arising from stored dispositional representations, as happens with records concerning identity and typical response patterns.

In our framework, the cognitive-neural self is the cognitive-neural instantiation of a concept, no different in its essence from the concept of a particular object whose representation relies on the segregated mapping of its properties (e.g., shape, size, color, texture, characteristic motion, etc.) in varied neural systems from where they can be conjointly retrieved as the concept is activated. But if the essence of the concept of self and of, say, orange, need not be different in basic cognitive and neural specifications, they are different in one important respect. Objects come and go from the vicinity of the organism and thus they come and go from the sensory sheaths that can signal their presence. Yet the body, its parts, and some of its operations, as well as the stable aspects of our autobiography, remain with us, the former signaling incessantly to the brain, the latter indelibly represented and ready to be reinstantiated.

We propose that the core components of the concept of self concern body structure (i.e., viscera, musculoskeletal frame) and fundamentals of one's identity, (i.e., usual activities, preferences, physical and human relationships, etc.). These core components change substantially during childhood and adolescence, and then less and more gradually throughout the remaining life span. The anchor for the concept of self lies with visceral states and with the neural mechanisms that represent and regulate basic biologic processes whose modifiability is minimal. The former are continuously signaled to brainstem structures and to the complex of somatosensory cortices in the insula, parietal operculum, and postrolandic parietal cortices (the signaling is bilateral, but a right hemisphere dominance effect exists in humans). The biological regulating machinery is represented in the brain core (hypothalamus, brain stem).

Skeptics may counter that we are usually unaware of our body states and that body signaling is thus an odd choice to anchor subjectivity. The objection is weak, however (A. R. Damasio, 1994). First, although our attention more often than not is centered in nonbodily signals, its focus may shift rapidly, especially in conditions such as pain and emotional upheaval. Second, the argument we are making is especially concerned with the historical development of the sense of self, in evolutionary and individual development terms, rather than with the situation of an adult. Third, since we all agree that the mechanisms behind the emergence of subjectivity are hidden, there is no reason why the body states we propose as their scaffolding should be easily revealed in consciousness. The important issue to decide is whether the mechanisms we propose are a plausible base, not whether we are or should be aware of them.

Subjective States

How do we see subjectivity emerging from the neural device described above? As images corresponding to a newly perceived entity (e.g., a face) are formed in early sensory cortices, the brain reacts to them. In our framework this happens for two reasons. First, signals arising in those images, rather than the images themselves, are relayed to several subcortical nuclei, for instance, the amygdala and the thalamus, and to several cortical regions in temporal, parietal, and frontal sectors. Second, those nuclei and cortical regions contain dispositions for response to certain classes of signals. The result is that dispositional representations in nuclei and cortical regions are activated and induce, as a consequence, some collection of changes in the state of the organism. In turn, those changes alter the body state momentarily, and thus perturb the current instantiation of the concept of self. In other words, the multifarious process of recognizing an object generates sets of responses—autonomic, hormonal, motor, imagetic—and those responses change the organism's state for a certain time interval. We propose that the essence of the neural mechanisms of consciousness resides with the perturbation of self states by newly occurring images.

Although this responding process implies knowledge, knowledge that is recorded in innate as well as experience driven dispositions throughout the brain, it certainly does not imply that any brain component "knows" that responses are being generated to the presence of an entity. In other words, when the organism's brain generates a set of responses to the image of an entity (e.g., a growling dog), the existence of a representation of self does not make that self know that its organism is responding. The self, as described, cannot *know*; it is not a homunculus.

Here we arrive at the critical question in this proposal. How can the current image of an entity, on the one hand, and a set of images of the organism's state, on the other, both of which exist as momentary neural activation patterns generate subjectivity? Our current answer is that (a) the brain creates

A. R. Damasio and H. Damasio

some kind of *description of the perturbation of the state of the organism* that resulted from the brain's responses to the presence of an image; (b) the description *generates an image of the process of perturbation*; and (c) the image of the *self perturbed* is displayed together or in rapid interpolation with the image that triggered the perturbation.

To perform this task the brain must possess neural structures that support the image of an object, neural structures that support the images of the self, and neural structures that support neither and yet are reciprocally interconnected with both. In other words, the brain must have available the kind of third-party neuron ensemble that we call a convergence zone, and that we invoke as the neural substrate for building dispositions in cortical regions and in subcortical nuclei.

Such a third-party ensemble receives signals from both the representation of an object as well as the representations of the self, as the latter are perturbed by the reaction to the object. In other words, the ensemble can build a dispositional representation of the self in the process of changing, while the organism responds to an object. This representation would be of precisely the same kind that the brain continuously holds, makes, and re-models. The information necessary to build it is readily available: shortly after we see an object and hold a representation of it in early visual cortices, we also hold many representations of the organism reacting to the object in varied somatosensory regions.

As is the case with all dispositions, the construction we envision has the potential, once formed, to reactivate an image in any early sensory cortex to which it is connected. The basic image in the description would be that of the organism's body in the process of responding to a particular object (i.e., a somatosensory image).

We propose that all ingredients described—an object that is being represented, an organism responding to the object of representation, and a description of the organism in the process of changing in response to the object— are held simultaneously in working memory and are placed side by side or in rapid interpolation in early sensory cortices. Subjectivity would emerge during this step, when the brain is simultaneously producing not just images of an entity, of self and of organism's responses, but also another kind of image: that of an organism in the act of perceiving and responding to an entity. In our hypothesis, the latter kind of image, is the source of subjectivity (A. R. Damasio, 1994).

The description we have in mind is neither created nor perceived by a homunculus, and it does not require language. The third-party disposition provides a nonverbal narrative document of what is happening to the main protagonists in the process, accomplished with the elementary representational tools of the sensory and motor systems.

Subjectivity would emerge in any brain equipped with some basic representation of self, with the capacity to form images and respond to them, and with the capacity to generate some kind of dispositional description in a third-party neuron ensemble.

The second-order narrative capacities provided by language would allow humans to engender verbal narratives out of nonverbal ones, and the refined form of subjectivity that is ours would emerge from the latter process. The virtual serial machine mechanism proposed by Dennett would operate at that high level rather than at the lower level we postulate here. It would not be the source of subjectivity, although it might contribute to important aspects of thinking and reasoning. In short, language would not be the source of the self, but it certainly would be the source of I.

This proposal is quite distinct from Crick's hypothesis (1994) for the neural basis of visual awareness and shares some important traits with Edelman's proposal (1992) for primary consciousness, namely, the notion of biological value and of a self rooted in homeostatic systems.

A machine equipped with image-making devices, with the ability to represent its physical structure and physical states imagetically, and with dispositional knowledge about its past, would probably not be capable of generating subjectivity. Even if it were to construct images of itself perturbed, as described above, it could not do that unless the machine's body were to be a living body, with properties derived from its precarious homeostatic balance, from its inherent necessity for survival, and from its inherent sense that what promotes survival is valuable. The neural device we propose to generate subjectivity serves to connect images with the process of life, and that is what we believe consciousness is most about.

ACKNOWLEDGMENTS

This manuscript follows closely the text of our proposal for a generator of subjectivity, as described in another article of ours, "Images and Subjectivity: Neurobiological Trials and Tribulations," in *The Churchlands and Their Critics*. Blackwell Scientific, Cambridge, 1995.

REFERENCES

Churchland PM. (1984). *Matter and consciousness*. MIT Press, Cambridge.

Churchland PM. (1995). *The engine of reason, the seat of the soul: A philosophical journey into the brain*. MIT Press, Cambridge.

Churchland PS. (1986). *Neurophilosophy: Toward a unified science of the mind-brain*. MIT Press, Cambridge.

Churchland PS, Sejnowski TJ. (1992). *The computational brain: Models and methods on the frontiers of computational neuroscience*. MIT Press, Cambridge.

Churchland PS, Sejnowski TJ, Ramachandran VS. (1994). The critique of pure vision. In: *Large-scale neuronal theories of the brain*. C Koch, ed. MIT Press, Cambridge.

Crick F. (1994). *The astonishing hypothesis: The scientific search for the soul*. Charles Scribner's Sons, New York.

Damasio AR. (1989a). Time-locked multiregional retroactivation: A systems level proposal for the neural substrates of recall and recognition. *Cognition* 33:25–62.

Damasio AR. (1989b). The brain binds entities and events by multiregional activation from convergence zones. *Neural Computation* 1:123–132.

Damasio AR. (1994). *Descartes' error: Emotion and reason in the human brain*. Putnam, New York.

Damasio AR, Damasio H. (1993). Cortical systems underlying knowledge retrieval: Evidence from human lesion studies. In: *Exploring brain functions: Models in neuroscience*. John Wiley & Sons, New York, 233–248.

Damasio AR, Damasio H. (1994). Cortical systems for retrieval of concrete knowledge: The convergence zone framework. In: *Large-scale neuronal theories of the brain*. C Koch, ed. MIT Press, Cambridge.

Damasio H, Grabowski TJ, Damasio AR, Tranel D, Boles-Ponto LL, Watkins GL, Hichwa RD. (1993a). Visual recall with eyes closed and covered activates early visual cortices. *Soc Neurosci* 19:1604.

Damasio H, Grabowski TJ, Frank RJ, Knosp B, Hichwa RD, Watkins GL, Boles-Ponto LL. (1993b). PET-Brainvox, a technique for neuroanatomical analysis of positron emission tomography images. In: *Proceedings of the PET 93 Akita: Quantification of brain function*. Elsevier, New York, 465–473.

Dennett DC. (1991). *Consciousness explained*. Little, Brown, Boston.

Edelman G. (1987). *Neural darwinism: The theory of neuronal group selection*. Basic Books, New York.

Edelman GM. (1992). *Bright air, brilliant fire*. Basic Books, New York.

Kagan J. (1989). *Unstable ideas: Temperament, cognition, and self*. Harvard University Press, Cambridge.

Kosslyn S. (1994). *Image and brain*. MIT Press, Cambridge.

Llinás R. (1993). Coherent 40-Hz oscillation characterizes dream state in humans. *Proc Natl Acad Sci USA* 90:2078–2081.

Singer W, Gray C, Engel A, Konig P, Artola A, Brocher S. (1990). Formation of cortical cell assemblies. *Symp Quant Biol* 55:939–952.

Tononi G, Sporns O, Edelman G. (1992). Reentry and the problem of integrating multiple cortical areas: Simulation of dynamic integration in the visual system. *Cerebral Cortex* 2:310–335.

Tootell RBH, Switkes E, Silverman MS, Hamilton SL. (1988). Functional anatomy of macaque striate cortex. II. Retinotopic organization. *J Neurosci* 8:1531–1568.

von der Malsburg C. (1986). Statistical coding and short-term synaptic plasticity: A scheme for knowledge representation in the brain. In: *Disordered systems and biological organization*, NATO ASI Series, Vol. F20. E Bienenstock, et al. eds. Springer-Verlag, Berlin, 247–272.

Zeki S. (1993). *A vision of the brain*. Blackwell Scientific Publications, London.

3 Illusions of Body Image: What They Reveal About Human Nature

V. S. Ramachandran, L. Levi, L. Stone,
D. Rogers-Ramachandran, R. McKinney, M. Stalcup,
G. Arcilla, R. Zweifler, A. Schatz, and A. Flippin

The social scientists have a long way to go to catch up, but they may be up to the most important scientific business of all, if and when they finally get to the right questions. Our behavior toward each other is the strangest, most unpredictable, and almost entirely unaccountable of the phenomena with which we are obliged to live.
—Lewis Thomas

In 1995 we not only celebrate the decade of the brain but also commemorate the 100th anniversary of Freud's project for a scientific psychology. As everyone knows, Freud was originally trained as a neurologist, but since his real interest was in the mysteries of the human mind, he quickly became disillusioned with the minutiae of neuroanatomy, which he saw as being somewhat remote from his ultimate goal. (His first paper was on the spinal ganglia of petromyzon, a primitive fish.) As a student of the eminent French neurologist Charcot, he became interested in hysteria, hypnosis, and, eventually, practically all aspects of human nature—dreaming, sexuality, religion, humor, laughter, psychoneuroses, anthropology, and even slips of the tongue. And although we are amused today by such ideas as penis envy and the Oedipus complex, there is a real danger of throwing the baby out with the bathwater, of failing to recognize Freud's monumental contributions to human thought. His basic idea, that consciousness is simply the tip of the iceberg and that our behavior is mostly governed by a cauldron of emotions and motives of which we are largely unconscious (the unconscious mind), is still a perfectly valid concept that is sure to continue to have a tremendous impact on both psychology and neurology. Modern reincarnations of this idea include such phenomena as blindsight (Weiskrantz, 1981) or the elicitation of changes in skin conductance in patients who have no conscious recognition of faces, or prosopagnosia (Damasio, 1994).

Even though Freud's own interests shifted from hard-core neuroanatomy to "soft" psychology, he never lost sight of his initial goal of providing a neural explanation for psychological phenomena, and he continued to pay lip service to this goal until the end. Surely, had he been alive today, he would have been delighted with the syndrome of anosognosia; the vehement denial of paralysis that one sees in some patients who have suffered a right hemisphere stroke. As we will see later in this chapter, this curious disorder may eventually allow us to anchor the airy abstractions of Freudian psychology in the physical flesh of the brain.

We have conducted experiments on two fascinating syndromes dealing with distortions of body image, phantom limbs, and anosognosia-somato-paraphrenia. In the case of phantom limbs, the patient has lost an arm in an accident or due to amputation, but continues to feel its presence vividly (Mitchell, 1871; Melzack, 1992; James, 1887; Sunderland, 1959; Ramachandran, 1993). Anosognosia, on the other hand, is usually seen in patients who have had a right hemisphere stroke, resulting in paralysis of the left side of the body. Some of these patients vehemently deny the paralysis and in extreme cases (somatoparaphrenia) may ascribe the arm to another person such as a spouse or even the examining physician (Galin, 1992; Edelman, 1989; Heilman, 1991; Damasio, 1994; Levine, 1990; McGlynn and Schacter, 1989; Critchley, 1962; Juba, 1949; Cutting, 1978; Weinstein and Kahn, 1950).

These illusions have been widely known for about a century, but there has been a tendency in the medical profession to regard them as enigmatic clinical curiosities. Despite many fascinating clinical case reports, almost no experimental work has been done on them. We will try to bring these syndromes into the mainstream of modern neuroscience and argue that far from being mere oddities, they illustrate certain important principles underlying the functional organization of the normal human brain.

PHANTOM LIMBS

A recurring theme in the vast clinical literature is that phantom limbs are a purely a psychological phenomenon; wishful thinking on the part of the patient, who wants to have the amputated limb back (Parkes, 1973; Szasz, 1975). Typically, however, these patients have a very vivid sensory experience with the phantom. For example, a person will report that the phantom seems to move about spontaneously, try to shake hands when greeting someone, or even try to break his or her own fall. Often a vivid and excruciating pain in the phantom is real enough to drive many to suicide.

But what exactly does it mean to say that a person has volitional control of a phantom arm? One possibility is that messages from the motor cortex in the front part of the brain continue to be sent to the muscles in the hand even though the hand is missing. After all, the part of the brain that controls movement does not "know" that the hand is gone. It is likely that these movement commands are simultaneously monitored by the parietal lobes that are concerned with body image. In a normal person, messages from the frontal lobe are sent either directly or through the cerebellum to the parietal lobes, which monitor the commands and simultaneously receive feedback from the arm about its position and velocity of movement. There is no feedback from a phantom arm, of course, but the monitoring of motor commands might continue to occur in the parietal lobes, and thus the patient vividly feels movements in the phantom.

Not all amputees experience movements in their phantoms. A subset (approximately 30–40%) do not feel any movement at all. They describe it as feeling frozen as if in a cement block, and they cannot generate any volitional movements in it, even with intense effort. At least some of these patients had a preexisting peripheral nerve paralysis in the arm before it was amputated; for example, the patient may have suffered an avulsion of the brachial plexus, the bundle of nerve fibers that connect the spinal cord to the arm. This results in paralysis, and very often, even after the arm is amputated, the phantom remains frozen in the same position that it was in before the operation.

But how can a phantom—a nonexistent limb—be paralyzed? One possibility is that during the months preceding amputation the brain "learned" that the arm was paralyzed; that is, every time the message went from the motor cortex to the arm, the brain received visual feedback that the arm was not moving. This contradictory information is somehow stamped into the neural circuitry of the parietal lobes so that the brain learns that the arm is fixed in that position. Hence, when the arm is amputated the brain still "thinks" the arm is fixed in the previous position and the net result is a paralyzed phantom limb (Ramachandran, 1993, 1994, 1995a).

Amputation of a Phantom Limb Using Virtual Reality

If this hypothesis of learned paralysis is correct, would it be possible to unlearn the phantom paralysis? To do this, every time the patient sends a message to the phantom arm, he would have to receive a visual feedback message that his arm is indeed moving correctly. But how can this happen when the patient does not even have an arm? To let the patient perceive real movement in a nonexistent arm, we constructed a virtual reality box. It is made by placing a vertical mirror inside a cardboard box the top of which is removed. The front of the box has two holes in it through which the patient inserts his good arm and his phantom arm. The patient is asked to view the reflection of his real hand in the mirror, thus creating the illusion of observing two hands, when in fact the patient is only seeing the mirror reflection of the intact hand. If he now sends motor commands to both arms to make mirror-symmetrical movements he will literally see his phantom hand resurrected and obeying his commands. That is, he receives the positive visual feedback informing his brain that his phantom arm is moving correctly.

This experiment was conducted with a patient who had had his left arm amputated 10 years earlier (table 3.1). For over a year before the amputation his arm had been paralyzed as a result of a brachial plexus avulsion and had been in a sling. The man also had extreme pain in the arm both before and after the amputation. For this experiment the man was first instructed to place both his normal arm and his phantom arm into the virtual reality box, close his eyes, and try to move both hands. He reported, as expected, that he

Table 3.1 Clinical details of patients tested

Patient	Age (yr)	Pathology	Location	Time of Testing after Amputation	Mobility of Phantom Arm with Eyes Closed	Comments
RL	56	Melanoma infiltrating brachial plexus	Right upper limb disarticulation at shoulder 1 yr after onset of melanoma	2 mo	No voluntary movements possible	Experienced frequent involuntary clenching spasms.
RT	55	Sarcoma infiltrating ulnar nerve	Left arm 6 cm above elbows	7 mo	No voluntary movements possible	Involuntary clenching spasms and muscle cramps in phantom. Sensation of "nails digging into palm."
DS	28	Brachial plexus avulsion	Left above elbow amputation 1 yr after avulsion	9 yr	No voluntary movements possible	Pain in elbow, 9 yrs' duration. Pain disappeared for first time after telescoping was induced by the mirror box. The arm was still telescoped 6 mo later.
BD	29	Brachial plexus avulsion	Right, above elbow, amputation 2 yrs after avulsion	3 mo	Completely fixed and immobile	Permanently clenched and painful fist could not be unclenched. Mirror box completely ineffective even with intense concentration.
KS	73	Car accident crush injury	Left arm 5 cm above elbow	2 yrs	Completely fixed and immobile	Mirror restored movements but did nothing for pain.
PNN	40	Airplane propeller cut off arm	Right arm above elbow	8 yrs 3 mo	Voluntary movements during the first 2 yrs but not after that	Arm became suddenly telescoped 2 yrs after amputation. Prosthesis did not make it untelescope, but mirror did.

All patients underwent a thorough neurological evaluation to rule out CNS pathology and to ensure that their mental status was normal. All patients were right handed. Patient DS had a left Horner's syndrome. Patient RL had a subdural hematoma 30 years ago but it did not leave any residual neurological deficits.

When patient DS was touched on the lower face region ipsilateral to the amputation, sensations were referred to the phantom fingers, as in some of the patients whom we studied previously (Ramachandran, 1993). This patient also had magnetoencephalographic evidence of remapping in the cortex (Ramachandran, 1993).

Patients RL, RT and BD also experienced frequent involuntary clenching spasms in the phantom. In two of them (RL and RT) the spasms were relieved when they used the mirror box (see text). In one (RT), the spasms caused "the fingernails to dig into my phantom palm," and this sensation also went away each time that the spasm went away. Perhaps the two sensations—clenching and nail digging—had been linked in RT's brain by a Hebbian learning mechanism, so that relieving one also relieved the other. Sensations that were apparently unrelated to the clenching (e.g., burning pain) were completely unaffected by the mirror procedure.

Patient BD could not generate any movements in the phantom, whether or not he used the box, and he had no relief from pain. ("Its frustrating: I can *see* it move; I want it to move, but it doesn't feel like it's moving.") In patient KS the mirror induced movements in the phantom, but the pain remained completely unabated. Thus, the procedure may not work in all patients, and the reasons for the variability remain to be explored.

could move his right hand inside the box but that his phantom was frozen. He was then asked to open his eyes, look at the reflection of his hand in the mirror, and try the same procedure so that he could "see" his phantom come to life and move in response to his commands. A few seconds later he exclaimed, with considerable surprise, "Mind-boggling. My arm is plugged in again; it's as if I am back in the past. All these years I have often *tried* to move my phantom several times a day without success, but now I can actually *feel* I'm moving my arm. It no longer feels like it's lying lifeless in a sling." The mirror was removed and it was verified that, as before, the man could no longer feel his phantom moving if he closed his eyes and tried mirror-symmetrical movements. ("It feels frozen again.")

The patient also tried moving his index finger and thumb alone while looking in the mirror but, this time, the phantom thumb and index finger remained paralyzed, they were not revived. This is an important observation, as it rules out the possibility that the previous result was simply a confabulation in response to unusual task demands. Thus it was as though there had been some temporary inhibition or block of the neural circuits that would ordinarily move the phantom, and visual feedback could be used to overcome this block. The remarkable thing is that these somatic sensations could be revived in an arm that had never experienced such sensations in the preceding 10 years.

The patient was asked to take the virtual reality box home and try the same procedure every day in the hope that he could eventually dispense with the mirror. After a week he reported the same phenomenon—with his eyes open he was able to move the phantom, but as soon as he closed his eyes it was paralyzed again. The man continued with the procedure and after three weeks reported that the phantom arm had completely disappeared. The entire arm was gone and he was left with just his phantom fingers dangling from his stump. This telescoping effect is a well-known clinical phenomenon, but the patient was unaware of it and was therefore quite surprised by this sudden change in his body image that had been induced by a simple optical trick. He actually claimed to enjoy the telescoping because the pain that he used to have in his phantom elbow also disappeared, since he now no longer had an elbow. Of interest, however, the pain in his phantom fingers persists (Ramachandran, 1994, 1995a).

The evidence from this experiment suggests that when the right parietal lobe is presented with conflicting signals, such as visual signals telling the patient that his arm is moving and muscles telling him that the arm is not there, the brain resorts simply to denying or gating the signals from the arm, to resolve the confusion, and hence the phantom disappears. (Perhaps the fingers do not disappear because they are overrepresented in the sensory cortex.) The bonus for this patient was that he lost the pain in the elbow, since it may be impossible to have a disembodied pain.

A New Treatment for Phantom Limb Pain?

After amputation of an upper limb many patients also experience a clenching spasm of the hand. The pain can be excruciating, occurring several times a week and lasting for an hour or more each time. One such patient had had his left arm amputated above the elbow six months before we tested him. He found that he could relieve the pain by unclenching the hand with intense voluntary effort, but this usually took half an hour. When looking in the virtual reality box, however, he could immediately unclench his hand by watching the mirror reflection of his normal hand, thus producing instant and dramatic relief from the clenching spasm. He repeated the procedure on four consecutive days with identical results.

It would be difficult to explain these results in terms of current concepts in neuroscience. We suggest that when commands are sent to the hand from the motor cortex they are normally damped by error feedback from propriocep-tion. In the absence of the arm, such damping is not possible, so that the motor output is amplified even further, thereby flooding the system with command signals that are themselves experienced as pain. What virtual real-ity does is provide an extraneous visual feedback signal to interrupt this loop. These ideas can be tested directly by using modern imaging techniques such as magnetic resonance imaging and position emission tomography.

Conclusions

The observations we made on these patients have at least two important implications. First, it is possible to revive volitional control and somatic sensations in a phantom arm by simply using a mirror, even when no sensa-tions have been experienced during the preceding 10 years. This implies a surprising degree of plasticity in the adult brain. Second, far from being mediated by completely autonomous modules that are insulated from each other, vision and touch must interact to a significant extent, much more so than anyone would have suspected.

The effect of the virtual reality box on the phantom, especially the revival of the movements, is sufficiently clear cut that it is unlikely to be merely the result of suggestion. Recall that the first patient could initially revive move-ments only in his elbow and wrist, but not in his fingers, a result that would be difficult to attribute to suggestion. Pain, however, is notoriously suscepti-ble to placebo effects, and until we have done additional experiments it is difficult to be sure that the disappearance of pain in these two patients was a specific result of the mirror therapy. (Recall that in ancient Rome, electric eels were placed on the side of the head to provide relief from pain!) As far as these patients were concerned, however, this distinction is somewhat academic—they did not really care whether the effect was a placebo or not. They had tried every available treatment, including large doses of morphine, and none of them was effective.

Touching the Phantom

Next we wondered whether other types of sensations could be referred from the normal hand to the phantom in the presence of visual feedback. Such intermanual transfer of sensations to the phantom can occasionally be seen even without visual feed back (Ramachandran, 1994b), but I wondered whether the effects might be enhanced by visually resurrecting the phantom.

A patient was instructed to place his phantom on the right side of the mirror and look into the mirror at the reflection of his left hand so that the reflection was superimposed on the felt position of the phantom. He then closed his eyes, and when we touched or stroked individual fingers of his left hand with a Q-Tip, he reported that he felt the touch only in his left hand, with no referral to his phantom. However, as soon as he opened his eyes and looked into the mirror, he exclaimed with some surprise that he clearly felt the tactile sensations in the exact mirror-symmetrical location on his phantom. (In a comparison of eight "eyes closed" trials interleaved with eight "eyes open" trials, the referral was seen in all of the former and none of the latter.) However, when ice-cold (0°) or hot water (86°) was dabbed on his normal hand he reported feeling only the dabbing on the phantom; the temperature was not carried over.

This is important, as it rules out confabulation as a possible explanation of these effects. If the patient was confabulating, why should touch be referred and not temperature? Therefore, this is clearly a genuine sensory phenomenon. Certain bimodal cells in the parietal cortex described by Graziano, Yapp, and Gross (1994) that have visual and tactile receptive fields superimposed on the hand might provide a neural substrate for these curious effects.

Control Condition

The mirror box procedure was used on four healthy control subjects. They were instructed to place their hands on either side of the box and to look at the mirror reflection of, say, the left hand superimposed on the right hand, which was hidden by the mirror. Each subject was asked to perform various types of movements with the left hand but they felt no movements at all in the right hand. Touching the left hand so that the subject could "see" the other hand being touched also did not produce any referred sensations. We conclude, therefore, that the referral of movement and touch sensations is unique to phantom limbs.

Visual Feedback Without Moving the Intact Arm   In all the experiments described so far, the patient simultaneously attempts mirror-symmetrical movements with both arms and this was effective in temporarily restoring voluntary control over the phantom. But notice that in this experiment there are also two other potential sources of information besides the visual feedback, the proprioceptive feedback from the intact limb and the motor commands to the intact limb. These could be conveyed by the corpus callosum to the hemisphere that controls the phantom and may therefore contribute to the revival of movements in the paralyzed phantom.

To explore this we adopted a simple modification of our basic procedure: instead of using the patient's intact hand, we used the experimenter's hand to produce the mirror reflection. For practical reasons we were able to try the experiment only on two patients (PNN and KS) and both of them vividly experienced movements in the phantom even though they did not send motor commands to either hand. Apparently the visual cue was sufficiently compelling that it created a vivid feeling of joint movements in the phantom whether or not the patient moved the contralateral hand (and even though no commands were sent to the phantom). One of the patients noted, however, that the joint sensations were less vivid when the experimenter's hand was used than when he himself moved his fingers. This was not because of a lack of perfect resemblance between the patient's hand and the experimenter's since a gloved hand produced the same result. We may conclude, therefore, that even though movements of the normal hand are not necessary for inducing movements in the phantom, they may nevertheless contribute to the sensations.

Induction of Anatomically Impossible Finger Positions in the Phantom

By using the experimenter's hand one can also convey the illusion that the patient's phantom fingers have adopted abnormal or anatomically impossible positions. What would be the feelings generated in the phantom by such a procedure?

We tried this in two patients (PNN and KS). Ordinarily, if the patient places her phantom on the right side of the mirror, the experimenter places his gloved left hand on the left side of the mirror. This creates the illusion of a resurrected gloved phantom. If the patient has "placed" her phantom palm down on the table, the experimenter would obviously place his left hand palm down. But consider what would happen if the experimenter places his gloved *right* hand with the palm up on the table. To the subject this will look almost identical to the left hand palm down. If the experimenter then flexes his index finger or adducts the thumb, the patient will see her phantom perform an anatomically impossible hyperextension of these fingers.

We tried this four times on PNN's index finger. Each time she said she distinctly felt—and not just saw—the finger bending backward. ("One would have thought that it should feel peculiar, but it doesn't. It feels exactly like the finger is bending backward, like it isn't supposed to.") It would be interesting to repeat this result with a larger number of patients and with other types of "impossible" movements. For example, would it be possible to induce an anatomically impossible lengthening of the arm using a Fresnel lens?

The result on patient KS was especially intriguing. When we did exactly the same experiment with the thumb bending backward he winced. ("That hurt; it felt like somebody was grabbing and pulling my thumb backward, producing a slight twinge of pain.") This is a remarkable result, for it suggests that at least under some conditions, even the mere visual appearance of a bending thumb can evoke pain in the phantom. This flatly contradicts the view held by the artificial intelligence community that the brain is composed of a number of autonomous modules that perform sequential computations on sensory input. Indeed, the result is much more consistent with the dynamic, interactive view of the brain proposed by Edelman (1989).

If these principles are valid, they may have very general implications not only for understanding how the brain works but also for the treatment of other types of neurological dysfunction in which visual feedback might be important (e.g., stroke, anorexia nervosa, apraxia, and focal dystonia). We recently tried the procedure on a patient with "pianist's cramp"—a form of focal dystonia—and found, to our amazement, that there was some improvement in the dystonic hand!

We must hasten to add, however, that our results certainly do not disprove the existence of specialized modules in the brain. It may be useful, in this context, to distinguish between facultative and obligatory modules, ones that can function autonomously when other cues are absent but usually interact with each other versus those that always function autonomously. We believe that the majority of brain mechanisms belong to the former rather than the latter category.

ANOSOGNOSIA

As mentioned, anosognosia is observed in patients with left-sided paralysis caused by damage to the right hemisphere, usually the result of a stroke.[1] Most patients with right hemisphere stroke acknowledge their paralysis, but a small proportion (approximately 5%) vehemently deny it. This syndrome was first described at the turn of the century by French neurologist Babinsky (1914). Since then numerous fascinating clinical cases of anosognosia have been described but the tendency has been to regard them as outlandish or bizarre. We attempted to bring this syndrome into the domain of modern cognitive neuroscience, and believe that it raises some fundamental questions concerning the organization of the human mind.

As an illustration of this syndrome, consider the following conversation we had with an elderly woman (FD) who had had a right hemisphere stroke eight days previously, resulting in a complete left hemiplegia (clinical details for this and other patients with anosognosia are described in appendix 3.1). She was unable to move without a wheelchair and had no use of her left arm.

VSR: Mrs. D, how are you feeling today?

FD: I've got a headache. I've had a stroke so they brought me to the hospital.

VSR: Mrs. D., can you walk?

FD: Yes.

(She had been in a wheelchair for the past two weeks. She could not walk.)

VSR: Mrs. D., hold out your hands. Can you move your hands?

FD: Yes.

VSR: Can you use your right hand?

FD: Yes.

VSR: Can you use your left hand?

FD: Yes.

VSR: Are both hands equally strong?

FD: Yes, of course they are.

This is quite typical of a person with anosognosia. At this point I wondered what would happen if I kept pushing the patient further. I did so with some hesitation, for fear of precipitating what Goldstein (1940) called a catastrophic reaction, which is simply medical jargon for the patient becoming depressed and starting to cry because her defenses crumble.

VSR: Can you point to my nose with your right hand?

FD: (She pointed to my nose.)

VSR: Point to me with your left hand.

FD: (Her hand lay paralyzed in front of her.)

VSR: Are you pointing to my nose?

FD: Yes.

VSR: Can you clearly see it pointing?

FD: Yes, it is about two inches from your nose.

At this point the woman produced a frank confabulation, a delusion about the position of her arm. She had no problems with her vision and could see her arm perfectly clearly, yet she created a delusion about her own body image. (I had verified previously that she had no left hemineglect, and also took the precaution of standing on her right side.)

VSR: Can you clap?

FD: Of course I can clap.

VSR: Will you clap for me?

FD: (She proceeded to make clapping movements with her right hand as if clapping with an imaginary hand near the midline.)

VSR: Are you clapping?

FD: Yes, I'm clapping.

Thus, here at last, we may have an answer to the Zen master's eternal riddle: what is the sound of one hand clapping? Mrs. D. obviously knew the answer!

What we saw in Mrs. D. was quite extreme. What is much more common in patients with anosognosia is a tendency to come up with all sorts of rationalizations to explain why the arm does not move; they do not usually say that they can actually see their arm moving. Consider the following conversation I had with another more typical patient. She too had sustained a right hemisphere stroke causing the left side of her body to be paralyzed.

VSR: Mrs. R., How are you doing?

LR: I'm fine.

VSR: Can you walk?

LR: Yes.

VSR: Can you use your arms?

LR: Yes.

VSR: Can you use your right arm?

LR: Yes.

VSR: Can you use your left arm?

LR: Yes, I can use my left arm.

VSR: Can you point to me with your right hand?

LR: (LR pointed to me with her right hand.)

VSR: Point to me with your left hand?

LR: (Her hand remained lying in front of her.)

VSR: Are you pointing?

LR: I have severe arthritis in my shoulder, you know that doctor. It hurts.

These patients often come up with ingenious excuses and poignantly comic euphemisms to evade the main thrust of the question.

Physician: How come you are not using your left arm?

LR: I've never been very ambidextrous.

There is a striking similarity between the strategies these patients use and what Sigmund and Anna Freud called psychological defense mechanisms (S. Freud, 1961; A. Freud, 1946). They are used when people are confronted with disturbing facts about themselves. Examples are rationalization, denial, repression of unpleasant memories, and reaction formation. People suffering from anosognosia do the same things but in a grossly exaggerated form (Ramachandran, 1994, 1995b). For example, a normal person who has peripheral nerve damage and is left with a paralyzed arm may downplay the extent of the deficit ("Oh, I think I'll recover soon"), but he is unlikely to declare that the arm does not belong to him or that he sees it pointing about two inches from your nose. Most people would not carry defense mechanisms to such absurd limits.

One interpretation of anosognosia would be in psychodynamic terms; the patient is confronted with something unpleasant, paralysis, and plays it down or even denies it. This explanation does not work for one simple reason—the disorder is rarely seen when the left hemisphere is damaged and results in right-sided paralysis. That paralysis ought to be just as unpleasant, yet patients rarely engage in denial. Such asymmetry suggests that anosognosia is a neurological rather than a psychological syndrome. Indeed, the reason that it is so fascinating is precisely because it straddles the borderline between neurology and psychiatry, between brain and mind.

Another more cognitive interpretation of the syndrome would be in terms of the hemineglect-heminattention that often accompanies denial. That is, one could argue that the patient neglects her paralysis in much the same way that she neglects everything else on the left side. This hypothesis is probably at least partially correct, but it does not account for why the denial usually persists even when the patient's attention is drawn to the paralysis. Nor does it explain why the patient does not intellectually correct her misconception even though she may be quite lucid and intelligent in other respects. Indeed, the reason anosognosia is so puzzling is that we have come to regard the intellect as primarily propositional in character, and we ordinarily expect propositional logic to be internally consistent. To listen to a patient deny ownership of her arm and yet, in the same breath, admit that it is attached to her shoulder is one of the most perplexing phenomena that a neurologist can encounter.

The Surreal Logic of Anosognosia

Several earlier attempts have been made to explain anosognosia but most of then are one variant or another of the two theories outlined above— the psychodynamic theory or the neglect theory. Here, we propose a new approach to this syndrome. To formulate the problem clearly, we consider two theoretical question:

1. Why do normal individuals have psychological defense mechanisms? Why should they hold false beliefs about themselves?
2. Why are these mechanisms grossly exaggerated in anosognosia?

A New Biological Theory of Self-Deception; Was Trivers Right?

Freudian defense mechanisms are essentially false beliefs about oneself, but what possible benefit could holding false beliefs confer on an organism? Indeed, on the face of it, they actually seem maladaptive.

The most popular theory of self-deception, currently in vogue, was proposed by the well-known evolutionary biologist Trivers (1985). According to him there are many occasions when a person needs to deceive someone else. Unfortunately, it is difficult to do this convincingly since one usually gives the lie away through subtle cues, such as facial expressions (Ekman, 1975) and tone of voice. Trivers proposed, therefore, that maybe the best way to lie to others is first to lie to oneself. Self-deception, he suggests, may have evolved specifically for this purpose: you lie to yourself to be able to deceive others more effectively.

Although his argument is ingenious and may contain some truth, it is not entirely convincing. When you lie to someone, your purpose is to withhold information that you do not want the other person to know. For example, suppose chimp A sees where a zoo keeper places a big bunch of bananas. Chimp A now points chimp B in the wrong direction so that he can have all the bananas to himself. Now, according to Trivers' argument, if chimp A wants to make sure that chimp B does not detect the lie, he engages in self-deception; that is, he really believes that the bananas are in the place that he points to. But if this were true, chimp A himself would also go look for the bananas in the false location. This would defeat the whole purpose of deception and be obviously maladaptive.

The real reason for the evolution of these defense mechanisms (confabulations, rationalization) we suggest is to create a coherent belief system to impose stability in one's behavior. To understand this alternative hypothesis, one must invoke the idea of hemispheric specialization. Popular psychology acknowledges that the left hemisphere is specialized for language and the right hemisphere engages in visual-spatial tasks. Yet many basic differences between the two hemispheres are overlooked.

In particular, we suggest each of us has a tremendous need to impose consistency, coherence, and continuity onto our behavior. In other words, we need a script, a thread of continuity in time. The left hemisphere is primarily responsible for imposing consistency onto the story line, and this would correspond roughly to what Freud calls the ego. At any given moment in out waking lives our brains are flooded with a bewildering variety of sensory inputs, all of which have to be incorporated into a coherent perspective that is based on what stored memories already tell us is true about ourselves and the world. To act, the brain must have some way of selecting from this superabundance of detail and ordering it into a consistent belief system, a story that makes sense of the available evidence. When something does not quite fit the script, however, we very rarely tear up the entire story and start from scratch. What we do instead is to deny or confabulate to make the information fit the big picture (this is preferable to saying that we try to "reduce dissonance," which does not really mean anything). Far from being maladaptive, such everyday defense mechanisms keep the brain from being hounded into directionless indecision by the combinational explosion of possible stories that might be written from the material available to the senses.

We can illustrate this concept with an analogy. Imagine a military general about to wage war on the enemy. It is late at night and he is in the war room planning strategies for the next day. Scouts keep coming into the room to give him information. They tell him that the enemy has 500 tanks, and since he has 600 tanks, the general decides to attack the next morning. He positions all of his troops in strategic positions and prepares to launch battle exactly at sunrise, 6 A.M. But imagine further that at 5:55 A.M. one scout comes running into the war room with a report that says that the enemy actually has 700 tanks, not 500! What does the general do? A good general would ask the scout to shut up and instruct him not tell anyone about what had been seen. Indeed, he may even shoot the scout and hide the report in a drawer. In doing so, he relies on the probability that the previous scouts' information was correct and this single new tank count is probably wrong. The likelihood seems to be small that this one source of information is right, and so the general sticks to his original position. Not only that, but for fear of mutiny, he might tell the scout to lie to the other generals and tell them that he only saw 500 tanks, which would be analogous to a confabulation. The purpose of all of this is to impose stability on behavior and to avoid vacillation, because indecisiveness does not serve any purpose. Any decision, as long as it is probably correct, is better than indecision. A perpetually indecisive general will never win a war.

By now the reader will have recognized that the general[2] is in the left hemisphere and that his behavior is analogous to the confabulations and delusions of both healthy individuals and patients with anosognosia. What we have to explain, however, is why these defense mechanisms are grossly exaggerated in the patients. This is where the right hemisphere comes into the picture.

The Devil's Advocate

To understand what the right hemisphere is doing we must push the analogy a step farther. Suppose that instead of the scout's report saying that the enemy has 700 tanks, it said that the enemy had nuclear weapons. The general would be very foolish if he adhered to his original plan. He must now abandon his original strategy and formulate a new one, as the consequences, if the scout is correct, are just too great. Once a certain threshold is reached, people must have a mechanism for revising their models completely, and that is where the right hemisphere becomes important.

The basic idea here is that the coping strategies of the two hemispheres are fundamentally different. The left hemisphere's job is to create a model and maintain it at all costs. If confronted with some new information that does not fit the model, it relies on Freudian defense mechanisms to deny, repress, or confabulate; anything to preserve the status quo. The right hemisphere's strategy is fundamentally different. I like to call it the "devil's advocate," for when the anomalous information reaches a certain threshold, the right hemisphere decides that it is time to force the organism to revise the entire model and start from scratch. The right hemisphere thus forces a Kuhnian paradigm shift in response to anomalies, whereas the left hemisphere always tries to cling to the original model.

V. S. Ramachandran et al.

In patients suffering from anosognosia, the left hemisphere is doing all of the confabulation and denial as it would in a normal person. The difference is that these patients have lost the mechanism in the right hemisphere that would ordinarily force them to generate a paradigm shift in response to conflicting information. Thus they fall into a delusional trap and continue to confabulate without switching paradigms. They may glibly explain away any anomaly or discrepancy, so that they are, on the whole, blissfully oblivious to their predicament.

A similar dichotomy between the two hemispheres was proposed by Kinsbourne (1989), not so much as an explanation for anosognosia, but as an attempt to account for laterality effects in depression seen in stroke victims. Although Kinsbourne does not discuss Freudian defense mechanisms or paradigm shifts, he makes the ingenious suggestion that the left hemisphere may be involved in maintaining continuing behavior, whereas the right hemisphere may interrupt behavior when the goal is not met, an idea that fits perfectly with what we have proposed.

A note of caution, however, is necessary concerning hemispheric specialization. We have been warned of the dangers of "dichotomania" (Bogen, 1975; Galin, 1976); that is, of ascribing any given cognitive function entirely to one hemisphere or the other. [Even the "mute" right hemisphere appears to be linguistically much more sophisticated than previously believed (Zaidel, 1985).] We must bear in mind not only that the specialization is probably relative rather than absolute, but that the human brain also has a front and back, and an up and down, and countless other subdivision, not just left and right. Thus the idea is that the right hemisphere is a left-wing revolutionary that generates paradigm shifts, whereas the left hemisphere is a die-hard conservative that clings to the status quo, is almost certainly a gross oversimplification.[3] Even so, if it leads to some interesting new experiments, it will have some adequately served its purpose. As noted by Charles Darwin (1871):

False facts are highly injurious to the Progress of Science for they often endure long; but false views do little harm, as every one takes a salutory pleasure in proving their falseness; and when this is done, one path towards error is closed and the road to truth is often at the same time opened.

What Darwin is arguing for here is that hopeful monsters and natural selection may be just as important for the evolution of ideas as it is for the evolution of the species.

The notion that mirror-symmetrical points in the two hemispheres might be specialized for complementary rather than identical functions is also attractive for another quite distinct reason. Throughout evolution, the exploitation of duplicate body parts to permit the emergence of new modules is the rule rather than the exception. It would be surprising, therefore, if the redundancy inherent in the two cerebral hemispheres had not been exploited in this manner (Ramachandran, 1989).

Implications for Mnemonic Functions

Another curious aspect of anosognosia that is rarely commented upon in the clinical literature concerns the patients' memories of their failure to use their left hand. When I asked a patient (Mrs. OS) on one occasion "Mrs. OS, can you use your left hand," her response was, "Yes, of course I can use my left hand. In fact, I used it to wash my face this morning." And when asked, "Can you walk," another patient replied, "Yes, I can walk; I just went to the rest room." I find it quite astonishing that an otherwise mentally lucid and intelligent person can instantly generate such an absurd confabulation— a false memory—from the recent past. A more intensive study of these phenomena will surely have implications for understanding how memories are "retrieved"—even in normal individuals—and how they are squeezed into one's preexisting belief systems.

This amnesia seems to affect only the *actions* of the left hand, but not other aspects of that hand. On one occasion the patient was surprised to notice that I had slipped a red hair band on her left hand. After removing the band, I started questioning her about the movements of that hand and—as expected—she vehemently denied the paralysis but with repeated questioning, she finally admitted that it "wasn't working." Yet a few minutes later she had no recollection of this "confession," even though she vividly remembered the hair band! Surprisingly, even on the one occasion when the patient had a "catastrophic reaction," she had no subsequent recollection of this.

Multiple Personalities, Fugue States, and Supernumerary Phantoms

We have considered how the coherencing of consciousness and the need to create a unified belief system may have evolved primarily to confer stability to one's behavior and may even help explain human self deception and Freudian defense mechanisms. The same principle might help account for two other clinical oddities: multiple personalities and supernumerary phantoms.

Instead of a single anomaly, if there are several anomalies inconsistent with the original belief system (A), but consistent with each other, they may coalesce—like soap bubbles—into a new belief system (B) that is insulated from (A), creating multiple personalities. I find the reluctance of cognitive psychologists to accept the reality of this phenomenon somewhat puzzling, given that even *normal* individuals have such experiences from time to time. I am reminded of a dream I once had in which someone had just been telling me a very funny joke which made me laugh—implying that there must have been at least two mutually amnesic personalities inside me during the dream. This could be regarded as an "existence proof" for the plausibility of multiple personalities!

Supernumerary phantoms—the patient's delusion that he has two left arms (after a right hemisphere stroke)—may have a similar origin. But before we explain this syndrome, let us recall briefly why a single phantom limb is experienced after amputation of an arm. As we have noted elsewhere the phantom limb experience has at least four sources: (1) Irritation of neuromas in the stump activating the original hand area in the cortex. (2) Sensory input from the face "invading" the deafferented hand area, so that spontaneous activity in the face might be felt in the phantom arm (Ramachandran, 1993). (3) Monitoring of "reafference" signals from motor commands sent to the phantom as we noted in the first part of this article. (4) "Memories" of sensory impressions that existed in the arm prior to amputation.

Now in a *real* arm there is, of course, also one other important source—namely, the visual image of the arm—that verifies its existence, and it is perhaps the continued absence of visual and proprioceptive confirmation in an amputee that leads to the eventual telescoping and disappearance of the phantom (Ramachandran, 1994b). The four sources cited above usually provide *consistent* information about the position of the arm, thereby conspiring to create a vivid illusion that the arm is still there. But what if one or more sources provide *inconsistent* information about the arm's position? One option could be to "split" the image, that is, to hallucinate a supernumerary phantom in a manner analogous to multiple personalities. We have recently seen striking example of this in a patient with a brachial plexus avulsion. The patient claiming that in addition to her senseless, paralyzed, lifeless left arm that she could *see*, she also *felt* a smaller hand that was "telescoped" and attached to her elbow even though she realized that this was absurd—"only an illusion." Similarly, in right-hemisphere injuries, if there has been damage to afferent white matter coming from the arm to the somatosensory cortex, "remapping" might occur in a manner analogous to what is seen after amputation or brachial avulsion (Ramachandran, 1993) and, again, if the information conveyed by the remapped zones is inconsistent with visual and "reafference" signals, the net result may be the perceptual illusion of a vividly felt extra left arm. If, in addition, there has been damage to other regions of the right hemisphere, the illusion may evolve into a full blown *delusion*—that is, an actual change in the patient's belief system to accommodate an extra arm, however bizarre that may seem to the examining physician.

EXPERIMENTS ON ANOSOGNOSIA

Experiment 1.   The Virtual Reality Box

Can anosognosia really be conceived of as failure to generate paradigm shifts in response to an anomaly? If so, would it be possible to test this idea experimentally? An alternative interpretation of anosognosia would be in terms of hemineglect of the left side of the body; that is, the patient's failure to orient to the left. I have already noted that I find this idea implausible, but to test the idea more directly I devised a new experiment. What would happen, I wondered, if one were temporarily to paralyze the right arm of a patient who already had anosognosia in association with left hemiplegia?

(Assume the paralysis is achieved by cutting peripheral nerves in the right arm.) Would the anosognosia now encompass his right arm as well? Note that the theory of anosognosia outlined above makes the counterintuitive prediction that he should now deny that his right arm is paralyzed, since his brain fails to initiate a paradigm shift, whereas the neglect theory makes the opposite prediction, since there is no neglect of his right side.

To "paralyze" a patient's (Mrs. FD) right arm, I once again used a simple optical trick. The technique is similar to one originally developed for studying intersensory conflict in normal subjects (Nielsen, 1963), but I realized that it might provide a valuable tool for probing the depth of anosognosia in patients with a right parietal lesions (Ramachandran, 1994a, b).

The virtual reality box was constructed out of cardboard and mirrors. The patient's gloved right hand was inserted through a window in front of the box and she peeked into the box from a hole in the top to look at what she thought was her own hand. Unbeknown to her, an accomplice inserted his gloved left hand through another opening in the box so that its mirror image was optically superimposed on the patient's right hand. Thus she was tricked into thinking that she was looking directly at her own right hand. The patient was then instructed to move her right hand up and down to the rhythm of a metronome. The accomplice held his hand completely steady so that the woman was fooled into thinking that her hand was absolutely still, as though it were paralyzed. I repeated the experiment on two consecutive days, and each time she maintained that she could clearly see her arm moving up and down[4] to the rhythm of the metronome, even though the view afforded to her through the virtual reality box was that of a paralyzed hand.

This simple experiment demolishes all neglect theories of anosognosia, since there was certainly no neglect of the right visual (or somatic) field in this patient, yet she was producing confabulations about her right hand. Clearly, at least in this one woman, what was critical was the presence of a discrepancy in sensory inputs; it is not critical whether the discrepancy arises from the left or from the right side of the body.[5]

Experiment 2.   Cocktail Glasses on a Tray

A second question that arises is how deeply a patient believes his or her own denials and confabulations. Is it simply a surface facade, or perhaps even an attempt at malingering? The vehemence of the patient's denials and her quasi-humorous, emphemistic remarks can themselves be taken as evidence that she is "aware" at some level that she is paralysed (e.g., "Yes, of course I can use my left hand; in fact I used it to wash my face this morning" or "Yes, I can walk. I just walked to the rest room" or "I am not very ambidextrous, doctor").

To question then becomes, for what sorts of behavior is this tacit knowledge available—if it exists? For example, would it be available for a spontaneous, nonverbal motor response? To explore this we confronted the patient with a large tray on which were placed cocktail glasses filled with water. If a healthy person were asked to reach out and take the tray, she would place one hand on either side and proceed to lift the tray. But if one hand was tied behind her back, she would obviously reach for the center of the tray and lift from there.

We asked two patients with right hemisphere stroke (left-sided paralysis) who did not deny the paralysis (i.e., who did not have anosognosia) to lift the tray and each one of them reached for the center of the tray as one might expect. Patients with anosognosia, however, when tested in exactly the same manner, reached straight for the right side with their good hand, even though this would obviously have made the glasses topple over. In one case I had to reach over and grab the other side of the tray so that it could be lifted without spilling the water. When asked if she lifted the tray herself, the patient replied with some surprise that she had. When asked if she used both hands, she replied, "Of course."

Experiment 3. Unimanual versus Bimanual Tasks

Another test we did was to give patients with anosognosia a choice between a simple unimanual task or a simple bimanual task that would be impossible to perform with one hand. The choice was either to thread a light bulb into a socket that was mounted on a heavy base (unimanual) or to tie a shoelace (bimanual) (table 3.2). If the patients threaded the light bulb they would receive a $2 reward and if they tied the shoelace they would receive $5. Normal people always go for the shoelace, which makes sense, because although they can do either task, they would rather earn $5 than $2. When we tried this test on stroke victims without anosognosia, they always went straight for the light bulb task, presumably because they realized that they could not tie the shoe and would rather earn $2 than nothing. Finally, we tested four patients with anosognosia, and on 27 out of 31 trials they went without hesitation straight for the bimanual task. Remarkably, they started trying to tie the laces and keep at it for several minutes without showing any signs of frustration. Even when given the same choice ten minutes later, they again went invariably for the bimanual task. In one patient the tests were repeated on seven consecutive occasions, always with the same result. Indeed, it looks as though these patients have no memory of their previous failures, a selective amnesia for their failed attempts.

Researcher: Mrs. R., do you remember a short while ago when we did some tests on you?

LR: Yes I do.

Researcher: What did you do?

LR: That nice Indian doctor...he asked me to tie shoelaces...I did it successfully *using both hands.*

Table 3.2 Complete list of bimanual and unimanual tasks used in the experiment

Tasks	Prizes
Bimanual	
Tie the laces of a baby shoe	$5
Sew yarn around a small card	Ceramic angel
Tie a bow around a large box	Large box of candy
Use scissors to cut a paper circle	
Unimanual	
Screw the nut onto the bolt (mounted on wood to remain perpendicular)	$2
	Bar of scented soap
Stack five blocks	Small box of candy
Pick up objects with a clamp and put them into a bag	
Pick up a toy octopus with a fishing hook and put it into a cup	

The tasks were paired randomly with different rewards on different trials.

The patients were confronted with a choice between a unimanual task or a bimanual task in a gamelike atmosphere. They had to choose only one of these and complete it successfully to obtain a reward. Before each trial, they were given careful demonstrations of both tasks and told that they would be given the corresponding prize. They were also told that if they were unable to accomplish the task successfully they would be given nothing. The combinations of bimanual and unimanual tasks were randomized, together with their prize pairs, but the larger or more valuable prizes were always coupled with the bimanual and the smaller or less valuable prizes with the unimanual tasks.

This patient had no problem carrying on a conversation or remembering me when I came to see her each day, yet she did not remember her failure with the shoelaces ten minutes earlier. Of interest, she volunteered the information "with both hands" when referring to her ability to tie the shoelace. It is difficult to imagine a normal person saying this, and it suggests that in some part of her brain the woman knew that she was paralyzed. She was exhibiting what Freud called "reaction formation," asserting the opposite of what one believes to be true. (A notable example comes from *Macbeth*, "Methinks the lady doth protest too much.")

Our experience with anosognosia suggests that Freudian psychology may actually have a neural basis that can be studied in these patients. The only previous attempt to link psychoanalysis to illusions of body image was made by Schilder (1950). Unfortunately, his ideas were not taken seriously by the scientific community. The reason for this is that he took a concrete neurological phenomenon, the sequelae of right parietal damage, and tried to explain it in terms of a nebulous theoretical framework—Freudian psychology. In science one rarely gets very far explaining the concrete in terms of the nebulous. Here we have attempted the opposite; we have tried to provide a neurological explanation of Freudian defense mechanisms.

An interesting question concerns the domain specificity of anosognosia. Do the patients deny only paralysis of body parts or do they deny other disabilities as well? This would probably depend on how anterior the lesion is; lesions that are toward the front may tend to produce a more global denial, whereas those in the parietal may generate denials that are confined to one's body image.[6] Indeed, some clinical evidence illustrates that patients with right frontal strokes tend to be blissfully indifferent to the gravity of their predicament; that is, they have a global anosognosia. Those with left frontal strokes, on the other hand, are often depressed (Robinson, Dubos, and Starr, 1984) perhaps because they lack even the minimum coping mechanisms that they need to get on with their lives.

Experiment 4. "Repressed" Memories in Anosognosia

Our experiments with anosognosia seem to suggest that the information that the patient is paralyzed is being held somewhere in the brain, but that access to this information is blocked. To demonstrate this more directly, we took advantage of an ingenious experiment performed by Italian neurologists on a patient with neglect and anosognosia (Bisiach, Rusconi, and Vallar, 1992). They took a syringe filled with ice cold water and irrigated the woman's left ear canal, a procedure that is usually used to test vestibular nerve function. Within a few seconds the patient's eyes started to move vigorously (caloric-induced nystagmus). The researchers then asked her if she could use her arms. Surprisingly, she replied that she had no use of her left arm. The cold water irrigation of the left ear brought about admission of her paralysis.

I tried this same experiment on my patient Mrs. BM, an elderly woman who had had a right parietal stroke that resulted in left side paralysis. My purpose was not only to confirm the observation of Bisiach et al, but also to ask questions specifically to test her memory, something that had not been done before on a systematic basis.

VSR: Mrs. M., can you walk?

BM: Yes, I can walk.

VSR: Can you use your right hand?

BM: Yes.

VSR: Can you use your left hand?

BM: Yes, I can.

VSR: Are both hands equally strong?

BM: Yes, of course they're equally strong!

I then irrigated her *right* ear with cold water and her eyes started moving in the characteristic way. After about a minute I began to question her.

VSR: How are you doing?

BM: My ear is cold, but I'm fine.

VSR: Can you use both of your arms?

BM: Yes, I can use both arms.

The next day, after going through the same questions and eliciting a vehement denial of paralysis, I irrigated the patient's left ear with cold water. I waited until her eyes started moving and then questioned her again about her paralysis.

VSR: Do you feel okay?

BM: My ear is very cold, but other than that I am fine.

VSR: Can you use your hands?

BM: I can use my right arm but not my left arm. I want to move it but it doesn't move.

VSR: (holding the arm in front of the patient) Whose arm is this?

BM: It is mine, of course.

VSR: Can you use it?

BM: No, it is paralyzed.

VSR: Mrs. M, how long has your arm been paralyzed? Did it start now or earlier?

BM: It has been paralyzed continuously for several days now.

After about one-half an hour later my assistant tested her.

Assistant: Mrs. M, can you walk?

BM: Yes.

A.: Can you use both your arms?

BM: Yes.

A.: Can you use your left arm?

BM: Yes.

A.: This morning, two doctors did something to you. Do you remember?

BM: Yes. They put water in my ear; it was very cold.

A.: Do you remember they asked some questions about your arms, and you gave them an answer? Do you remember what you said?

BM: I said my arms were okay.

Thus, even though BM had denied her paralysis every time I had seen her in the clinic since the stroke, the information about her failed attempts had been nevertheless getting into her brain. It seems as though the access to these memories is ordinarily blocked, but cold water removes the block. The memories then come to the surface and the patient "confesses" her paralysis. Yet after the effect from the water wears off, the patient flatly denies her earlier admission of paralysis, as though she were completely rewriting her "script." Indeed, it was almost as if we had created two separate conscious human beings who were mutually amnesic: the "cold water" Mrs. BM who is intellectually honest, who acknowledges and is disturbed by her paralysis, and the Mrs. BM without the cold water who has anosognosia and completely denies her paralysis.

These results suggest, therefore, that anosognosia might provide a new experimental paradigm for studying mnemonic functions in the human brain, especially the question of how new memories are seamlessly incorporated into one's preexisting cognitive schemata. Such experiments would be especially easy to carry out in conjunction with caloric-induced reversible hyperamnesia, if this effect is confirmed on additional patients. However, since patients with this syndrome tend to recover spontaneously over a period of several days, the experiments could also in principle be carried out, even without caloric testing, by simply interviewing the patients repeatedly about their memories as they gradually regain insight. For example, four months after her repeated denial of paralysis and repeated failure with bimanual tasks (e.g., tying shoelaces), another patient (Mrs. OS) had recovered completely from anosognosia and she now complained that her left arm was paralyzed. Her memory for various irrelevant details of the early testing sessions were quite vivid, but when asked if she had always been paralyzed, she said yes. When asked whether she remembered denying the paralysis,[7] she said, "Well, if I did I must have been lying and I don't usually lie" (Ramachandran, 1995b).

The question arises as to why cold water produces these apparently miraculous effects, acting almost like a truth serum, as it were. One possibility is that it arouses the right hemisphere. Connections from the vestibular nerve project to the vestibular cortex in the right parietal lobe as well as other parts of the right hemisphere. Arousal of the right hemisphere makes the patient pay attention to the left side. Thus the patient pays attention for the first time to her arm that is lying lifeless and recognizes that she is paralyzed.

This interpretation is probably at least partly correct, but an alternative hypothesis is that this phenomenon is related to rapid-eye-movement (REM) sleep. People spend one-third of their lives sleeping; 25% of that time their eyes are moving and that is when they have vivid, emotional dreams. In both the cold water state and in REM sleep noticeable eye movements occur and unpleasant memories come to the surface, and this may not be a coincidence. Freud believed that in dreams we pull out material that is ordinarily censored. At the risk of pushing the analogy too far, we can refer back to our general who is now sitting in his bedroom late the night before battle sipping a glass of cognac. He has time to engage in leisurely inspection of the report brought to him by the one scout at 5:55 A.M., and this is what we call dreaming. If the material makes sense, he may decide to incorporate it into his battle plan for the next day, but if it does not make sense or is too disturbing for him, he will put it back into his drawer and try to forget about it. This is what happens 90% of the time in dreaming, which is why we cannot remember most of our dreams. Perhaps the vestibular stimulation partly activates the same circuitry that generates REM sleep, thereby allowing the patient to pull out unpleasant, disturbing facts about herself including her paralysis, which is usually repressed when she is awake.[8] This is obviously a highly speculative conjecture and I would give it only a 25% chance of being correct. (My colleagues would probably give it 10%!) But it does lead to a simple testable prediction; patients with anosognosia should *dream that they are paralyzed*. In fact, if they are awakened during a REM episode they may continue to admit their paralysis for several minutes before reverting to denial again. (Recall that the effects of caloric-induced nystagmus lasted for at least 30 minutes.)

A THEORY OF DREAMS: NATURE'S OWN VIRTUAL REALITY

Developing this theme a little further, we suggest that during ordinary waking life the left hemisphere engages in "on-line" processing of sense data, including the temporal ordering of experiences and the imposition of consistency and coherence. This would necessarily involve the kinds of censoring, repressions, denials, and rationalizations that characterize most of our conscious lives. In dream sleep, on the other hand, your brain is allowed to tentatively bring some of the repressed memories[9] out for an "improv" rehearsal on the main stage to see if they can be incorporated coherently into the main script without penalty to your ego. If the new script does not make sense, the material gets repressed again unless you wake up accidentally, in which case it emerges in disguised form but is not incorporated into your psyche. But if it does work, then it gets incorporated seamlessly into the conscious self in the left hemisphere so that your personality becomes progressively more refined and less encumbered by unnecessary defenses. (This might explain why psychoanalysis is so notoriously difficult. What the therapist tries to do during wakefulness is precisely what nature has evolved to avoid during wakefulness and allows to occur only during REM sleep.)

The reason you cannot carry out these rehearsals in your imagination— when awake—is not obvious, but two possibilities come to mind. First, for the rehearsals to be effective, they must look and feel like the real thing, and this may not be possible when you are awake since you know that the images are internally generated. (As Shakespeare said, "You cannot cloy the hungry edge of appetite with bare imagination of a feast." It makes good evolutionary sense that imagery cannot substitute for the real thing.) Second, unmasking disturbing memories when awake would defeat the very purpose of repressing them in the first place and may have a profound destabilizing effect on the system, whereas unmasking them during REM sleep may permit realistic and emotionally charged simulation in a part of your mind/brain that is informationally insulated from your ordinary conscious mind that is active during wakefulness.

HUMOR AND LAUGHTER: A BIOLOGICAL HYPOTHESIS

Let us now consider how essentially the same dichotomy between the two hemispheres may help explain another major biological puzzle—the origin of humor and laughter. Theories of humor and laughter go all the way back to Kant (1790) and Schopenhauer (1819), two singularly humorless German philosophers. Typically, humor involves taking someone along a garden path of expectation so that the left hemisphere (in our scheme) is allowed to construct a story or model and then introducing a sudden unexpected twist at the end so as to generate a *paradigm shift*; that is, a completely new model is invoked to explain the same data. Of course the twist is necessary but certainly not sufficient to generate humor; for example, if my plane were about to land in San Diego and one of the engine fails unexpectedly, I would not regard this as very funny. They key idea here is that the twist has to be novel but *inconsequential*. Thus, we may regard humor as a response to an inconsequential anomaly.

Incongruity theories of humor have a long history (Gregory, 1991). We can take these early ideas can be taken a step farther by invoking hemispheric specialization and by proposing a specific explanation for the loud, explosive, stereotyped quality of the sound associated with laughter. I suggest that humor emerges when a dialogue between the consistency-imposing tendencies in the left hemisphere and the anomaly detector in the right hemisphere leads to a paradigm shift whose consequences are trivial. Imagine you are in a dimly lit room late at night and you hear some annoying sounds. Ordinarily you interpret this to be the wind or something equally innocuous. If it gets a little louder you continue to ignore it, following the left hemisphere's strategy of ignoring evidence contrary to its preexisting model. But now the sound is really loud and your right hemisphere forces a paradigm shift; you decide it must be a burglar and orient to the presumed anomaly. Your limbic system is activated so that you are both aroused and angry, preparing to fight or flee. But then you discover that it is in fact your neighbor's cat and so you laugh and harmlessly displace the emotion that has been built up.

But why laughter? Why the particular loud, explosive, repetitive sound? Freud's view that it is during laughter that you discharge pent-up psychic energy does not make much sense without recourse to an elaborate hydraulic metaphor. Instead, laughter may have evolved specifically to alert others in the social group that the anomaly is inconsequential; they need not bother orienting. For example, if someone slips and falls and hurts herself, you do not laugh; in fact, you rush to her aid. But if she is not hurt you do laugh (the basis of all slapstick humor), thereby signaling to others that they need not rush to her aid. Thus laughter is nature's false alarm signaling mechanism.

Notice, however, that although this view explains the logical structure of humor, it does not explain why humor itself is sometimes used as a psychological defense mechanism. One possibility is that jokes are an attempt to trivialize what would otherwise by genuinely disturbing anomalies. In other words, when an anomaly is detected, it is ordinarily dealt with by orienting or, when appropriate, by denial or repression. But if, for some reason, it becomes more conspicuous and starts clamoring for attention, an alternative strategy would be to pretend that it is a trivial anomaly by using a joke (i.e., you set off your own false alarm mechanism). Thus, a mechanism that originally evolved specifically as an ethological signal to appease others in the social group has now become internalized to deal with cognitive anomalies in the form of a psychological defense mechanism. (Hence the phrase "nervous laughter.")

SUMMARY AND CONCLUSIONS

The ideas proposed here have article have much more in common with biologically based theories of cognition and perception (Crick, 1994; Edelman, 1989) than it does with the central tenets of classical artificial intelligence (AI). As we pointed out in the past (Ramachandran, 1988, 1989), classic AI ignores the relevance of the neural machinery in the brain and the evolutionary history of the organism, both of which can provide vital clues to understanding the functional organization of complex biological systems such as the human brain.

We conclude with a note of caution followed by a note of optimism. The need for caution arises because we are dealing here with single case studies. There is nothing against single case studies per se. The majority of syndromes in neurology that have stood the test of time (e.g., major aphasias, anterograde amnesia, etc.) were in fact originally discovered by insightful studies of a single or a small handful of patients, not by mindless screening of thousands of patients. A single afternoon spent with a patient with a split-brain (commissurotomy) can reveal more about the mind-brain than several years of quantitative studies on large groups of patients who do not have such clean lesions. Yet, having said that, let us add that our work on the reversible amnesia and hyperamnesia with cold water and the effects of virtual reality on phantom limbs has to be repeated on a large number of subjects, and it would not be at all be surprising if the effects are seen only in a subset of patients. (E.g., neglect can occur due to frontal, cingulate, parietal, and even thalamic lesions, and only some of these might be reversible by caloric stimulation.)

On a more optimistic note, however, many of these questions can now be addressed directly by the new imaging techniques that are currently available, such as magnetic resonance imaging, magnetoencephalography, and position emission tomography. What type of activation is seen in a brain of a stroke victim who denies her paralysis? When she says that she can see herself touching your nose with her left hand, is she confabulating or hallucinating? If the latter is correct, would there be activity in the visual areas? Does the supplementary motor area "light up" when a person tries to move her phantom limb? And would the virtual reality device activate only the visual area and motor cortex (as expected) or the somatosensory areas as well? All these questions can now be answered with currently available technology.

Talking to a patient with anosognosia can be an uncanny experience. The reason the disorder seems so peculiar to us is because it brings us face to face with some of the most fundamental questions that one can ask as a conscious human being. What is the self? What brings about the unity of my conscious experience? What does it mean to will an action? Such questions are often considered to be outside the scope of legitimate scientific enquiry, and neuroscientists usually shy away from them. What we have tried to argue, however, is that patients with anosognosia afford a remarkable opportunity for experimentally approaching these seemingly intractable problems. As we have seen, they may even help us answer the eternal riddle, what is the sound of one hand clapping?

ACKNOWLEDGMENTS

This essay is based on the inaugural "Decade of the Brain lecture" which I gave at the 25th annual meeting of The Society of Neuroscience, (1995). I thank C. Gillin, L. McClure, D. Galin, J. Bogen, R. Bingham, J. Saek, R. Rafael, F. H. C. Crick, P. S. Churchland, A. Starr, M. Kinsbourne, J. Smythies, D. Presti, O. Sacks, and J. Ramachandran for stimulating discussions. Each coauthor of this article participated in at least one of the experiments, but I assume sole responsibility for data interpretation and theoretical speculations. I also thank J. Shreeve for the many interesting conversations I had with him. His 1995 article is based on my paper published in *Consciousness and Cognition* (1995b) and I, in turn, borrowed some of his more colorful metaphors in writing this chapter. Finally, I am grateful to the National Institutes of Mental Health for funding this research, and to the San Diego Rehabilitation Institute (Alvarado), Sharpe Memorial Hospital, and Kaiser Hospital for providing facilities.

NOTES

1. Throughout this chapter the word anosognosia is restricted to denial of hemiplegia, not to its generic use to indicate denial of other types of deficits.

2. The general is not unlike Freud's ego or the language-based "interpreter" (Gazzaniga, 1992) that was postulated to account for the occasional rationalizations of the left hemisphere in patients with split brain disorder. What I try to make clear, however, is the biological rationale, in Darwinian terms, for having such a mechanism in the brain, and also postulate a complementary mechanism in the right hemisphere that serves as a counterbalance.

3. The dialectic between the opposing tendencies of the two hemispheres that we are proposing also bears a tantalizing resemblance to what physicists refer to as the "edge of chaos" in dynamical systems: the emergence of "complexity" at the boundary between stability and chaos. Chaos arises in deterministic systems that show a highly sensitive dependence on initial conditions. This is not unlike the sensitivity to perturbation (or "anomalies") that I have postulated for the cognitive style of the right hemisphere. In marked contrast, the left hemisphere is relatively *insensitive* to change and tries to preserve stability. "Interesting" or "complex" types of behavior, on the other hand, seem to emerge spontaneously at the boundary between the two—a place where there is just enough novelty to keep things interesting and unpredictable but also just enough stability to avoid complete anarchy and instability. And it is precisely these little eddies of "complexity" at the border zone that may correspond roughly to what we call human caprice, innovation, and creativity.

4. Similar confabulations occurred when the patient was asked to keep her right hand still while the accomplice's hand moved up and down to the rhythm of the metronome. This time

the patient insisted that she was not seeing her hand move, that it looked perfectly stationary. We are still a long way from understanding the neural basis of such delusions, but the important recent work of Graziano, Yap, and Gross (1994) may be relevant. They found single neurons in monkey supplementary motor area that had visual receptive fields that were superimposed on somatosensory fields on the monkey's hand. Curiously, when the monkey moved its hand, the visual receptive field moved with the hand, but eye movements had no effect on the receptive field. These hand-centered visual receptive fields ("monkey see, monkey do" cells) may provide a neural substrate for the kinds of somatoparaphrenic delusions I have seen in patients.

5. Contrary to what the term "neglect" implies, the syndrome must surely involve much more than merely ignoring the sensory input from the left side of the world. For if that were the case how does one account for the common observation that, when asked to draw a flower, the patient will often *draw* only half a flower—even with her eyes closed?

   E. Altschuler, K. McClain, and I recently asked a patient to look into a mirror hanging on her right. Standing on her left (neglected) side, I then showed her a candybox, the reflection of which was clearly visible to her. Remarkably, instead of reaching leftward to accept the candy, she kept reaching repeatedly into the mirror complaining that the candybox was outside her reach!

6. Such exquisite domain specificity is, of course, not restricted to anosognosia, it shows up in many areas of neurology. What are we to make of selective loss of vegetable names with sparing of fruits? Or, of loss of inanimate object names but not of animate ones? Such findings pose a serious challenge for any theory of knowledge representation in the brain (Damasio, 1994). I hasten to add that the theory of hemispheric specialization I am proposing certainly is not the only explanation for all forms of anosognosia; e.g., the anosognosia of Wernicke's aphasia probably arises because the very part of the brain that would ordinarily represent beliefs about language is itself damaged. The unawareness of the blind spot or of scotomas of cortical origin is different yet again, since the subject certainly does not deny the blindness *once it is pointed out to him*.

7. Not all patients rewrite the script to match their current beliefs. For example, I recently interviewed a patient 12 years after he had recovered form a massive right hemisphere infarct. He vividly remembered denying his paralysis, asking his wife what "Ken" (as in Ken and Barbie dolls) was doing in bed with him, and denying that his left arm belonged to him. Thus the extent to which memories are accurately recollected by any given patient after the acute effects have worn off may itself depend on the presence or absence of residual neurological deficits.

8. Soon after we wrote this chapter it was pointed out to me that a fad therapy, popular among some psychologists, uses eye movements to enhance patients' "insight" and uncover repressed memories. Although I would ordinarily be inclined to dismiss this as bizarre, it makes perfect sense from the point of view of my theory!

9. These ideas about dreams raise an interesting new question: what do amnesics dream of? Patients with medial temporal lobe/hippocampal amnesia (such as HM) have a profound anterograde amnesia, intact immediate memory, and a relative sparing of "old" premorbid memories. If a patient had developed sudden-onset anterograde amnesia (say) three years ago, and she were to be woken up during REM episodes, would all her dreams be only about premorbid events from her life or would she also dredge up events from the recent past—*even though she cannot remember them when awake*?

   C. Gillin, L. McLure and I tried this experiment recently on a single patient (SM) who had all the classic signs of medial temporal amnesia but was otherwise intact neurologically. Interestingly, on three successive REM awakenings she vividly remembered salient events from the recent past even though she did not remember the events in the morning! (We checked with her husband that these events had indeed occurred well after the onset of her amnesia.)

The implication is that amnesia results not from a failure of acquisition or a "consolidation" but from a failure of *retrieval*. Since the hippocampus is intimately linked to the limbic system, we suggest that its main function might be to serve as a "sorting office" in conjunction with the cortex; that is, it serves to tag episodic memories, labeling them with the appropriate value or significance. If the hippocampus is damaged, the information does get in but is *misfiled*. These mislabeled memories might be inaccessible during ordinary recollection but might be spontaneously dredged up in the bizarre, uncensored world of dreams where value-labels are largely irrelevant. Surprisingly, there is only one previous study on the dreams of amnesics, but the investigators did not specifically look for *postmorbid* memories, which is critical for my argument (Turola, 1964).

10. Another fascinating question concerns the extent to which a patient with anosognosia will acknowledge the paralysis of *another patient*. I explored this a few years ago on three patients. All of them were mentally quite lucid and none of them had any apraxia, autotopagnosia, or radiological evidence of left hemisphere damage. To my amazement when I performed a neurological exam on another hemiplegic patient in the adjacent wheelchair—and demonstrated the hemiplegia—two of my anosognosic patients denied that the other patient was paralyzed (Ramachandran, 1995b)! This curious result implies that at least in some situations, one may need to access one's own body schema even when making judgments about someone else's movements.

REFERENCES

Babinski MJ. (1914). Contribution a l'etude des troubles mentaux dans l'hemiplegie organique cerebrale. *Rev Neurol* 1:845–848.

Bisiach E, Rusconi ML, Vallar G. (1992). Remission of somatophrenic delusion through vestibular stimulation. *Neuropsychologia* 29:1029–1031.

Bogen JE. (1975). The other side of the brain. *UCLA Education* 17:24–32.

Critchley M. (1962). Clinical investigation of disease of the parietal lobes of the brain. *Med Clin North Am* 46:837–857.

Critchley M. (1966). *The parietal lobes*. Hafner, New York.

Crick FHC. (1994). *The astonishing hypothesis*. Charles Scribner's Sons, New York.

Cutting J. (1978). Study of anosagnosia. *J Neurol Neurosurg Psychiatry* 41:548–555.

Damasio AR. (1994). *Descartes' error: Emotion and reason in the human brain*. Putnam, New York.

Darwin C. (1871). *The descent of man*. John Murray, London.

Edelman GM. (1989). *The remembered present*. Basic Books, New York.

Ekman P. (1975). *Unmasking the face; a guide to recognizing emotions from facial clues*. Prentice-Hall, Englwood Cliffs, NJ.

Freud A. (1946). *The ego and the mechanisms of defense*. International Universities Press, New York.

Freud S. (1961). *The standard edition of the complete works of Sigmund Freud*, Vols. 1–23. Hogarth Press, London.

Galin D. (1976). Two modes of consciousness in the two halves of the brain. In: *Syposium on consciousness*. PR Lee, RE Ornstein, D Gallin, eds. Viking Press, New York.

Galin D. (1992). Theoretical reflections on awareness, monitoring and self in relation to anosagnosia. *Consciousness and Cognition* 1:152–162.

Gazzaniga M. (1992). *Nature's mind*. Basic Books, New York.

Geschwind N, Galaburda A, eds. (1984). *Cerebral dominance*. Harvard University Press, Cambridge.

Goldstein K. (1940). *Human nature*. Harvard University Press, Cambridge.

Graziano MSA, Yap GS, Gross C. (1994). Coding of visual space by premotor neurons. *Science* 266:1051−1054.

Gregory RL. (1991). *Odd perceptions*. Routledge, Chapman, & Hall, New York.

Heilman J. (1991). In: *Awareness of deficits after brain injury*. G Prigatano, D Schacter, eds. Oxford University Press, New York and Oxford.

James W. (1887). The consciousness of lost limbs. *Proc Am Soc Psychical Res* 1:249−258.

Juba A. (1949). Beitrag zur struktur der ein- und doppelseitigen korperschemastorungen. *Monatsschr Psychiatrie Neurol* 118:11−29.

Kant I. (1790). Unteilskraft, Berlin.

Kinsbourne M. (1989). A model of adaptive behavior relates to cerebral participation in emotional control. In: *Emotions and the dual brain*. G Gainnotti, C Caltagrione, eds. Springer-Verlag, Heidelberg.

Levine DN. (1990). Unawareness of visual and sensorimotor defects: A hypothesis. *Brain Cogn* 13:233−281.

McGlynn SM, Schacter DL. (1989). Unawareness of deficits in neuropsychological syndromes. *J Clin Exp Neuropsychol* 11:143−205.

Melzack R. (1992). Phantom limbs. *Sci Am* 266:120−126.

Mitchell SW. (1871). Phantom limbs. *Lippincott's Magazine of Pop Lit & Sci* 8:563−569.

Nielsen TI. (1963). Volition: A new experimental approach. *Scand J Psychol* 4:215−230.

Parkes T. (1973). Factors determining the persistance of phantom pain in the amputee. *J Psychosomat Res* 17:97−108.

Ramachandran VS. (1988). Perception of depth from shading. *Sci Am* 269:76−83.

Ramachandran VS. (1989). Vision; a biological perspective. Presidential lecture given at the annual meeting of the Society for Neuroscience, Phoenix, Arizona.

Ramachandran VS. (1993). Behavioral and MEG correlates of neural plasticity in the adult human brain. *Proc Natl Acad Sci USA* 90:10413−10420.

Ramachandran VS. (1994a). How deep is the denial (anosagnosia) of parietal lobe syndrome. *Soc Neurosci Abstr*.

Ramachandran VS. (1994b). Phantom limbs, somatoparaphrenic delusions, repressed memories and Freudian psychology. In: *Neuronal group selection. International review of neurobiology*. O Sporns, G Tononi, eds. Academic Press, San Diego.

Ramachandran VS. (1995a). Amputation of a phantom limb using virtual reality. Presented at the annual meeting of the Cognitive Neuroscience Society, San Francisco.

Ramachandran VS. (1995b). Anosognosia in parietal lobe syndrome. *Conciousness and Cognition* 4:22−51.

Robinson RG, Dubos KL, Starr IB. (1984). Mood disorders in stroke patients. *Brain* 107:81−93.

Schilder P. (1950). *The image and appearance of the human body; studies in the constructive energies of the psyche*. International Press, New York.

Schopenhauer A. (1819). *Die welt als wille und*. Vorstellung, Leipzig.

Shreeve J. (1995). The brain that misplaced its body. *Discover* 82–91.

Sunderland S. (1968). *Nerves and nerve injuries*. Williams & Wilkins, Chicago.

Szasz TS. (1975). *Pain and pleasure*. Basic Books, New York.

Trivers R. (1985). *Social evolution*. Benjamin/Cummings, Menlo Park, CA.

Turda C. (1964). Dreams of subjects with loss of memory for recent events. *Psychophysiology*. 6:358–365.

Weinstein EA, Kahn RL. (1950). The syndrome of anosagnosia. *Arch Neurol Psychiatry* 64:772–791.

Weiskrantz L. (1986). *Blindsight*. Oxford University Press, Oxford.

Zaidel E. (1985). Academic implications of dural brain theory. In: *The dual brain*. D Benson, E Zaidel, eds. Guilford Press.

APPENDIX 1

Case Reports

The five patients who participated in our anosognosia study were elderly women who had recently sustained a right hemisphere stroke causing left hemiplegia. No formal neuropsychological tests (WAIS-R, CVLT) were administered, but they did have a routine neurological work-up, including a mental status examination. At the time our experiments were conducted, they did not have any obvious signs of dementia, aphasia or amnesia, and they were able to understand my instructions clearly. Patients 2, 3, and 4 were sometimes somnolent and/or distractible, but I tried to confine my experiments to lucid periods when they were alert and willing to participate. Whenever possible a computerized tomographic (CT) scan and/or magnetic resonance imaging (MRI) was performed.

Patient No. 1   Patient LR, a 78-year-old, right-handed, Caucasian woman with 16 years of schooling and a degree in journalism, was admitted after the sudden onset of loss of strength in her left limbs. She was alert, cooperative, and conversed fluently with the experimenters and hospital staff. She had no gross deficits in her memory and orientation; for example, when I saw her on two consecutive days, she clearly recognized me the second time and even remembered the tests that were administered. Touch sensation was partially spared on the left side and clear signs of severe left hemiplegia were present. The patient had left hemispatial neglect, as seen in line cancellation and bisection tasks, and also had right head and gaze deviation. She denied any motor or visual impairments, yet admitted she had come to the hospital for treatment of a stroke.

The CT scan performed on admission revealed a right frontoparietal cerebrovascular accident.

Patient No. 2   Patient BM, a 76-year-old, right-handed woman with three years of schooling. She initially appeared slightly somnolent and easily distractible, but was able to communicate successfully through a Spanish-English interpreter. She had no obvious sign of aphasia or dementia, but she did experience difficulty with serial subtraction. Touch and pain sensations were absent on the left side, and she showed clear signs of severe left hemiplegia. Extreme left hemispatial neglect was evident from her line cancellations and bisections, and her head, gaze, and trunk were deviated to the right. The woman denied having any motor or visual deficits, and when questioned about the ownership of her left hand, she falsely ascribed it to either the experimenter or to her son.

An MRI performed one month after admission revealed a large infarct involving much territory of the right middle cerebral artery, especially in the right parieto-occipital region. There was also an area of hemorrhage in the head of the caudate nucleus.

Patient No. 3   Patient OS, a 65-year-old, right-handed, Caucasian woman was easily distracted and somnolent three days after the stroke, but after a week she became more lucid, mentally alert, and personable. Her memory functions seemed intact, but she exhibited some left-right confusion. The patient had almost complete left hemiplegia with some limited preservation of sensations. Left unilateral neglect and denial of motor or visual impairments were present, as well as somatoparaphrenic delusions. When questioned about her left arm, she reported it belonged to either her son or to her husband.

A CT scan performed five days after admission revealed a right temporoparietal infarct.

Patient No. 4   Patient LH was a 77-year-old, right-handed, Caucasian woman who developed a left hemiplegia after coronary bypass surgery. In addition to hemiplegia, she had a left hemispatial neglect. When we first saw her she was drowsy, confused, and inattentive, but two weeks later, when we conducted our experiment, she had improved considerably and was able to converse slowly but fluently with us. Even during the initial work-up she was able to state that she was "in a place where people come to get back on their feet" and that she had "developed a stroke following heart surgery." Also, at that time she was able to count slowly backward from 20 to 1; was able to spell the word "world" forward but not in reverse, and had a digit span of 4. Furthermore, she could see that a hat and coat were similar because they were both clothes, a rose and tulip were both flowers, and watch and ruler were measures. She could not clearly classify the words happy and sad, however.

A CT scan without contrast revealed a subacute right middle cerebral artery and left cerebellar artery infarct.

Patient No. 5   Patient FD was a 77-year-old, right-handed woman who developed a complete left hemiplegia after right hemisphere stroke. At the time when I saw her eight days after the stroke, she had complete paralysis of left upper and lower limbs, no visual hemineglect (line bisection, line cancellation), and no visual extinction. Touch sensations were partly spared in her left hand, but she showed mild tactile extinction. Visual fields were apparently normal.

Patient FD was very alert and had no obvious signs of dementia or aphasia: in fact, her intelligence seemed above average. She could do a serial subtraction by 2s from 100 without difficulty, and was clearly oriented in time and place. When questioned about her family, she provided detailed and accurate descriptions of her son and daughter. She also described the circumstances that led to her hospitalization and was aware that she had had a stoke.

Despite the fact that she was mentally lucid, Mrs. FD was densely anosognosic and denied her paralysis every time she was questioned. When asked whether she could point with her left hand she insisted that she could. A CT scan performed on the day of admission showed and infarct involving the territory of the right middle cerebral artery and the right cerebellar artery.

4 Neural Representations, Experience, and Change

M. M. Merzenich and R. C. deCharms

We support the view that the mind is expressed in physical form as the brain, that it can in principle be studied to any level of detail, and that ultimately this study will lead to the solutions of many of its great unsolved mysteries. Here we will convey something of our vision of how this study program might unfold and what it might mean. Our view is that the nervous system, particularly the cerebral cortex, is best understood in terms of ensembles of neurons that are used to represent the perceived world. These ensembles function dynamically and in relation to one another, providing both the content and the context of our experiences. They are continually formed, reformed, and maintained by simple competitive rules operating throughout life. We believe that the rules that govern changes in the brain that account for learning can be understood, and that these rules underlie the creation of cognitive functions, experiences, and human behaviors.

We will discuss several aspects of brain activity processes that have been insufficiently studied, and that are crucial to explore to relate brain mechanisms to cognitive functions and behaviors. We will briefly summarize the principles of cortical representational plasticity as they are understood at the present time. Finally, we will consider some aspects of what these principles mean for our limited understanding of the functioning of the mind in terms of the brain.

PERSPECTIVES FOR EXPLORING NEURAL REPRESENTATION

Five themes are largely underrepresented in contemporary neurophysiology. These themes are not new, and most would agree with the themes at least in part, but they do not yet hold a central position in current neurologists thinking about brain operations, and in some cases, have been almost entirely neglected.

(a) *The cerebral cortex is always changing*, so its most fundamental functions will be fully understood *only* by models and experiments that seek to explain how specific properties develop and are maintained over time, rather than by attempting to explain cortical functions as if they were innate or static. (b) The cerebral cortex is not a passive machine that waits for inputs, but an active, dynamic system that constructs and maintains our complex internal world through its activities. *All perceptions, choices, actions, and representations take place against the backdrop of an internal context* that is formed from experience and is maintained with the cortical system. (c) *A key element in cortical processing is temporal structure*, meaning both the use of temporal information by the nervous system as a representational strategy, and the fact that most of the percepts and actions that we experience throughout life proceed moment by moment through time, as opposed to being discrete events. (d) *The cortex represents the world through the use of interconnected networks of neurons or neuronal ensembles*, and these ensembles can be fully understood only when observed as such, and not by observing individual neurons in isolation. (e) *Coding in the cortex is probably relational* rather than strictly combinatorial, meaning that the system uses relations between elements and ensembles to establish reliable and flexible representations.

Cortical Representations Are Constantly Changing

It is now clear that the brain is malleable throughout life, but the implications of this have not yet permeated deeply into the general understanding of neural representation in experimental neuroscience. On the short time scale of a particular experience, as an individual pays attention to a stimulus object, the neurons that represent this object can show increased activation in a number of sensory cortical areas. In addition, the *pattern* of activity of neurons in sensory areas can be altered by patterns of attention, leading to measured shifts in receptive fields or tuning of individual neurons. This means that the computational meaning within the cortex of a signal carried by an individual neuron is changed by the attentional state of the organism, and thus that individual neurons cannot be relied on to be carrying the same sensory information signal in different circumstances.

The fact that the tuning of individual neurons is shifted in systematic ways by attention and expectancy suggests that entire spatial maps across the cortical surface are systematically distorted by attention. Again, this implies a rapid remapping of the representational functions of cortex, and suggests that representation cannot be based on the assumption that a given stimulus object will be represented by a fixed pattern across a given sensory map in different circumstances. In particular, expectant attention seems to shift receptive fields in the direction of the expected object or event, or in the direction of the attentional focus.

On the longer time scales of repetitive learning, long-lasting changes to the pattern of cortical maps can be created by repeated practice and learning, as will be elaborated in detail below. It seems very likely that the two phenomena of short-term and long-term dynamics of neuronal tuning and cortical spatial mapping are closely related. We hypothesize that as a map is stretched by attention, then stimulated by afferent input in the behavioral context of learning, this new form is made stable and enduring by synaptic or morphologic modification. Since the patterns of cortical activation by sensory

M. M. Merzenich and R. C. deCharms

objects change over time as cortical maps change their shape but many objects themselves are static, the cortical system must use some other strategy to represent the constancy of objects over time than fixed representational patterns. This raises the issue of how perceptual constancy is maintained in a changing cortex, which will be addressed below.

These facts suggest that the function of cortical neurons can only be understood when both the present activity and the past history of the neuron is understood, and understood within the context of the entire cortical population. Although it is now widely appreciated that global cortical activity is changed by attention and by experience, many experimental studies continue to ignore these facts. Attempting to understand the function of a cortical area by studying single neurons in isolation, without considering how they interact or how they have developed their functions through learning is an impoverished method. It is akin to trying to learn how a team of people function to perform a task without realizing that some of the people may be professionals at the task and others newcomers, what effect experience and training of the team may have on the members' performance, or how the team as a whole can interact to complete the task even though the individuals could not do it alone. One common approach is to study functional representation in a cortical field without any direct behavioral assessment of the area's capacities. This is akin to studying the performances of team members one at a time, with no knowledge of how any individuals or the team as a whole can actually perform the task, and with no knowledge of their experiences that might affect their performance in any event. Another approach is to overtrain the team at the task until an asymptotic performance level is achieved. Overtraining in a strictly contextually controlled behavior creates a highly artificial picture of functional representation in any cortical area under study, reflecting circumstances that scarcely ever occur in real life.

Our general approach has been to try to control what practice our hypothetical team has had, comparing the performance of the individuals in a presumed naive state with that in a trained state, discovering that a given ability or function can be created and shaped by experience in the ways that the data show. We believe that the ideal approach, which still has not been accomplished in more than a limited sense, is to record the progress of many individuals and preferably much of the whole team simultaneously at various stages of practice, to try to figure out what they can do individually and as a team, and how they came to be able to do it through practice. We believe this will ultimately explain what cortical elements do in the context of how they came to be able to do it. Short of this approach, we will keep missing major elements of cortical function and plasticity.

The Cortex Is a Dynamic System in Which all Representations Occur Against a Backdrop of a Continuing, Internally Generated Content

We all know that our perceptions, decisions, actions, and so on take place against a backdrop of what is going on in our minds at the time; for example, the extent to which we see what we are looking for while we ignore much of the rest of incoming information. The effects of what we have experienced and learned in the past are often expressed through these processes of attention and expectation. In a parallel fashion, the brain also operates with incoming and outgoing information existing within an ever-changing context of internal representations, which are rarely studied. Since a whole psychological literature is dedicated to this subject,[1-5] and an entire subfield of philosophy is dedicated to its implications,[6-8] it is clearly worthy of our experimental time.

Traditionally, this territory was put off limits by behaviorism, which said that mental states did not exist if they could not be perceived by an outside observer, and more recently by what we call neurobehaviorism, which similarly suggests that subjective mental phenomena are too hard to measure with current techniques, or even that they are impossible to measure, as the behaviorists thought. Studies that began to address this issue showed that this is not true,[9-17] that there is no absolute barrier that prevents us from gaining significant insights into subjective mental phenomena, and that the techniques to continue this pursuit are already in hand. For example, if traditional experiments can systematically hold the behavioral context of an observer constant and present different stimuli, then parallel experiments can hold the stimuli constant while systematically changing the behavioral context, and thereby changing their meaning to the observer.

The internal context supplied by the nervous system includes such things as attention, expectancy, mental semblancy, planning, emotion, and motivation, and it determines the qualities of our awareness of an object, our choices of how to act, and our actions themselves. It is our belief that object and context hold equally important causal roles that lead to perception and onward through action, that each is represented by continuing activity patterns in the brain, that mentation can only be fully understood as the interaction of these two processes, and that the tools to begin to test this view rigorously are now available.

The Nervous System Functions Over Time

Serial order is typical of the problems raised by cerebral activity .... We can, perhaps, postpone the fatal day when we must face them, by saying that they are too complex for present analysis, but there is a danger here of constructing a false picture of those processes that we believe to be simpler.
—Karl Lashley 1951[18]

In the early 1950s Lashley made a point that most everyone agreed with in principal, but that has still not been embraced by the field of neuroscience as a whole. He contended that real understanding of the neural basis of the mind will depend critically on how neural processes take place in context and through time.[18] These comments went against the prevailing behaviorist winds of his time, which almost entirely ignored dynamic temporal questions such as motor control and language, or the context within which perception and action take place. Lashley stressed that behavior is a continuing process, not a discrete series of responses to isolated stimuli, and that it takes place against an ongoing background of activity. The neurobehaviorist version of this wind still blows, and it is that discrete, rapid onset stimuli produce the most robust neural firing rate responses—in other words, that they are the observables—and that these are therefore the most important types of phenomena for us to study. There has been very little exploration of how neural responses progress through time during perceptual streams (see McAdams and Bregman, this volume). Even the most basic issues of representation in the time domain, such as how one stimulus conditions the cortical representation of a following stimulus, have yet to be explored systematically.

One of the central questions to be answered here is how streams of perception are held together through time and held separate from one another. Another is whether temporal coding is time locked to external events and so can be averaged across instances, or is commonly locked to internal events and so would be completely lost by averaging. We know there are powerful neural mechanisms for temporal smoothing, completing, and conditioning of responses across time, but their mechanistic origins are not yet clearly understood, and it has still to be determined how they can account for time-continuous percepts.

Stimulus Representation Is by Neuronal Ensembles

Many convincing arguments contend that individual neurons in the cortex are not the units of representation: there are not enough of them to code stimuli individually (the grandmother cell argument); their activity patterns show broad tuning and maps of coordinated activity (the argument of inadequate specificity); individual events, such as percepts, activate cortical systems widely, and focal lesions do not knock out focal functions but diminish overall performance (the distributed representation argument); cortical connectivity is sufficiently dense and synapses sufficiently weak that most cortical neurons probably cannot activate other neurons when they fire individually (the argument of weak connectivity); and so on. An assessment of these findings and our own cortical plasticity results lead to the obvious conclusion that the cortex has to be investigated by measuring the neural structures that it creates and then uses for representation, distributed neuronal ensembles. Several classes of studies have shown that important aspects of neural representation take place only through the combined actions or interactions or parts of neuronal ensembles, and are not understandable by the activities of the individual neurons alone.[18-21]

Furthermore, representational ensembles clearly span cortical and subcortical systems, with objects represented simultaneously across broadly separated cortical areas. Only a few direct attempts have been made thus far to learn about how single representations simultaneously span several brain areas,[22-24] and therefore no direct studies of how dramatic plasticity can occur within representations with the maintenance of appropriately associated linkages between them.

Representations Are in Part Relational

Cortical neuronal representations must be understood as being relational, rather than merely combinatorial. By relational representation we mean something conceptually separate from traditional combinatorial ensemble representation. The static view of neuronal ensembles is that each neuron in a large population carries its own small signal of a distinct feature, and that by combining many of these signals together a single distributed representation is formed. Our relational view suggests that the signal carried by a single neuron can vary with the functioning of the whole population, that it need not represent the same distinct feature at different times, and that it only has computational meaning with relation to the context of the remainder of the population. In cases where the responses of neurons in a cortical map are changing over time, the significance of a given neuron's signal can only be interpreted by the brain in terms of its relation to the activity of other neurons, not with respect to a fixed system whereby each neuron indicates a distinct feature.

In a relational representation, information is carried in the relations between elements and ensembles. For a spatial metaphor of this, if all of the people in a football stadium hold up red and yellow cards to form a pattern that spells out the word "mind," then each person passes his or her card three people to the left and then all hold up their new cards, the same word is still represented, although the individuals might all be doing something different. It is heuristically more useful to consider the information borne by the relations in the group, and not merely the combination of all the members' activities. For a temporal metaphor, imagine that all of the people in the crowd are clapping about four times per second. Now imagine that all of the people near the midline of the field continue clapping at the same rate but that all begin to clap in unison, or that each person claps just after the person to his or her left, so that there are moving waves of clapping and silence. Again, the activity of each individual and even the combined activity of the population do not adequately represent what is happening. What is taking place might become clear only by reconstructing relationships. The representation of such an event certainly requires a population to take place, but it requires a relational reconstruction of that population to be understood.

We believe that relational coding must apply in a dynamically changing cortex for two reasons. First, only the representational relations among a group of neural elements can be isomorphic across changing patterns of activity and effective connectivity, and thereby can accomplish representational constancy. Second, a representational system based on relations is hypothetically a powerful one for creating novel complex representational combinations that have not been directly experienced or practiced. Neural representation is virtually certain to make use of the relations between elements of ensembles, for example, distributed temporal synchrony and other timing relations (see Singer and von der Malsburg, this volume).[22-24] These relations will be understood only when significant parts of ensembles are sampled together. To understand the principles of network self-organization and learning and the distributed representations of learned stimuli and behaviors in general, we believe that we must use multiple-site recording methods that probe the instantaneous relations across and between engaged ensembles. In our view, although relational coding may indeed be involved in solving the binding problem, a presently important idea, it is likely to have a fundamental role in all cortical representation, a role that goes well beyond the issue of how local features are grouped together into objects.

Summary

These five themes suggest a study program of neurophysiology that we believe will have to be met, sooner or later, before a full understanding of cortical processing can be reached. They point to new areas of research that should bear fruit once they are addressed in earnest. This perspective in expanded form represents our attempt to put forward testable ideas of how experience and neural representation might be brought together into a unified and empirical understanding of awareness and action.

SOME NEUROLOGICAL PRINCIPLES OF LEARNING AND CORTICAL PLASTICITY

Over the past decade we focused our experimental studies on the definition of the principles and mechanisms of cortical plasticity. Here we turn to these more detailed facets of cortical function. This section presents many of the complex issues of cortical processing and plasticity in a highly condensed and schematic form, with references to more detailed treatments of these topics. From our work and the work of many others we now understand a great deal about many aspects of the operations of dynamic cortical networks. A brief summary of what we understand about these processes constitutes collective testimony about the fundamentally dynamic nature of the forebrain's representations of perceptions and behaviors. It also further illustrates how we have been led inescapably to study cortical neuronal ensembles, the representations and dynamics of input sequences, internal knowledge-based and modulatory control system contexts, and relational aspects of representation.

Some Basic Features of Cortical Representational Plasticity

Experimental results from many lines of study collectively demonstrate that cortical representational changes recorded in plasticity experiments involve processes of coincident input coselection.[25-31] In other words, behaviorally important inputs that are delivered together in time to given cortical network locations change positively together in their excitatory effects. These coincident input coselection mechanisms account for details of cortical neuronal response specificity and for representational topographies. Considered in detail, cortical neuronal response specificity—that subset of possible inputs that neurons actually respond to—and orderly cortical maps are functionally emergent constructs created by the time-order histories of afferent inputs.[6-29,32,33] In this coincidence-based self-organizing machine, the effectiveness of synapses from inputs that excite neurons nearly simultaneously in time come to be represented in closely adjacent cortex. A result of this is that over time cortical areas will function to *map out* topographically any inputs they receive based on the source's input relations and anatomical connectivity.

These anatomical input sources and projection overlaps enable change and establish the limits for change. Since every cortical field has specific anatomically delivered extrinsic and intrinsic input sources with defined spreads of connectivity, these limit its combinatorial, dynamic input-selection capacities.[29,32,33] At lower system levels the anatomical constraints are tighter, so more limited combinatorial results are possible. At the top of system hierarchies, the anatomical projection topographies are nearly all-to-all, and incredibly rich combinations of inputs are generated from a large number of cascaded cortical sources. There, the full combinatorial power of coincidence-dependent input coselection is revealed by neurons that can come to respond to very many of the specific abstracted features of highly complex experiences.[34,35]

The laws of coincident input coselection contain time constants that govern the capacity of individual inputs to generate representational changes based on the particular pattern of temporal relations found within those inputs. Given the short time constants governing synaptic plasticity in the cortex (milliseconds to tens of milliseconds), temporally coincident, coherent inputs are highly effective in driving representational changes. More temporally dispersed or consistently nonsynchronous inputs must have less power for inducing positive synaptic effectiveness changes.

Different cortical areas contain different functional structures—ensembles of neurons that respond to field-specific input relations. These representational structures are created within individual cortical areas by field-specific sources, relations, and distributions of synchronizable inputs. These field-specific differences are very marked across system levels.[26,27,29] For example, compare the statistics of the afferent inputs from retina, or skin, or cochlea into the primary cortical receiving areas VI, SI, and AI (17, 3b, and 43), which are all strictly topographically wired, with the statistics of afferent inputs to the high-level inferotemporal (visual), insular (somatosensory), and dorsolateral temporal (auditory) cortical fields, which are highly diffused. In the former cases, very heavy schedules of repetitive and highly temporally coher-

M. M. Merzenich and R. C. deCharms

ent inputs are delivered during perception by highly redundant projections from the strictly topographically ordered, mainline thalamic nuclei. In inferotemporal, insular, and dorsolateral temporal cortices, afferent input projections are maximally dispersed, highly repetitive inputs are uncommon, several inputs from other cortical sources are proportionally more powerful, and considerably more varied and complex input combinations are the rule. These differences in spreads, combinations, and schedules of input presumably account for much of the dramatic differences in the patterns of representation of behaviorally important stimuli that are created at lower versus higher cortical levels.[26,27,29,34-39]

For this reason, at lower system levels, the cortical areas are occupied by topographically ordered representations of the retina, cochlea, or skin, and during learning it is possible for large, continuous, strongly interconnected neuronal ensembles to emerge and represent behaviorally important stimuli. At higher system levels, whereas neighboring neurons can share some response properties and can be more strongly coupled than are more distant neurons, the representations of behaviorally important stimuli are sparse. Neurons or very small neuron clusters that respond selectively to a learned input are separated, share much less information with their neighbors, and are scattered widely across these higher cortical zones. Therefore, it is likely that during learning the representational constructs that emerge from practice are also more widely distributed.

Change mechanisms are competitive, so another contributor to differences in the expression of plasticity within different cortical areas is the difference in the powers of vying competitors. In behavioral conditioning, behaviorally important inputs rapidly come to dominate cortical neuronal responses in a process by which they can displace formerly dominant afferent inputs over large cortical sectors.[19,40-48] Even more dramatic representational substitutions and translocations take place if one of the inputs is taken out of competition completely. This takes place, for example, after somatosensory peripheral deafferentation, during which a major competitive input source, the thalamic zone representing the deafferented skin, remains anatomically intact but has been silenced (see Ramachandrau et al, this volume).[49-53] Similar large-scale competitive representational reorganizations occur after induction of restricted cochlear or retinal lesions.[54-57] In primary cortical receiving areas such as somatosensory area 3b or auditory cortical area A1, an epoch of repetitive training or microstimulation can result in the expansion of neuronal populations selective for specific skin or cochlear site many-fold in neuron number.[26-28,58] In higher cortical areas, very large populations of neurons, probably numbering in the hundreds of thousands or millions, can come to be selective for the specific sensory input combinations that guide the learned behavior, or that are demonstrated to be remembered in it.[26-28,59-62]

Representational plasticity takes place within cortical nets, as well as on extrinsic inputs. Researchers often think of representational competition in terms of a vying of competing extrinsic inputs, but intrinsic projections from neurons within the local cortical network itself have also been demonstrated to be major players in this competitive mechanism. The majority of input to cortical neurons actually comes from other neurons in the local network neighborhood. When viewed in this way, the importance of the plasticity of intrinsic patterns of connectivity is clear.

Strongly correlated afferent bombardment leads to changes in the connections among neighboring neurons, thereby creating cooperating neuronal groups that, because of their strengthened, positive interconnections, appear to discharge as members of a neuronal syncitium.[26-28,61-65] That is, neurons in these cooperative (coupled) groups operate together to select specific input subsets that they all share. That sharing is apparently accomplished primarily by their strong positive coupling to other group members, and it results in their strong, mutual exchange of coselected inputs.[64,65]

These cooperatively operating neuronal groups are themselves strong competitors for neuronal response domination, with the strongest competition near group borders.[58,61-65] For example, as cortical neurons come to be selective for a new set of specific inputs, tightly locally coupled cell assemblies grow progressively in their neuron memberships, and thereby provide progressively more numerous and more temporally coherent inputs to the immediately neighboring cortical zones. The more statistically consistent and temporally coincident the representation of important stimulus features, and the larger the neuronal membership in the expanding neuronal groups that constitute parts of its representation, the more dominant is the representation's competitive power and the greater its influences on the response properties of neurons of nearby groups. For several simple behaviors, we now have evidence that these plastic changes in intrinsic connections conferred into a surrounding cortical network zone account in part for learning generalization. Thus learning an exercise that directly engages a limited cortical zone induces positive changes in a wide surround that accounts for behavioral improvements for other inputs, for example, skin surfaces surrounding the skin that is directly behaviorally engaged during a learning paradigm.[19,20] It might be noted that intergroup competition effects will have a radically different expression at higher cortical representational levels, where a wider dispersion of competitive inputs results in their sparser representation and, consequently, in correspondingly weaker and more diffused neighboring intergroup competition effects.

As the local strengths of connections between cortical neurons increase as they are excited by behaviorally important inputs, progressively stronger positive coupling in cortical nets generates progressively more synchronous responses from the progressively more strongly syncytially interconnected neuronal populations.[19-26,28,64,66,67] This finding has at least two major implications. First, whereas neurophysiologists have long emphasized neuron discharge rate as the appropriate index of the power of output from cortical neurons, for a machine that is organizing itself on the basis of coincidence-based mechanisms, the temporal coherence of distributed outputs from a cortical zone is a main determinant of their effectiveness at inducing plastic changes downstream.[33] Thus, the generation of progressively more coincident firing across neuronal ensembles as a consequence of learning amplifies representational power and effects, both locally, as noted above, and within the projection targets of a reorganizing cortical area. Second, we believe with others that distributed temporal response synchrony likely constitutes a fundamental aspect of stimulus representation by neuronal ensembles, and a main basis of separating object representations in our nervous systems.[19–24]

Modulatory Control of Cortical Plasticity

Many studies have now collectively demonstrated a powerful behavioral-state modulation of plastic change.[19,41–45,67–69] Cortical plasticity is induced by learning, but not when equivalent stimuli are delivered to a nonattending animal, or when there is not an appropriate source of cognitive drive (reward, punishment, novelty, etc.) in the behavior. The specific enabling conditions for behavioral change and their relative modulatory powers have been studied exhaustively in experimental psychology, and it is reasonable to suppose that the weights of these effects measured behaviorally will be paralleled by modulatory effects measured electrophysiologically. However, up to this point, the neurophysiological effects of this modulation by learning context are known only on a very superficial level.

As an aside, it has also been shown that at least some cortical maps apparently generate completely different representational constructs from the same input sources because of powerful input gating effects.[33,65] For example, inputs delivered into specific skin surface or auditory representations are shut down during hand or head movements in specific cortical areas, but are gated on during these behavioral epochs in other areas.[70,71] As a consequence of this modulation, the former cortical fields would appear to generate use-driven representations that apply specifically for the static hand or head condition, and the latter would be hypothetically specialized for the moving hand or head condition, or accommodate aspects of both static and moving hand and head behaviors.

Another important and as yet little-studied contributor to cortical representational plasticity comes from cognitive sources representing expectations. Relatively powerful backward-projecting inputs have been recorded in the superficial layers of the cortex in behaving animals that presumably make a major contribution to the genesis of representational ensembles and their plasticity. Strong intermodal behavioral and neuronal effects have been recorded in experiments that might be interpreted as shaping expectations, for example in a monkey trained to touch objects that are geometrically related to visually presented patterns, or in a monkey trained to respond to felt objects while viewing those or other object patterns on a screen.[16,17]

Representational Changes with Overlearning

A common progression in skill learning goes from a closely attended behavior to a stereotyped automatic or little-attended behavior. In the cortex, changes appear to fade when practiced behaviors are not attended.[26] In this respect, the cortex operates as a learning machine. It appears that cortical plasticity supports a well-learned skill in a kind of homeostatic manner, by coming into play whenever the recovery or refinement or elaboration of the skill again requires directed attention, which would reenable positive representational change. We would expect the emergence of representations of other competitive, attended behaviors to erode progressively at least the cortical parts of the global representations of nonattended, automatic behaviors. Consistent with that view, we have shown that positive representational changes apparently reverse slowly when a learned behavior is not practiced.[19,40] However, it should also be noted that consistently weak or nonassociated inputs can actively produce negative changes in excitatory synaptic effectiveness.[67,69] Consistent with these findings is growing evidence for the operation of long-term depression of excitatory synapses for nonassociated or weak inputs.[26,27,67,73,74] By this process, which Pavlov argued many decades ago must happen,[75] affected neurons become less sensitive and meaningless applied stimuli are deselected.[69]

We have described cortical plasticity up to this point in terms of positive and negative changes in the effectiveness of excitatory synapses, but it must be remembered that cortical response specificity is a complex product of cortical excitatory and inhibitory processes. In all tested cortical areas, local administration of γ-aminobutyric acid (GABA)-receptor blockers results in the revelation of a wide set of excitatory inputs in addition to those that directly excite neurons in the normal state, which were being held in active, profound suppression. A change in cortical response selectivity in learning logically requires both a change in the identity of effective excitatory responses and a closely linked change in specific, always-present afferent inputs that are being inhibited.[2,27,29,33]

Plastic Changes Underlying the Representations of Temporal Features of Stimuli

Cortical plasticity studies almost exclusively focused on representational changes induced by brief transient stimuli. We have more recently begun to evaluate plastic changes to representations of temporal features of stimuli, and stimulus input sequences and streams. However, a substantial body of physiological, psychophysical, and computational modeling evidence indicates that temporal integration, segmentation, and sequence features will all be subject to representational remodeling.[26,76,95] In our own studies, we showed that neuronal ensembles engaged by a monkey performing a frequency discrimination or signal detection task come to be more strongly

M. M. Merzenich and R. C. deCharms

synchronous in their discharges, presumably because they are becoming progressively more strongly positively coupled.[19,20,76] This results in a sharper event-by-event representation of stimuli taking place over time by the responding neuronal ensemble. Such a change could plausibly account for our abilities to distinguish sequence orders at faster and faster sequence presentation rates with practice. In human subjects, several-fold gains in temporal segmentation capabilities can be achieved for a variety of specific sequenced input behavioral tasks with several days to weeks of practice.[76-80] At the very least, our studies show that this practice would result in the generation of a progressively more coherent and more sharply separated representation of individual stimulus events resulting from such practice.

In studies in progress, our colleague Christoph Schreiner recorded a several-fold degradation in neuronal integration and temporal segmentation periods in animals that were sensorially deprived compared with normals, and recorded a several-fold improvement in animals that were behaviorally trained (C Schreiner, K Kruger, B Calhum, R Snyde, S Rebscher, unpublished observation). This is a physiological finding that is again consistent with human psychophysical evidence that this aspect of temporal input representation can be easily altered by behavioral practice,[77-80] and is degraded in human subjects who have a history of sensory deprivation.[76] Finally, earlier investigators, but principally Roy Johns and colleagues, conducted a number of studies showing that neurons can become selective for specific temporal input sequences in learning.[81]

We are just beginning our experimental consideration of the creations of representations of complex input streams. In theory, coincident input coselection mechanisms must operate moment by moment, and almost certainly must create a plastic representational structure in time. Moreover, computational cortical network models indicate that these changes in the representations of temporal stimulus features may account for aspects of perceptual generalization of temporal stimulus features.[82]

In considering how events are represented that take place over time, it is important to consider that the cortical system temporally enriches the representations of stimulus input streams by its intrinsic processes and extrinsic feedback projections, and these in turn affect coincidence-dependent plasticity mechanisms. In the representation and plasticity of stimulus input sequences and streams, any specific input will dramatically alter the engaged cortical zone for its receipt of subsequent inputs. Excitation of the cortex sets the cortical machinery in gear, engaging excitatory-inhibitory cycling and paired pulse facilitation and depression, resetting cortical oscillators, and pairing together pieces of information that arose originally at different times and in separate cortical and subcortical areas. Temporal modulation created by intrinsic oscillators will temporally alter distributed neuronal population responses, thereby making them potentially more powerful sources for generating downstream plastic change, and increasing the possibilities for relational representation.

Enduring Brain Representations of Learned Behaviors and Memories

What specific plastic changes are induced in short-, intermediate-, and long-term learning and memory tasks? This is a complex subject founded on a massive literature, but it is important to note several aspects of cortical plasticity phenomenology that short-, intermediate-, and long-term mechanisms must account for. First, it is well established that input effectiveness changes are generated input by input, and progressively over long training epochs. Thus, in a powerful behavioral context in which rewards are great or punishments are severe, an animal can be conditioned with the application of just one or a few stimuli.[93,60,61,83,84] Such training appears to generate conditioning-stimulus-specific changes that apply to many thousands or hundreds of thousands of neurons in engaged cortical areas. These changes endure for as long as the animal can be demonstrated to remain conditioned, for example, for at least many weeks thereafter.[85] They can be quickly reversed at any point by a period of behavioral extinction training.[86-88] If an animal is trained in an operant behavior at which it improves day by day, changes in stimulus representations appear to progress day by day, in parallel with, and we believe accounting for, the animals behavioral gains with practice.[19,20]

We know logically that changes probably sit in impermanent form in cortex, available for contributions to priming, posthoc reinforcement, and so on,[32,33] commonly fading over time and over the subsequent sleep period, simply because that is a fundamental quality of many types of learning and memory. In addition, intriguing evidence indicates that in the cortex, the conversion from temporary to permanent change may occur in part largely in nonbehavioral periods, including the subsequent sleep period.[89]

Enduring cortical changes are probably accounted for by local changes in neuropil anatomy. Dramatic changes in synapse turnover, synapse number, synaptic active zones, dendritic spines, and the elaboration of terminal dendrites are all demonstrated to occur in a behaviorally engaged cortical zone, and in several models, in parallel with changes in synaptic effectiveness.[90-92] Although specific, detailed morphological changes accounting for connectional changes in learning have not been documented in any mammalian model, changes in synapse numbers, active zones, spines, and in dendritic arborization are all very likely to contribute to observed functional remodeling.

Some Implications for System Organization and Coordination

Cortical representational plasticity must be viewed as arising from multiple-level systems that are broadly engaged in learning, perceiving, remembering, thinking, and acting. Any important input or behavior engages many cortical areas and probably drives at least most of them to change. Whereas experiments designed to evaluate the progression of change usually focused on one cortical area at a time, such studies have now been conducted in many auditory, somatosensory, motor, and higher-level cortical areas.[44,59-61,83,93,94] All showed rapid emergence of representations selective for the stimuli or motor behavior applied in behavioral training. Other somatosensory, motor, and auditory cortical areas were examined before and after a period of behavioral training.[19,20,40,41,44-48,95] Again, in all of them, very substantial representational changes emerged that were related specifically to behaviorally important stimuli or responses. Taken together, such studies indicate that real-world input representations are subject to continuous change across all system levels and within parallel cortical streams.

It should be noted that in this kind of continuously evolving representational machine, perceptual constancy cannot be accounted for by locationally constant brain representations,[22,32,33,50] and relational representational principle must probably be invoked to account for it. Moreover, changes must be related level by level.[29,33] Consider, for example, the consequences of a change in the location of representation of a finger created by a learned behavior or injury. The meaning of outputs from the newly occupied area has now changed. If the identity of the digit is important for the creation of representational constructs within other cortical zones, which must be the case, then their representations must generate new level-to-level associations. Cortical representations must logically change together to retain correct relations.

Finally, it must be remembered that plastic changes are also induced in a multitude of extracortical sites that we have not considered here, and that many extracortical structures contribute to the plastic change that is recorded at the cortical level. During experience, the brain must function and change as an integrated whole.

SUMMARY

We considered three main themes. First, studies of the principles of cortical plasticity have made us very aware that much of what is the most important to understand about our dynamic learning, perceiving, thinking, and acting brains remains to be explored. Representations of temporally sequenced inputs and temporal input streams, neuronal bases of temporal and spatial binding and distinction, operations of neuronal ensembles in learning and in brain operations, documentation of relational forms of representation, more specific elucidation of the roles of modulating and gating process-control inputs, influences of context and expectations derived from prior knowledge, and other subjective operations of the mind must now be brought directly into play in future experiments.

Second, we wanted to make clear that a large and indisputable body of experimental evidence shows that representational plasticity is a fact of cortical life. Its dynamics and consequences must be considered more directly and more seriously in the designs of forebrain studies undertaken to understand the brain origins of learning, memory, perception, cognition, and action. Finally, although we have not considered this explicitly, we hope that the information and perspectives provided here might give some insight into a number of more general issues, such as learning, recovery from injury, and the representation of experience in the broadest sense.

CONCLUSION

Functional activity and plasticity are inseparable, and can be fully understood only when explored together. Many current approaches treat these processes as largely autonomous, and conduct experiments accordingly. We believe that questions of change and of function are so closely related that they cannot be dissociated one from the other. Connectivity leads to activity and activity to connectivity. Fortunately, modern approaches are integrating these two questions more and more.

We believe that mind is the product of an environment expressed in the nervous system and manifested by it through actions; it is a circular and relational interaction among an incoming world, an experiential context, and outgoing activity. To a large extent we choose what we will experience, then we choose the details that we will pay attention to, then we choose how we will react based on our expectations, plans, and feelings, and then we choose what we will do as a result. This element of choice and the relational nature of awareness in general have almost never been considered in neurophysiological experiments. We realize now that experience coupled with attention leads to physical change in the structure and future functioning of the nervous system. This leaves us with a clear physiological fact, a fact that is really just a mechanistic confirmation of what we already know experimentally: moment by moment we choose and sculpt how our ever-changing minds will work, we choose who we will be the next moment in a very real sense, and these choices are left embossed in physical form on our material selves.

We have reached the point in experimental neuroscience at which we should bring this experiential aspect of our minds more directly into our studies of brain operations. We must begin to explore more specifically how the brain operates in real life, with fewer of the artificial behavioral restraints that are applied in almost all neurophysiological experiments, but rarely in our own human existence.

ACKNOWLEDGMENTS

This research is supported by a grant from the National Institutes of Health, Hearing Research, Inc., the Francis A. Sooy Fund, and the Coleman Memorial Fund.

REFERENCES

1. Farah MJ. (1989). Mechanisms of imagery-perception interaction. *J Exp Psychol* 15:203–211.

2. Kinchla RA. (1992). Attention. *Annu Rev Psychol* 43:711–742.

3. Naatanen R. (1988). Implications of ERP data for psychological theories of attention. *Biol Psychol* 26:117–163.

4. Posner M, Rothbard MK. (1991). *Attentional mechanisms and conscious experience*. Academic Press, New York.

5. Moray N. (1970). *Attention: Selective processes in vision and hearing*. Academic Press, New York.

6. Feyerabend PK. (1965). *Beyond the edge of certainty*. NJ.

7. Churchland PM. (1979). *Scientific realism and the plasticity of mind*. Cambridge University Press, New York.

8. Feyerabend PK. (1981) *Problems of Empiricism*. Cambridge University Press, Cambridge.

9. Farah JM, Peronnet F, Gonon MA, Giard MH. (1988). Electrophysiological evidence for a shared representational medium for visual images and visual percepts. *J Exp Psychol (Gen)* 117:248–257.

10. Farah MJ. (1989). The neural basis of mental imagery. *Trends Neurosci* 12:395–399.

11. Finke RA. (1989). *Principles of mental imagery*. MIT Press, Cambridge.

12. Georgopoulos AP, Lurito JT, Petrides M, Schwartz AB, Massey JT. (1989). Mental rotation of the neuronal population vector. *Science* 243:234–236.

13. Kosslyn SM. (1988). Aspects of a cognitive neuroscience of mental imagery. *Science* 240:1621–1626.

14. Eskandar EN, Richmond BJ, Optican LM. (1992). Role of inferior temporal neurons in visual memory. I. Temporal encoding of information about visual images, recalled images, and behavioral context. *J Neurophysiol* 68:1277–1295.

15. Haenny PE, Schiller PH. (1988). State dependent activity in monkey visual cortex. I. Single cell activity in V1 and V4 on visual tasks. *Exp Brain Res* 79:225–244.

16. Haenny PE, Maunsell JH, Schiller PH. (1988). State dependent activity in monkey visual cortex. II. Retinal and extraretinal factors in V4. *Exp Brain Res* 69:245–259.

17. Hsiao SS, O'Shaughnessy DM, Johnson KO. (1993). Effects of selective attention on spatial form processing in monkey primary and secondary somatosensory cortex. *J Neurophysiol* 70:444–457.

18. Lashley K. (1951). The problem of serial order in behavior. In: *Cerebral mechanisms in behavior*. LA Jeffress, ed. John Wiley & Sons, New York.

19. Recanzone GH, Merzenich MM, Schreiner CE. (1992). Changes in the distributed temporal response properties of SI cortical neurons reflect improvements in performance on a temporally based tactile discrimination task. *J Neurophysiol* 67:1071–1091.

20. Jenkins WM, Beitel R, Xerri C, Peterson B, Wang X, Merzenich MM. (1993). Behavioral measurements of vibrotactile frequency response and temporal response properties of neurons in SI cortex of trained owl monkeys: Threshold shifts and duration effects. *Soc Neurosci Abstr* 19:162.

21. Wang X, Beitel R, Schreiner CE, Merzenich MM. (1993). Representations of natural and synthetic vocalizations in the primary auditory cortex of an adult monkey. *Soc Neurosci Abstr* 19:1422.

22. Ribary U, Ionnides AA, Singh KD, Hasson R, Bolton JP, Lado F, Mogilner A, Llinás R. (1991). Magnetic field tomography of coherent thalmocortical 40-Hz oscillations in humans. *Proc Natl Acad Sci USA* 88:11037–11041.

23. Engel AK, Kreiter AK, Konig P, Singer W. (1991). Synchronization of oscillatory neuronal responses between striate and extrastriate visual cortical areas of the cat. *Proc Natl Acad Sci USA* 88:6048–6052.

24. Murthy VN, Fetz EE. (1992). Coherent 25- to 35-Hz oscillations in the sensorimotor cortex of awake behaving monkeys. *Proc Natl Acad Sci USA* 89:5670–5674.

25. Hebb DO. (1949). *The organization of behavior: A neuropsychological theory.* John Wiley & Sons, New York.

26. Merzenich MM, Jenkins WM. (1994). Cortical representation of learned behaviors. In: *Memory concepts.* P. Anderson, O Hvalby, O Paulsen, B Hökfelt, eds. Elsevier, Amsterdam.

27. Merzenich MM, Sameshima K. (1993). Cortical plasticity and memory. *Curr Opin Neurobiol* 3:187–196.

28. Merzenich MM, Recanzone GM, Jenkins WM, Grajski KA. (1990). Adaptive mechanisms in cortical networks underlying cortical contributions to learning and nondeclarative memory. *Cold Spring Harbor Symp Quant Biol* 55:873–887.

22. Edelman GM. (1987). *Neuronal Darwinism: The theory of neuronal group selection.* Basic Books, New York.

30. Bear MF, Kirkwood A. (1993). Neocortical long-term potentiation. *Cur Opin Neurobiol* 3:197–202.

31. Asanuma H, Keller A. (1991). Neuronal mechanisms of motor learning in mammals. *Neuroreport* 2:217–224.

32. Merzenich MM, Jenkins WM, Middlebrooks JC. (1984). Observation and hypotheses on special organizational features of the central auditory nervous system. In: *Dynamic aspects of neocortical function.* GM Edelman, WE Gall, WM Cowan, eds. John Wiley & Sons, New York.

33. Merzenich MM, Recanzone GH, Jenkins WM, Allard T, Nudo RJ. (1988). Cortical representational plasticity. In: *Neurobiology of neocortex.* P Rakic, W Singer, eds. John Wiley & Sons, New York.

34. Tanaka K. (1992). Inferotemporal cortex and higher visual functions. *Curr Opin Neurobiol* 2:502–505.

35. Miyashita Y. (1993). Inferior temporal cortex: Where visual perception meets memory. *Annu Rev Neurosci* 16:245–263.

36. Young MP, Yamane S. (1992). Sparse population coding of faces in the inferotemporal cortex. *Science* 256:1327–1331.

37. Rolls ET. (1992). Neurophysiological mechanisms underlying face processing within and beyond the temporal cortical visual areas. *Proc R Soc Lond* (B) 335:11–20.

38. Gochin PM, Miller EK, Groos CG, Gerstein GL. (1991). Functional interactions among neurons in inferior temporal cortex of the awake macaque. *Exp Brain Res* 84:505–516.

39. Gawne TJ, Richmond BJ. (1993). How independent are the messages carried by adjacent inferior temporal cortical neurons? *J Neurosci* 13:2758–2771.

40. Jenkins WM, Merzenich MM, Ochs MT, Allard T, Guic RE. (1990). Functional reorganization of primary somatosensory cortex in adult owl monkeys after behaviorally controlled tactile stimulation. *J Neurophysiol* 63:82–104.

41. Recanzone GH, Merzenich MM, Jenkins WM. (1992). Frequency discrimination training engaging a restricted skin surface results in an emergence of a cutaneous response zone in cortical area 3a. *J Neurophysiol* 67:1057–1070.

42. Woody CD, Engel J. (1972). Changes in unit activity and thresholds to electrical microstimulation at coronal-pericruciate cortex of cat with classical conditioning of different facial movements. *J Neurophysiol* 36:230–252.

43. Weinberger NM, Ashe JH, Metherate R, McKenna TM, Diamond DM, Bakin J. (990). Retuning auditory cortex by learning: A preliminary model of receptive field plasticity. *Concepts Neurosci* 1:91–122.

44. Kossut M. (1992). Plasticity of the barrel cortex neurons. *Prog Neurobiol* 39:389–422.

45. Recanzone GH, Schreiner CE, Merzenich MM. (1993). Plasticity in the frequency representation of primary auditory cortex following discrimination training in adult owl monkeys. *J Neurosci* 13:87–103.

46. Milliken GW, Nudo RJ, Grenda R, Jenkins WM, Merzenich MM. (1992). Expansion of distal forelimb representations in primary motor cortex of adult squirrel monkeys following motor training. *Soc Neurosci Abstr* 18:506.

47. Pascual-Leone A, Torres F. (1993). Plasticity of the sensorimotor cortex representation of the reading finger in Braille readers. *Brain* 116:39–52.

48. Pascual-Leone A, Cammarota A, Wassermann EM, Brasil-Neto JP, Cohen LG, Hallett M. (1993). Modulation of motor cortical outputs to the reading hand of Braille readers. *Ann Neurol* 34:33–37.

49. Merzenich MM, Jenkins WM. (1993). Reorganization of cortical representations of the hand following alterations of skin inputs induced by nerve injury, skin island transfers, and experience. *J Hand Ther* 8:89–104.

50. Merzenich MM, Nelson RJ, Stryker MP, Cynader MS, Schoppmann A, Zook JM. (1984). Somatosensory cortical map changes following digit amputation in adult monkeys. *J Comp Neurol* 224:591–605.

51. Pons TP, Garraghty PE, Ommaya AK, Kaas JH, Taub E, Mishkin M. (1991). Massive cortical reorganization after sensory deafferentation in adult macaques. *Science* 252:1857–1860.

52. Ramachandran VS. (1993). Behavioral and magnetoencephalographic correlates of plasticity in the adult human brain. *Proc Natl Acad Sci USA* 90:10413–10420.

53. Ramanchandran VS, Stewart M, Rogers-Ramachandran DC. (1992). Perceptual correlates of massive cortical reorganization. *Neuroreport* 3:583–586.

54. Chino YM, Kaas JH, Smith EI, Langston A, Cheng H. (1992). Rapid reorganization of cortical maps in adult cats following restricted deafferentation in retina. *Vision Res* 32:789–796.

55. Gilbert CD, Wiesel TN. (1992). Receptive field dynamics in adult primary visual cortex. *Nature* 356:150–152.

56. Robertson D, Irvine DRF. (1989). Plasticity of frequency organization in auditory cortex of guinea pigs with partial unilateral deafness. *J Comp Neurol* 282:456–471.

57. Rajan R, Irvine DRF, Wise LZ, Heil P. (1993). Effect of unilateral partial cochlear lesions in adult cats on the representation of lesioned and unlesioned cochleas in primary auditory cortex. *J Comp Neurol* 338:17–49.

58. Recanzone GH, Dinse HA, Merzenich MM. (1991). Expansion of the cortical representation of a specific skin field in primary somatosensory cortex by intracortical microstimulation. *Cerebral Cortex* 2:181–196.

59. Mitz AR, Godschalk M, Wise SP. (1991). Learning-dependent neuronal activity in the premotor cortex: Activity during the acquisition of conditional motor associations. *J Neurosci* 11:1855–1872.

60. Kobatake E, Tanaka K, Wang G, Tamori Y. (1992). Effects of adult learning on the stimulus selectivity of cells in the inferotemporal cortex. *Soc Neurosci Abst* 19:975.

61. Li L, Miller EK, Desimone R. (1993). The representation of stimulus familiarity in anterior inferior temporal cortex. *J Neurophysiol* 69:1918–1929.

62. Edelman GM, Finkel L. (1984). Neuronal group selection in the cerebral cortex. In: *Dynamic aspects of neocortical function*. GM Edelman, E Gall, M Cowan, eds. MIT Press, Cambridge.

63. Pearson JC, Finkel LH, Edelman GM. (1987). Plasticity in the organization of adult cerebral cortical maps: A computer simulation based on neuronal group selectrion. *J Neurosci* 7:4209–4223.

64. Dinse H, Recanzone GH, Merzenich MM. (1993). Alterations in correlated activity parallel ICMS-induced representational plasticity. *Neuroreport* 5:173–176.

65. Merzenich MM, Recanzone GM, Jenkins MM. (1990). How the brain functionally rewires itself. In: *Natural and artificial parallel computations*. M Arbib, JA Robinson, eds. MIT Press, Cambridge.

66. Abeles M. (1991). *Corticonics: Neural circuits in the cerebral cortex*. Cambridge University Press, New York.

67. Ahissar E, Vaadia E, Ahissar M, Bergman H, Arieli A, Abeles M. (1992). Dependence of cortical plasticity on correlated activity of single neurons and on behavioral context. *Science* 257:1412–1415.

68. Woody CD. (1986). Understanding the cellular basis of memory and learning. *Annu Rev Psychol* 37:433.

69. Weinberger NM. (1993). Learning-induced changes of auditory receptive fields. *Curr Opin Neurobiol* 3:570–577.

70. Nelson RJ, Smith BN, Douglas VD. (1991). Relationships between sensory responsiveness and premovement activity of quickly adapting neurons in areas 3b and 1 of monkey primary somatosensory cortex. *Exp Brain Res* 84:75–90.

71. Brugge JF. (1985). Patterns of organization in auditory cortex. *J Acoust Soc Am* 78:353–359.

72. Haier RJ, Siegel BV, MacLachlan E, Soderling E, Lotenberg S, Buchsbaum MS. (1992). Regional glucose metabolic changes after learning a complex visuospatial/motor task: A positron emission tomographic study. *Brain Res* 570:134–143.

73. Clothiaux EE, Bear MF, Cooper LN. (1992). Synaptic plasticity in visual cortex: Comparison of theory with experiment. *J Neurophysiol* 77:1785–1804.

74. Dudek SM, Bear MF. (1993). Bidirectional long-term modification of synaptic effectiveness in the adult and immature hippocampus. *J Neurosci* 143:2910–2918.

75. Pavlov IP. (1927). *Conditioned reflexes. An investigation of the physiological activity of the cerebral cortex*. Oxford University Press, London.

76. Merzenich MM, Schreiner CS, Jenkins W, Wang X. (1993). Neural mechanisms underlying temporal inegration, segmentation, and input sequence representation: Some implications for the origin of learning disabilities. *Ann NY Acad Sci* 682:1–22.

77. Ball K, Sekular R. (1987). Direction-specific improvement in motion discrmination. *Vision Res* 27:953–965.

78. Karni A, Sagi D. (1991). Where practice makes perfect in texture discrmination: Evidence for primary visual cortex plasticity. *Proc Natl Acad Sci USA* 88:4966–4970.

79. Ahissar M, Hochstein S. (1993). Attentional control of early perceptual learning. *Proc Natl Acad Sci USA* 90:5718–5722.

80. Gibson EJ. (1969). *Principles of perceptual learning.* Appleton-Century-Crofts, New York.

81. John ER, Schwartz EL. (1978). The neurophysiology of information processing and cognition. *Annu Rev Psychol* 29:1–29.

82. Buonomano D, Merzenich M. (1993). A cortical neural network model of temporal information processing. *Soc Neurosci Abstr* 19:1609.

83. Edeline JM, Pham P, Weinberger NM. (1993). Rapid development of learning-induced receptive field plasticity in the auditory cortex. *Behav Neurosci* 107:539–551.

84. Woody CD, Gruen E, Birt D. (1991). Changes in membrane currents during Pavlovian conditioning of single cortical neurons. *Brain Res* 539:76–84.

85. Weinberger NM, Javid R, Lepan B. (1993). Long-term retention of learning-induced receptive-fleld plasticity in the auditory cortex. *Proc Natl Acad Sci USA* 90:2394–2398.

86. Disterhoft JF, Stuart DK. (1976). Trial sequence of changed unit activity in auditory system of alert rat during conditioned response acquisition and extinction. *J Neurophysiol* 39:266–281.

87. Diamond DM, Weinberger NM. (1986). Classical conditioning rapidly induces specific changes in frequency receptive fields of single neurons in secondary and ventral ectosylvian auditory cortical fields. *Brain Res* 3672:357–360.

88. Aou SJ, Woody CD, Birt D. (1992). Changes in the activity of units of the cat motor cortex after rapid conditoning and extinction of a compund eye blink movement. *J Neurosci* 12:549–559.

89. Karni A, Sagi D. (1993). The time course of learning a visual skill. *Nature* 365:250–252.

90. Rosenzweig MR, Bennett EL, Diamond MC. (1978). In: *Studies on the development of behavior and the nervous system.* Vol. 4. *Early influences.* G Gottlieb, ed. Academic Press, New York.

91. Greenough WT, Chang FF. (1988). In: *Cerebral cortex.* Vol. 7. *Development and maturation of cerebral cortex.* A Peters, EG Jones, eds. Plenum Press, New York, 335–392.

92. Keller A, Arissian K, Asanuma H. (1992). Synaptic proliferation in the motor cortex of adult cats after long-term thalamic stimulation. *J Neurophysiol* 68:295–308.

93. Aizawa H, Inase M, Mushiake H, Shima K, Tanji J. (1991). Reorganization of activity in the supplementary motor area associated with motor learning and functional recovery. *Exp Brain Res* 84:778–671.

94. Frafton ST, Mazziota JC, Presty S, Friston KJ, Frackowiak RS, Phillips ME. (1992). Functional anatomy of human procedural learning determined with regional cerebral blood flow and PET. *J Neurosci* 12:2542–2548.

95. Suner S, Gutman D, Gaas G, Sanes JN, Donoghue JP. (1993). Reorganization of monkey motor cortex related to motor skill learning. *Soc Neurosci Abstr* 19:775.

5 Neurotransmitter Receptor Regulation and Its Role in Synaptic Plasticity and Stabilization

P. W. Hickmott and M. Constantine-Paton

All cognitive and behavioral abilities of an organism depend on the properties of its neurons and the ways that these neurons are assembled into neural circuits. During development of the nervous system, individual neurons must make specific connections with their target cells so as to form these relatively stereotyped neural pathways. To accomplish this, the axons of the neurons must grow, sometimes for long distances, to their target region, find their appropriate targets, and form synapses on the appropriate region of those cells. During early stages of development young axon terminals branch profusely, and the potential to form any of a variety of connections between sets of presynaptic and postsynaptic neurons is high. Adult local circuitry arises during this dynamic period of synaptogenesis as a result of the structural plasticity that allows some synapses to be stabilized while others are withdrawn. After this period of synaptogenesis, many central nervous system (CNS) connections lose the potential for structural plasticity, presumably because the fundamental wiring of the brain must become relatively stable. However, assemblies involved in the cognitive processes of learning and memory must maintain their ability to modify synaptic efficacy and their output patterns throughout life. Neural activity is, by definition, the agent of synaptic plasticity during learning and memory. However, since early ground-breaking experiments (Hubel and Wiesel, 1963, 1965) it has become increasingly clear that neural activity is also critical in determining which synapses will survive the developmental period of structural plasticity.

A considerable amount of recent work implicated Ca^{2+} fluxes mediated by postsynaptic neurotransmitter receptors in both adult and developmental forms of synaptic plasticity. In some instances, the same receptor seems to be involved in both adult and developmental plasticity. These findings, suggesting similar molecular mechanisms, raise the question of how the brain manages independently to regulate the two forms of plasticity. In this speculative overview, we propose that an important factor in the developmental process is the activity-dependent down-regulation of the function of the transmitter receptors themselves. Work from our own laboratory, and that of many others showing that down-regulation of receptors occurs and that it is correlated with decreases in synaptic plasticity during development supports this hypothesis. However, this link between down-regulation of receptors and developmental synaptic plasticity does not answer a question of equal importance to the cognitive neuroscientist: how do some regions of the brain retain plasticity throughout life, whereas others restrict plasticity?

NEUROMUSCULAR PLASTICITY AND THE NICOTINIC CHOLINERGIC RECEPTOR

The neuromuscular junction (NMJ) constitutes the best understood synapse in terms of the trophic and activity-dependent interactions that regulate innervation and the restructuring of synaptic connections (Hall and Sanes, 1993; Scheutze and Role, 1987). Synaptic activity across the NMJ is important for these processes in both mature and developing systems. For example, in the mature animal, activity blockade of a motor nerve leads to motoneuron sprouting (Brown and Ironton, 1977) and extrajunctional nicotinic acetylcholine receptor (AChR) expression (Brockes and Hall, 1975; Merlie et al, 1984). An inappropriate motoneuron (i.e., one that would not normally innervate the muscle) can be made to form functional synapses at these nonjunctional sites (Frank et al, 1975; Weinberg, Sanes, and Hall, 1981). Such inappropriate connectivity is never seen in normally innervated muscle, and it can be prevented on denervation if the muscle is electrically stimulated in a pattern that mimics normal motoneuron activity patterns (Jansen et al, 1973). The development of extrajunctional AChR expression has also been shown to occur in normally innervated muscle after muscle activity has been blocked by the irreversible AChR antagonist α-bungarotoxin (Berg and Hall, 1975). Thus, it appears that muscle activation is a critical factor in the adult maintenance of specific connections at the NMJ.

How does this adult plasticity relate to the early development of neuromuscular connections? Early in mammalian development, many motoneurons innervate a single muscle fiber. Over time, most of these motoneurons are eliminated, leading to the adult pattern of a single motoneuron innervating a given muscle fiber (Thompson, 1985; Van Essen et al, 1990). Increasing activity at the NMJ accelerates this process (Thompson, 1985), and blockade of activity retards it (Brown, Holland, and Hopkins, 1980; Thompson, Kuffler, and Jansen, 1979). These experiments suggest that activity across the NMJ drives the normal developmental program of synapse selection and elimination, as has been observed in the regenerating system.

Recent in vitro experiments on *Xenopus* spinal neuron-myocyte cocultures provide a better understanding of the interaction among the early numerous inputs to developing muscle. These studies indicate that the temporal coincidence between activity arriving through motoneurons and postsynaptic Ca^{2+} fluxes mediated by AChRs determine changes in synaptic efficacy. Brief tetanic stimulation of one spinal neuron synapsing on a given myocyte decreases the efficacy of another less active spinal neuron synapsing on that same myocyte. Such changes in function are probably the first phase of physical synapse elimination. If the spinal neurons are tetanized simultaneously, however, the decreases in efficacy are not reliably observed (Lo and Poo, 1991). In addition, repetitive application of acetylcholine (ACh) to a myocyte with either no activation or asynchronous activation of the spinal neuron leads to a decrease in the spinal neuron-myocyte synapse efficacy. Since this decrease occurs even when the myocyte membrane is voltage clamped to prevent depolarization, it is not merely due to postsynaptic depolarization.

That postsynaptic Ca^{2+} is a critical mediator of these synaptic interactions was demonstrated by infusing the myocyte with the Ca^{2+} buffer BAPTA. This treatment blocks the effect. Furthermore, it appears that this competitive decrease in synaptic efficacy is brought about by a decrease in transmitter release from motoneurons that are not coactive with the postsynaptic rise in Ca^{2+} (Dan and Poo, 1992).

In vivo studies paint a similar picture of nerve-muscle interaction mediated through the AChR. This work used fluorescent dyes to label different motoneuron terminals and postsynaptic receptors at the same developing junctions. When multiply innervated end plates are studied in successively older animals, the physical withdrawal of presynaptic terminals is associated with a loss of AChR-rich patches on the postsynaptic membrane (Balice-Gordon and Lichtman, 1993).

In short, available data suggest that the process of activity-dependent synapse elimination at the NMJ entails at least two stages of presynaptic and postsynaptic interaction. Initially, Ca^{2+} current flow through the nicotinic receptor triggers a rapid retrograde effect that decreases transmitter release from nonactive inputs. At a later stage, the potential for reinnervation at that synapse is lost, both because the presynaptic structure is withdrawn, and because the AChR is lost from the postsynaptic membrane. This loss removes the means of generating a postsynaptic Ca^{2+} influx, which consequently prevents other inputs from being stabilized on the muscle fiber. Multiple or inappropriate innervation can be reintroduced in the adult by denervation, presumably because the normal suppressive effect of muscle activity on AChR expression is removed, leading to an increase in AChR expression across the muscle membrane, reactivation of this competitive process, and return of the potential to make novel connections.

Thus, the AChR at the NMJ occupies a central role in controlling the plasticity of neuromuscular connections, in terms of both synaptic efficacy and the structural integrity of the synaptic contact. This superficially simple scheme masks a complex set of interactions in which an intrinsic developmental program for AChR subunit expression is modulated by both activity-dependent and activity-independent factors arising from the motoneuron (Martinou and Merlie, 1991). These interactions regulate the function, the amount of expression, and the distribution across the muscle membrane of AChRs. Activity-induced Ca^{2+} influx appears to increase the lifetime of junctional AChRs while simultaneously reducing the overall synthesis of the receptor (Hall and Sanes, 1993). These effects of activity on AChR turnover probably occur because extrajunctional expression of the AChR subunits α, β, γ, and δ is specifically decreased by activity (Berg et al, 1985; Burden, 1977). The transcription of the ε subunit, which, when substituted for the γ subunit, switches the AChR's immature properties of long open time and low conductance to short open time and high conductance, is dependent on the nerve (both activity-dependent and -independent processes) for a short postnatal period (Martinou and Merlie, 1991; Scheutze and Vicini, 1984). Therefore, the AChR, the major mediator of the postsynaptic Ca^{2+} influx that controls synapse elimination and thus innervation by the appropriate motoneuron, is itself controlled by this innervation. These observations emphasize the complex interrelationships among activity at the NMJ, synapse stabilization, and the properties of the AChR.

A point of particular importance here, because it will reappear in the discussion of central synaptic plasticity, is why bother to use a complex pattern of gene activation to produce a mature AChR with shorter but larger conductance synaptic currents? One possibility is that, due to the immature properties of young muscle fibers, longer-duration synaptic currents are better at causing these muscles to contract, because postsynaptic summation of postsynaptic potentials (PSP) can occur more readily (Jaramillo, Vicini, and Scheutze, 1988). Since propagation of the effects of a synapse are greatly facilitated by contraction, this ability to integrate activity over a longer time could be very important for controlling development across the entire fiber.

Why switch to the channels with faster kinetics? One possibility is that channels with slower kinetics would admit more Ca^{2+} than channels with fast kinetics. As maturation proceeds, motoneuron activity increases and motoneuron synapses become more effective. If the AChR retained slow kinetics, these changes might cause a prolonged end plate current, which could admit toxic levels of Ca^{2+} into the muscle. Evidence supporting this possibility was obtained at the adult NMJ: when end plate currents are artificially prolonged by blocking acetylcholinesterase the muscle in the region of the NMJ degenerates. This can be prevented by removing extracellular Ca^{2+} (Leonard and Salpeter, 1982). Thus, as NMJ synapses mature and become more effective, it could become necessary to decrease the duration of the end plate current to prevent excessive Ca^{2+} influx and muscle death.

CENTRAL SYNAPTIC PLASTICITY AND GLUTAMATERGIC SYNAPTIC TRANSMISSION

Compared with the neuromuscular junction, much less is known about the molecular mechanisms underlying activity dependent plasticity in the CNS. This lack of knowledge is partly because of the complexity of the network in which central synapses are embedded, partly because much less is known about the native composition and control of most central neurotransmitter receptors, and partly because the central target cells are both heterogeneous and small, thereby prohibiting the types of detailed biochemical and spatial analyses of receptor distribution and functional type that have been carried out at the NMJ. Nevertheless, there is ample evidence that forms of structural and functional plasticity quite similar to those observed at the NMJ occur in many brain regions, and that, in some regions, the N-methyl-D-aspartate (NMDA) subtype of glutamate receptor may play a role analogous to that of the nAChR at the neuromuscular junction in mediating structural and functional plasticity.

In the mammalian CNS, activity is involved in a competitive synaptogenic mechanism. This mechanism uses temporal summation of converging excitatory input to determine which synapses made by these converging inputs survive. It appears that synapses that are active when the target cell is significantly depolarized, are retained (Constantine-Paton, 1990; Goodman and Shatz, 1993). For example, suturing one eye shut in a newborn kitten, thus greatly decreasing the activity in that eye, causes a decrease in the number of cortical area 17 neurons that respond to the closed eye, and a corresponding increase in the number responding to the open eye (Hubel and Wiesel, 1963). Conversely, if the two eyes are rendered incapable of converging on the same object in the early postnatal period, the number of neurons in visual cortex that can respond to both eyes is greatly reduced (Hubel and Wiesel, 1965). However, dark rearing, or suturing both eyes shut, thereby equally reducing activity in both, decreases the responsiveness, but causes little change in the response properties of these neurons.

These changes in the physiology of visual cortical neurons are reflected in the anatomy of afferents from the lateral geniculate nucleus (LGN) to visual cortex. In normal animals, afferents from each eye segregate into eye-specific regions of layer IV, referred to as ocular dominance columns. Monocular deprivation causes a decrease in the amount of cortex that is innervated by afferents from the deprived eye and a concomitant increase in the amount innervated by the other eye. Thus, it appears that the patterns of activity in the afferents, rather than the overall amount of activity, are important for development of orderly projections.

This idea was confirmed in the cat by blocking activity in both eyes with tetrodotoxin (TTX) and then imposing patterns of electrical stimulation on the optic nerve. Synchronous activation prevents the formation of zones of eye-specific dominance among cortical neurons, whereas asynchronous stimulation leads to their formation (Stryker and Strickland, 1984). Furthermore, TTX injected prenatally into the eyes of developing cats prevents the proper segregation of retinal ganglion cell (RGC) axons in the LGN (Dubin, Stark, and Archer, 1986; Shatz and Stryker, 1988). When TTX is applied postnatally it prevents the segregation of the geniculocortical axons into ocular dominance columns in the input layer of visual cortex (Stryker and Harris, 1986).

How does activity lead to stabilization of appropriate synapses? In 1949 Hebb proposed a "neurophysiological postulate" of learning that states that presynaptic and postsynaptic cells that fire nearly synchronously tend to increase the efficacy of their connections. Stent (1973), after reviewing the visual cortical and neuromuscular data available, proposed a correlate of that hypothesis suggesting that connections between cells that fire asynchronously tend to become weaker. These postulates have been applied to activity-dependent map refinement, usually with the assumption that when the efficacy of a connection decreases below some threshold value, it is physically withdrawn (Constantine-Paton, Cline, and Debski, 1990; Shatz, 1991; Stent, 1973; Udin and Fawcett, 1988). Action potentials, both spontaneous and evoked, in RGCs of similar response types are well correlated only if their cell bodies lie in the same retinal locale (Arnett, 1978; Maffei and Galli-Resta, 1990; Mastronarde, 1983a,b; Meister et al, 1991). Thus, a Hebblike rule could lead to activity-dependent stabilization of ganglion cell inputs arising from the same region of the retina (i.e., from neighboring RGCs) on the same central neurons.

A form of adult, rather than developmental, plasticity, which follows Hebblike rules in some regions of the CNS, is found in several brain regions, particularly hippocampus and neocortex, and is known as long-term potentiation (LTP) (Bliss and Lomo, 1973; Brown et al, 1988; Kuba and Kumamoto, 1990; Madison, Malenka, and Nicoll, 1991; Tsumoto, 1992). It may be associative, as well as homosynaptic or heterosynaptic (Brown, Kariss, and Keenan, 1990). In addition, different patterns of stimulation can produce long-lasting depression (LTD) of these same synapses (Lynch, Dunwiddie, and Gribkoff, 1977; Stanton and Sejnowski, 1989; Tsumoto and Suda, 1979; Brown, Kariss, and Keenan, 1990; Tsumoto, 1992). For example, associative LTD can be induced by stimulating an input at a low frequency that is negatively correlated in time with another, high-frequency input (Stanton and Sejnowski, 1989). Thus, mechanisms exist, at least at these adult synapses, that allow the efficacy of these synapses to be up- or downregulated depending on patterns of activity.

The mechanisms underlying LTP are not fully known; however, in all carefully investigated areas it appears to depend on postsynaptic Ca^{2+} influx (Madison, Malenka, and Nicoll, 1991). In some regions, much of this influx, and hence LTP, can be blocked by antagonists of the NMDA receptor. Furthermore, the NMDA receptor has properties that make it a good candidate to act as a detector of correlated activity (Mayer and Westbrook, 1987). To be activated, the NMDA receptor must bind glutamate and the postsynaptic cell must be depolarized sufficiently to relieve the Mg^{2+} block of the channel (Mayer, Westbrook, and Gutherie, 1984; Nowak et al, 1984). Thus, NMDA receptor-mediated postsynaptic Ca^{2+} flux will be increased, with increases in the amount of temporal summation of excitatory synaptic potentials that occur across a region of postsynaptic membrane. Moreover, the NMDA receptor current is long lasting, thereby facilitating temporal summation.

In addition, as postulated for the NMJ, substantial evidence suggests that postsynaptic increases in Ca^{2+} can trigger a set of signals that cause active synapses to be stabilized and inactive synapses to be reduced in efficacy and ultimately lost. Some of these signals, moreover, must act as retrograde messengers and cause changes in presynaptic terminals. For example, increases in presynaptic release of glutamate were documented at hippocampal synapses after the induction of LTP (Bekkers and Stevens, 1990; Dolphin, Errington, and Bliss, 1982; Malinow and Tsien, 1990). In addition, an increase in the number of postsynaptic non-NMDA-type glutamate receptors at these synapses was shown in some experiments (Lynch and Baudry, 1984). Conversely, at least at neocortical and hippocampal synapses, evidence exists for heterosynaptic depression at synapses that are inactive when there is postsynaptic Ca^{2+} influx at other, converging synapses (Tsumoto, 1992). This observation is similar to the depression seen at the spinal cord-myoblast synapse in *Xenopus*.

Long-term application of NMDA receptor antagonists to developing regions of neuropil (Constantine-Paton, 1990; Constantine-Paton, Cline and Debski, 1990; Fox and Daw, 1993; Udin and Fawcett, 1988) has been used to show that NMDA receptor function is also involved in developmental plasticity and synapse elimination. Treatment of the frog optic tectum with the NMDA-receptor antagonist DL-2-amino-5-phosphonovaleric acid (APV) causes desegregation of eye-specific stripes (Cline, Debski, and Constantine-Paton, 1987). Long-term APV application also decreases the precision of the normal retinotopic map in amphibians (Cline and Constantine-Paton, 1989) and the regenerating retinotectal projections in goldfish (Schmidt, 1990). This same treatment prevents the indirect retinotectal map from aligning with the rotated, direct retinotectal map in *Xenopus* (Scherer and Udin, 1989). In the mammalian CNS, APV treatment blocks the refinement of the retinocollicular map in neonatal rats (Simon et al, 1993), the elimination of multiple climbing fiber inputs to cerebellar Purkinje cells (Rabacchi et al, 1992), and the segregation of on and off sublaminae in the ferret LGN (Hahm, Langdon, and Sur, 1991). Similar long-term treatment in both visual cortex (Bear, Kleinschmidt, and Singer, 1990; Kleinschmidt, Bear, and Singer, 1987) and the barrel field of somatosensory cortex (Schlagger, Fox, and O'Leary, 1993) blocks the expansion of the cortical representation of active inputs that normally occurs when the activity in a set of converging inputs is blocked or eliminated.

All of these results are consistent with the idea that Ca^{2+} changes produced largely, but not necessarily exclusively, by NMDA-receptor activation trigger the structural retention of some developing synapses and the loss of others.

This hypothesis has been challenged, however, because the contribution of the NMDA receptor to postsynaptic responses is maximum during periods of synapse rearrangement and elimination in many regions of the CNS (Fox and Daw, 1993). Whereas this observation would be expected if Ca^{2+} influx through the NMDA receptor is central to the selective elimination process, it also means that activation of the NMDA receptor causes significant postsynaptic depolarization in these neurons. This depolarization could trigger Ca^{2+} influx through voltage-gated Ca^{2+} channels. Thus, the source of the influx responsible for changes in synaptic efficacy in CNS neurons is not certain, particularly for these young synapses.

Influx of Ca^{2+} can occur through NMDA channels (Cline and RW, 1991; Regehr and Tank, 1990), through voltage-gated Ca^{2+} channels (Alford et al, 1993; Miyakawa et al, 1992), and through Ca^{2+}-activated Ca^{2+} release from internal stores (Alford et al, 1993). Indeed, in the CA3 region of hippocampus, LTP is not dependent on NMDA receptor activation (Harris and Cotman, 1986), but apparently on voltage-gated Ca^{2+} channel activation. In cocultures of dorsal root ganglion and ventral spinal cord neurons, activity-dependent changes in synapse strength is mediated by Ca^{2+} influx that is not necessarily mediated by NMDA receptors (Fields, Yu, and Nelson, 1991). In short, it is difficult experimentally to separate specific NMDA-receptor blockade from decreases in postsynaptic depolarization caused by the blockade (Fields and Nelson, 1992).

These arguments should not obscure a critical point: changes in the amount of postsynaptic Ca^{2+} in neurons in the CNS, as at the neuromuscular junction, appear to be central to induction of selective synapse reinforcement and structural survival. In many central neurons, these increases in cytoplasmic Ca^{2+} result from glutamate receptor activation, and, in the regions of the CNS where the issue has been investigated, much of that Ca^{2+} change results from the activation of the NMDA receptor subtype (Alford et al, 1993; Regehr and Tank, 1990). Since depolarization of the postsynaptic neuron is necessary for NMDA receptor activation, a number of developmental alterations in non-NMDA glutamate receptors may contribute to large glutamate-gated Ca^{2+} fluxes in young CNS neurons. There may also be instances where other excitatory inputs to a postsynaptic cell are so low that the NMDA-mediated Ca^{2+} flux is not sufficient to trigger plastic synaptic changes. However, there is also little doubt that for many regions of the brain, during normal development, activation of the NMDA receptor is a necessary component of the activity-dependent mechanism that selectively prunes synapses and tunes developing connections.

Recently, the central importance of the NMDA receptor in organization of the CNS was elegantly demonstrated by a study of mice in which functional NMDA receptors were genetically eliminated. The trigeminal sensory projection within the hindbrain of this mouse strain was severely disorganized even though there was no apparent change in the ability of the inputs to the hindbrain to depolarize the postsynaptic neurons (Li et al, 1994).

DEVELOPMENTAL CHANGES IN GLUTAMATE RECEPTORS

If the NMDA receptor is a necessary part of a system that detects correlation among inputs and triggers events that lead to selective synapse stabilization, then turning down the functional efficacy of that receptor should make it more difficult to detect correlations among inputs and stabilize new connections. Thus, the potential for synaptic reorganization should be reduced.

Additional support for the hypothesis that the NMDA receptor is a critical detector of correlated activity and mediator of which synapses will survive into adulthood comes from the tight correlation between the down-regulation of NMDA receptor function and the end of developmental periods in which synapses can show dramatic activity-dependent structural rearrangements or changes in efficacy. For example, the receptors are more effective during the critical period for plasticity in the visual cortex. In cortical layers 4, 5, and 6, their relative contribution to visual responses in cat visual cortex decreases over the interval between about three and six weeks postnatally (Fox, Sato, and Daw, 1989; Tsumoto et al, 1987). This decrease corresponds to the period of geniculocortical afferent segregation in layer 4.

In rat cerebellum, Purkinje cells lose their sensitivity to NMDA starting at about postnatal day (PN) 14, and reach low adult levels by about PN 21 (Garthwaite, Yamini, and Garthwaite, 1987). At birth, rat Purkinje cells are innervated by several climbing fibers. The process of climbing fiber synapse elimination, which can be blocked by NMDA-receptor antagonists, extends from birth to about PN 14 (Mariani and Changeux, 1981). Similarly, in rat superior colliculus the process of retinotopic map refinement, which also can be blocked by NMDA-receptor antagonists (Simon et al, 1993), extends from PN to about PN 12 (Simon and O'Leary, 1992). Decreases in the NMDA receptor contribution to the excitatory synaptic currents generated by optic tract stimulation in collicular neurons are first apparent at PN 13 and become more pronounced in successive weeks until low adult levels of NMDA receptor current are reached (Hestrin, 1992).

Similar parallels are apparent between NMDA receptor function and the ease with which LTP can be induced. In rat visual cortex, a developmental decrease in the NMDA-mediated contribution to the excitatory postsynaptic potential (EPSP) parallels a decrease in the susceptibility of synapses to LTP (Kato, Artola, and Singer, 1991). In hippocampus the efficacy of the NMDA receptor decreases with development (Kleckner and Dingledine, 1991; Morrisett et al, 1990), and this decrease is associated with the decreasing ability to induce LTP. In addition, in the amphibian optic tectum, it was possible experimentally to reduce the level of NMDA receptor function by treating tectal lobes with long-term, nontoxic levels of NMDA (Debski et al, 1991; Hickmott and Constantine-Paton, 1991, 1993). The treatment induces selective down-regulation of NMDA (relative to AMPA) receptor currents (Hickmott and Constantine-Paton, 1991). In direct support of the prediction that the NMDA receptor is a critical component of the correlated activity detector-stabilization system, this down-regulation of the receptor's function is also associated with a loss of synaptic contacts in regions of neuropil where correlations in activity among converging afferents are low (Cline and Constantine-Paton, 1990).

The idea that the developmental down-regulation of the NMDA receptor is involved in the down-regulation of synaptic plasticity as the CNS matures essentially parallels the findings in the NMJ showing that the potential for polyneuronal innervation is tightly associated with the expression of extrajunctional AChR of the low-conductance long open time (immature) type.

Since the extrajunctional sensitivity of muscle to ACh can be suppressed by muscle activity, it is relevant to ask whether the down-regulation of NMDA receptors is also induced by activity. The data on frog tecta treated for extensive periods with agonist suggest that such is the case in this system where receptor function (and plasticity) would normally remain high for extended periods of time. We have few similar data on mammalian CNS, but the existing studies suggest that the normal developmental decreases in NMDA receptor function can be delayed by suppressing activity.

Thus, dark rearing prevents the normal developmental decrease in NMDA receptor effectiveness in the deep layers of cat visual cortex, and also prolongs the critical period for synaptic plasticity in layer IV (Fox et al, 1991). In rat visual cortex, a developmental decrease in the NMDA receptor contribution to synaptic currents in cortical neurons occurs between two and three weeks postnatally. This decrease can be delayed by dark rearing or by applying TTX to the cortex (Carmignoto and Vicini, 1992). The decrease in NMDA receptor function in rat cortex is similar to that beginning around the same time in rat superior colliculus (Hestrin, 1992), and, since rats normally open their eyes around PN 14, it seems highly likely that the decrease is brought about by the great increase in visual activity resulting from the beginning of patterned vision.

What is the molecular basis of these developmental decreases in NMDA receptor function? Several lines of evidence suggest that at least some of the decreases are associated with changes in the receptor protein. First, although decreases in receptor number have been documented in many brain regions as neuropil matures, these changes are not invariably associated with functionally detected changes in the NMDA receptor contribution to synaptic transmission. Second, in the frog, the experimentally induced decreases in NMDA receptor function are not associated with decreases in receptor-binding sites (Debski et al, 1991) or with the dispersion of receptors away from subsynaptic membrane (Hickmott and Constantine-Paton, 1991). Finally, isolated patch recordings indicate that, in striking parallel with the cholinergic receptor at the NMJ, the functional decreases in the NMDA receptor in rat cortex and colliculus appear to reflect a decrease in mean channel open time (Carmignoto and Vicini, 1992; Hestrin, 1992).

The number and complexity of modulatory sites on the NMDA receptor make the possibility of posttranslational changes in the protein enormous (Mayer and Westbrook, 1987). However, given the precedent of subunit switching of the AChR at the NMJ and the fact that different subunit combinations may facilitate different posttranslational modifications (Hollmann and Heinemann, 1994), activity-dependent regulation of the pattern of NMDA receptor gene expression could provide a more fundamental mechanism of long-term changes in receptor protein.

The recent cloning and characterization of five NMDA receptor subunit genes facilitated the experimental investigation of this issue. The first NMDA subunit cloned, NR1, exists in at least eight different isoforms depending on which splice variant of the gene is translated (Durand et al, 1992; Hollmann et al, 1993; Nakanishi, Schneider, and Axel, 1990). The NR1 gene, when expressed as a homomer in *Xenopus* oocytes, has all the characteristics of the native NMDA channel (e.g., glutamate- and glycine-binding sites, and voltage gating). However, it requires coexpression of NR2 subunits to show conductances of the magnitude found for native receptors (Moriyoshi et al, 1991). In situ hybridization studies reveal that the NR1 gene is broadly distributed in the brain, and that the four NR2 subunits are expressed in patterns that vary across different brain regions and different developmental stages (Watanabe et al, 1992). Thus, the potential structural and functional diversity of possible heteromers composed of any of the NR1 splice variants and four NR2 gene products is enormous (Hollmann and Heinemann, 1994; Li et al, 1994; Nakanishi, Schneider, and Axel, 1990; Seeburg, 1993).

In situ analysis of messenger (mRNA) distributions for mouse NMDA-receptor subunits reveals that only NR2B and NR2D are present in embryonic brain: NR2B disappears from the midbrain and hindbrain during development, and NR2D disappears throughout the brain; NR2A appears throughout the brain during development, and NR2C appears only in the cerebellum (Watanabe et al, 1992). The important question is whether any of these changes in NMDA receptor gene expression can be closely related to changes in receptor function or instances of synaptic plasticity.

Our laboratory has begun to explore this question using quantitative Northern blot analyses of transcript levels for NMDA and non-NMDA glutamate receptor subunits in the rat superior colliculus (SC). In the superficial visual layers of the SC, the amount of NR1 mRNA increases significantly between PN 6 and PN 19, and then decreases to adult levels. In addition, the amount of NR2B mRNA is initially high, but decreases to adult levels between PN 6 and PN 12. During the same developmental interval the dominant splice variant of NR1 expressed in SC neurons changes (Hofer, Prusky, and Constantine-Paton, 1994). These changes coincide with the completion of the refinement of retinocollicular projections (Simon and O'Leary, 1992), an increase in the synaptic density in the superficial layers of the SC (Warton and McCart, 1989), and the development of visually evoked spike activity (Molotchnikoff and Itaya, 1993).

Thus, during an initial period of collateral sprouting and elaboration of arbors in inappropriate regions of SC, the level of NR2B is relatively high, but it decreases during the period when mistargeted axons are being withdrawn to form the adult projection. Although levels are relatively low during these early periods, NR1 is nevertheless present in greater quantities than NR2B, quantities sufficient to form a functional receptor with the NR2B subunits. During the peak of removal of mistargeted RGCs, SC levels of NR1 are rising rapidly; when refinement is complete and the eyes open, thus allowing high levels of afferent activity, the subunit composition changes. It seems likely that the functional decreases in NMDA receptor function that have been detected in collicular neurons beginning precisely at this time reflect these and probably other, as yet undetected, subunit changes, and that these events are brought about by the increased retinotopy and increased excitatory drive of the visual input.

Considerable evidence suggests that subunit changes in non-NMDA glutamate receptors also occur in many brain regions during development (Hollmann and Heinemann, 1994) and some of these changes alter channel kinetics and Ca^{2+} permeability when investigated in *Xenopus* oocytes (Hollmann, Hartley, and Heinemann, 1991). In contrast to the NMDA-receptor subunits we have explored to date, however, the relative levels of expression of the non-NMDA receptor subunits the AMPA/Kainate receptor GluR2 (Hofer, Prusky, and Constantine-Paton, 1994) and the metabotropic glutamate receptor mGluR1 (Hofer and Constantine-Paton, 1993) do not show a tight correlation with the major synaptogenic changes in the superficial visual layers of the SC, even though all the glutamate receptor subunits we have studied have their highest levels of expression just around eye opening.

CONCLUSION

Clearly, much more work on patterns of NMDA and non-NMDA glutamate receptor genes must be undertaken before any general statements can be made about whether particular subunits are responsible for mature versus immature receptor properties. Nevertheless, in systems as disparate as the NMJ and the CNS, similar cellular mechanisms appear to underlie developmentally regulated activity-dependent plasticity. This implies that, if molecular analyses of glutamate receptor composition are undertaken in brain regions where the developmental time course of both functional and structural synaptic plasticity are well understood, we will discover which subunit characteristics are responsible for which functional changes, and we may discover whether particular subunits are regulated either quantitatively or qualitatively by activity.

For cognitive neuroscience, however, a central developmental question is how the brain preserves the potential for plastic change in some circuits while limiting that change in others.

In attempting to answer the question, the molecular characterization of receptors that provide the potential for synaptic plastic is only the beginning. If activity brings about the patterns of receptor gene expression that make synaptic plasticity unlikely, then defining how some circuits are protected from the increasing barrage of activity as ascending sensory projections mature is likely to be critical for understanding the brain regions involved in learning and memory. It now seems likely that the same pharmacologically defined receptors are involved in both developmental plasticity and the plasticity that is retained throughout life. Thus, circuitry lying between the inputs to a region and those synapses that remain plastic in the adult could gate or filter incoming activity to ensure that these synapses retain the molecular mechanism of activity-dependent synaptic change (Kirkwood and Bear, 1994).

If this reasoning is correct, it is the development of this circuitry, still poorly defined in most regions of the adult brain, that must ultimately be understood before we truly comprehend the ontogenetic expression and maintenance of cognition, and the potential for adaptive behavioral changes in the nervous system throughout life.

REFERENCES

Alford S, Frenguelli B, Schofield J, Collingridge G. (1993). Characterization of Ca^{2+} signals induced bin hippocampal CA1 neurones by the synaptic activation of NMDA receptors. *J Physiol* 469:693–716.

Arnett DW. (1978). Statistical dependence between neighboring retinal ganglion cells in goldfish. *Exp Brain Res* 32:49–53.

Balice-Gordon P, Lichtman J. (1993). In vivo observation of pre- and postsynaptic changes during the transition from multiple to single innervation at developing neuromuscular junctions. *J Neurosci* 13:834–855.

Bear M, Kleinschmidt A, Gu Q, Singer W. (1990). Disruption of experience-dependent modifications in striate cortex by infusion of an NMDA receptor antagonist. *J Neurosci* 10:909–924.

Bekkers JM, Stevens CF. (1990). Pre-synaptic mechanism for long-term potentiation in the hippocampus. *Nature* 346:724–729.

Berg D, Hall Z. (1975). Increased extrajunctional acetylcholine sensitivity produced by chronic post-synaptic blockade. *J Physiol* 224:659–676.

Berg DM, Jacob M, Margiotta M, Nishi R, Stollberg J, Smith M, Lindstrom J. (1985). Cholinergic development and identification of synaptic components for chick ciliary ganglion neurons in cell culture. In: *Molecular basis of neural development*. GM Edelman, WE Gall, WM Cowan, eds. John Wiley & Sons, New York, 363–383.

Bliss TVP, Lomo T. (1973). Long-lasting potentiation of synaptic transmission in the dentate area of the anesthetized rabbit following stimulation of the perforant path. *J Physiol (Lond)* 232:331–356.

Brockes J, Hall Z. (1975). Synthesis of acetylcholine receptor by denervated rat diaphragm muscle. *Proc Natl Acad Sci USA* 4:1368–1372.

Brown M, Holland R, Hopkins W. (1980). Restoration of focal multiple innervation in rat muscles by transmission block during a critical stage of development. *J Physiol* 318:355–364.

Brown MC, Ironton R. (1977). Motor neurone sprouting induced by prolonged tetrodotoxin block of nerve action potentials. *Natures* 265:459–461.

Brown TH, Chapman PFE, Kairiss K, Keenan CL. (1988). Long-term synaptic potentiation. *Science* 242:724–728.

Brown TH, Kariss EW, Keenan CL. (1990). Hebbian synapses: Biophysical mechanisms and algorithms. *Annu Rev Neurosci* 13:475–511.

Burden S. (1977). Development of the neuromuscular junction in the chick embryo: The number, distribution, and stability of acetylcholine receptors. *Dev Biol* 57:317–329.

Carmignoto G, Vicini S. (1992). Activity-dependent decrease in NMDA receptor responses during development of the visual cortex. *Science* 258:1007–1011.

Cline HT, Constantine-Paton M. (1989). NMDA receptor antagonists disrupt the retinotectal topographic map. *Neuron* 3:413–426.

Cline HT, Constantine-Paton M. (1990). NMDA receptor drug treatment alters RGC terminal morphology in vivo. *J Neurosci* 10:1197–1216.

Cline HT, Debski E, Constantine-Paton M. (1987). NMDA receptor antagonist desegregates eye specific strips. *Proc Natl Acad Sci USA* 84:4342–4345.

Cline HT, Tsien RW. (1991). Glutamate induced increases in intracellular Ca^{++} in cultured frog tectal cells medicated by direct activation of NMDA receptor channels. *Neuron* 6:259–267.

Constantine-Paton M. (1990). The NMDA receptor as a mediator of activity-dependent synaptogenesis in the developing brain. *Cold Spring Harbor Symp Quant Biol* 55:431–444.

Constantine-Paton M, Cline HT, Debski EA. (1990). Patterned activity, synaptic convergence and the NMDA receptor in developing visual pathways. *Annu Rev Neurosci* 13:129–154.

Dan Y, and Poo M-M. (1992). Hebbian depression of isolated neuromuscular synapses in vitro. *Science* 256:1570–1573.

Debski EA, Cline HT, McDonald JW, Constantine-Paton M. (1991). Chronic application of NMDA decreases the NMDA sensitivity of the evoked potential in the frog. *J Neurosci* 11:2947–2957.

Dolphin AC, Errington ML, Bliss TVL. (1982). Long-term potentiation in vivo is associated with increased glutamate release. *Nature* 297:496–498.

Dubin MW, Stark LA, Archer SM. (1986). A role for action-potential activity in the development of neuronal connections in the kitten retinogeniculate pathway. *J Neurosci* 6:1021–1036.

Durand G, Gregor P, Zheng X, Bennet MVL, Uhl GR, Zukin RS. (1992). Cloning of an apparent splice variant of the rat *N*-methyl-D-aspartate receptor NMDAR1 with altered sensitivity to polyamines and activators of protein kinase C. *Proc Natl Acad Sci USA* 89:9359–9363.

Fields RD, Yu C, Nelson PG. (1991). Calcium, network activity and the role of NMDA channels in synaptic plasticity in vitro. *J Neurosci* 11:134–146.

Fields RD, Nelson PG. (1992). Activity-dependent development of the vertebrate central nervous system. *Int Rev Neurobiol* 34:133–214.

Fox K, Daw NW. (1993). Do NMDA receptors have a critical function in visual cortical plasticity? *Trends Neurosci* 16:116–122.

Fox K, Daw N, Sato H, Czepita D. (1991). Dark-rearing delays the loss of NMDA receptor function in the kitten visual cortex. *Nature* 350:342–344.

Fox K, Sato H, Daw N. (1989). The location and function of NMDA receptors in cat and kitten visual cortex. *J Neurosci* 9:2443–2454.

Frank E, Jansen J, Lømo T, Westgaard R. (1975). The interaction between foreign and original motor nerves innervating the soleus muscle of rats. *J Physiol* 247:725–743.

Garthwaite G, Yamini BJ, Garthwaite J. (1987). Selective loss of Purkinje and granule cell responsiveness to *N*-methyl-D-aspartate in rat cerebellum during development. *Dev Brain Res* 36:288–292.

Goodman CS, Shatz CJ. (1993). Developmental mechanisms that generate precise patterns of neuronal connectivity. *Neuron* 10(suppl):77–98.

Hahm J-O, Langdon RB, Sur M. (1991). Disruption of retinogeniculate afferent segregation by antagonists to NMDA receptors. *Nature* 351:568–570.

Hall ZW, Sanes JR. (1993). Synaptic structure and development: The neuromuscular junction. *Neuron* 10(suppl):99–121.

Harris E, Cotman C. (1986). Long-term potentiation of guinea pig mossy fiber responses is not blocked by N-methyl-D-aspartate antagonists. *Neurosci Lett* 70:132–137.

Hebb DO. (1949). *Organization of behavior*. John Wiley & Sons, New York.

Hestrin S. (1992). Developmental regulation on NMDA receptor-mediated synaptic currents at a central synapse. *Nature* 357:686–689.

Hickmott PW, Constantine-Paton M. (1991). Quantitative analysis of agonist-evoked currents in identified tectal neurons of *Rana pipiens*. *Soc Neurosci Abstr* 17:1134.

Hickmott PW, Constantine-Paton M. (1993). Effects of chronic N-methyl-D-aspartate treatment on spontaneous EPSCs recorded from *Rana pipiens* optic tectum. *Soc Neurosci Abstr* 19:452.

Hofer M, Constantine-Paton M. (1993). Regulation of glutamate receptors during retino-collicular map formation. *Soc Neurosci Abstr* 19:42.

Hofer M, Prusky GT, Constantine-Paton M. (1994). Regulation of NMDA receptor mRNA during visual map formation and after receptor blockade. *J Neurochem* 62:2300–2307.

Hollmann M, Boulter J, Maron C, Beasley L, Sullivan J, Pecht G, Heinemann S. (1993). Zinc potentiates agonist-induced currents at certain splice variants of the NMDA receptor. *Neuron* 10:943–954.

Hollmann M, Hartley M, Heinemann S. (1991). Ca^{++} permeabilities of KA-AMPA-gated glutamate receptor channels depends on subunit composition. *Science* 252:851–853.

Hollmann M, Heinemann S. (1994). Cloned glutamate receptors. *Annu Rev Neurosci* 17:31–108.

Hubel DH, Wiesel TN. (1963). Single-cell responses in striate cortex of kittens deprived of vision in one eye. *Neurophysiol* 26:1003–1017.

Hubel DH, Wiesel TN. (1965). Binocular interaction in striate cortex of kittens raised with artificial squint. *J Neurophysiol* 28:1041–1059.

Jansen J, Lømo T, Nicolaysen K, Westgaard R. (1973). Hyperinnervation of skeletal muscle fibers: Dependence on muscle activity. *Science* 181:559–561.

Jaramillo F, Vicini S, Scheutze S. (1988). Embryonic acetylcholine receptors guarantee spontaneous contractions in rat developing muscle. *Nature* 335:66–68.

Kato N, Artola A, Singer W. (1991). Developmental changes in the susceptibility to long-term potentiation of neurones in rat visual cortex slices. *Dev Brain Res* 60:43–50.

Kirkwood A, Bear M. (1994). Hebbian synapses in visual cortex. *J Neurosci* 14:1634–1645.

Kleckner NW, Dingledine R. (1991). Regulation of NMDA receptors by magnesium and glycine during development. *Mol Brain Res* 11:151–159.

Kleinschmidt A, Bear MF, Singer W. (1987). Blockade of NMDA receptors disrupts experience-dependent plasticity of kitten striate cortex. *Science* 238:355–358.

Kuba K, Kumamoto E. (1990). Long-term potentiations in vertebrate synapses: A variety of cascades with common subprocesses. *Prog Neurobiol* 34:197–269.

Leonard J, Salpeter M. (1982). Calcium-induced myopathy at neuromuscular junctions of normal and dystrophic muscle. *Exp Neurol* 76:121–138.

Li Y, Erzurumlu RS, Chen C, Jhaveri S, Tonegawa S. (1994). Whisker-related neuronal patterns fail to develop in the trigeminal brainstem nuclei of NMDAR1 knockout mice. *Cell* 76:427–437.

Lo YJ, Poo M-M. (1991). Activity-dependent synaptic competition in vitro heterosynaptic suppression of developing synapses. *Science* 254:1019–1022.

Lynch G, Baudry M. (1984). The biochemistry of memory: A new and specific hypothesis. *Science* 221:1057–1063.

Lynch G, Dunwiddie TV, Gribkoff VK. (1977). Heterosynaptic depression: A postsynaptic correlate of long-term potentiation. *Nature* 266:737–739.

Madison DV, Malenka RC, Nicoll RA. (1991). Mechanisms underlying long-term potentiation of synaptic transmission. *Annu Rev Neurosci* 14:379–397.

Maffei L, Galli-Resta L. (1990). Correlation in the discharges of neighboring rat retinal ganglion cells during prenatal life. *Proc Natl Acad Sci USA* 87:2861–2864.

Malinow R, Tsien RW. (1990). Presynaptic enhancement shown by whole-cell recordings of long-term potentiation in hippocampal slices. *Nature* 346:177–180.

Mariani J, Changeux J. (1981). Ontogenesis of olivocerebellar relationships. I. Studies by intracellular recordings of the multiple innervation of Purkinje cells by climbing fibers in the developing rat cerebellum. *J Neurosci* 1:696–702.

Martinou J-C, Merlie J. (1991). Nerve-dependent modulation of acetylcholine receptor epsilon-subunit gene expression. *J Neurosci* 11:1291–1299.

Mastronarde DN. (1983a). Correlated firing of cat retinal ganglion cells. I. Spontaneously active inputs to X- and Y-cells. *J Neurophysiol* 49:303–324.

Mastronarde DN. (1983b). Correlated firing of cat retinal ganglion cells. II. Responses of X- and Y-cells to single quantal events. *J Neurophysiol* 49:325–349.

Mayer ML, Westbrook GL. (1987). The physiology of excitatory amino acids in the vertebrate central nervous system. *Prog Neurobiol* 28:197–276.

Mayer ML, Westbrook GL, Gutherie PB. (1984). Voltage-dependent block by Mg^{++} of NMDA responses in spinal cord neurons. *Nature* 309:261–263.

Meister M, Wong R, Baylor DA, Shatz CJ. (1991). Synchronous bursts of action potentials in ganglion cells of the developing mammalian retina. *Science* 252:939–943.

Merlie J, Isenberg K, Russell S, Sanes J. (1984). Denervation supersensitivity in skeletal muscle: Analysis with a cloned cDNA probe. *J Cell Biol* 99:332–335.

Miyakawa H, Ross WW, Jaffe D, Callaway JC, Lasser-Ross N, Lisman JE, Johnston D. (1992). Synaptically activated increases in Ca^{2+} concentration in hippocampal CA1 pyramidal cells are primarily due to voltage-gated Ca^{2+} channels. *Neuron* 9:1163–1173.

Molotchnikoff S, Itaya SK. (1993). Functional development of the neonatal rat retinotectal pathway. *Dev Brain Res* 72:300–304.

Moriyoshi K, Masu M, Ishii T, Shigemoto R, Mizuno N, Nakanishi S. (1991). Molecular cloning and characterization of the rat NMDA receptor. *Nature* 354:31–37.

Morrisett TA, Mott DD, Lewis DV, Wilson WA, Swartzwelder HS. (1990). Reduced sensitivity of the N-methyl-D-aspartate component of synaptic transmission to magnesium in hippocampal slices from immature rats. *Dev Brain Res* 56:257–262.

Nakanishi N, Schneider NA, Axel R. (1990). A family of glutamate receptor genes. Evidence for the formation of heteromultimeric receptors with distinct channel properties. Neuron 5:569–581.

Nowak L, Bregestovshi P, Ascher P, Herbet AP. (1984). Magnesium gates glutamate-activated channels in mouse central neurones. Nature 307:462–465.

Rabacchi S, Bailly Y, Delhaye-Bouchaud N, Mariani J. (1992). Involvement of the *N*-methyl-D-aspartate (NMDA) receptor in synapse elimination during cerebellar development. *Science* 256:1823–1825.

Regehr WG, Tank DW. (1990). Postsynaptic NMDA receptor-mediated Ca^{++} accumulation in hippocampal CA1 pyramidal cell dendrites. *Nature* 345:807–810.

Scherer WJ, Udin SB. (1989). *N*-methyl-D-aspartate antagonists prevent interaction of binocular maps in *Xenopus* tectum. *J Neurosci* 9:3837–3843.

Scheutze S, Role L. (1987). Developmental regulation of nicotinic acetylcholine receptors. *Annu Rev Neurosci* 10:403–457.

Scheutze S, Vicini S. (1984). Neonatal denervation inhibits the normal postnatal decrease in endplate channel open time. *J Neurosci* 4:2997–2302.

Schlagger BL, Fox K, O'Leary DDM. (1993). Postsynaptic control of plasticity in developing somatosensory cortex. *Nature* 364:623–626.

Schmidt JT. (1990). Long-term potentiation and activity dependent retinotopic sharpening in the regenerating retinotectal projection of goldfish: Common sensitive periods and sensitivity to NMDA blockers. *J Neurosci* 10:233–246.

Seeburg PH. (1993). The molecular biology of mammalian glutamate receptor channels. *Trends Neurosci* 16:359–364.

Shatz C. (1991). Impulse activity and the patterning of connections during CNS development. *Neuron* 5:745–756.

Shatz CJ, Stryker MP. (1988). Prenatal tetrodotoxin infusion blocks segregation of retinogeniculate afferents. *Science* 242:87–89.

Simon DK, O'Leary DDM. (1992). Development of topographic order in the mammalian retinocollicular projection. *J Neurosci* 12:1212–1232.

Simon DK, Prusky GT, O'Leary DDM, Constantine-Paton M. (1993). NMDA receptor antagonists disrupt the formation of a mammalian neural map. *Proc Natl Acad Sci USA* 89:10593–10597.

Stanton PK, Sejnowski TJ. (1989). Associative long-term depression in the hippocampus induced by Hebbian covariance. *Nature* 339:215–218.

Stent GS. (1973). A physiological mechanism for Hebb's postulate of learning. *Proc Natl Acad Sci USA* 70:997–1001.

Stryker MP, Harris WA. (1986). Binocular impulse blockade prevents the formation of ocular dominance columns in cat visual cortex. *J Neurosci* 6:2117–2133.

Stryker MP, Strickland SL. (1984). Physiological segregation of ocular dominance columns depends on the pattern of afferent electrical activity. *Invest Ophthalmol Vis Sci* 25:278.

Thompson W. (1985). Activity and synapse elimination at the neuromuscular junction. *Cell Mol Neurobiol* 5:167–182.

Thompson W, Kuffler D, Jansen J. (1979). The effect of prolonged, reversible block of nerve impulses on the elimination of polyneuronal innervation of new-born rat skeletal muscle fibers. *Neuroscience* 4:271–281.

Tsumoto T. (1992). Long-term potentiation and long-term depression in the neocortex. *Prog Neurobiol* 39:209–228.

Tsumoto T, Hagihara K, Sato H, Hata Y. (1987). NMDA receptors in the visual cortex of young kittens are more effective than those of adult cats. *Nature* 327:513–514.

Tsumoto T, Suda K. (1979). Cross depression: An electrical manifestation of binocular competition in the developing visual cortex. *Brain Res* 168:190–194.

Udin SB, Fawcett JW. (1988). Formation of topographic maps. *Annu Rev Neurosci* 11:289–327.

Van Essen D, Gordon H, Soha J, Fraser S. (1990). Synaptic dynamics at the neuromuscular junction: Mechanisms and models. *J Neurobiol* 21:223–249.

Warton SS, McCart R. (1989). Synaptogenesis in the stratum griseum superficial of the rat superior colliculus. *Synapse* 3:136–148.

Watanabe M, Inoue Y, Sakimura K, Mishina M. (1992). Developmental changes in distribution of NMDA receptor channel subunit mRNAs. *Neuroreport* 3:1138–1140.

Weinberg C, Sanes J, Hall Z. (1981). Formation of neuromuscular junctions in adult rats: Accumulation of acetylcholine receptors, acetylcholinesterase, and components of synaptic basal lamina. *Dev Biol* 84:255–266.

6 Neuronal Synchronization: A Solution to the Binding Problem?

W. Singer

Evidence is growing that both perceptual and motor functions of the neocortex are based on distributed processes. These occur in parallel at different sites and always involve vast numbers of neurons that, depending on the complexity of the task, may be disseminated throughout the whole cortical sheath. In the visual system, for example, even simple sensory stimuli evoke highly fragmented and widely distributed activity patterns. Neurons preferring the same features or coding for adjacent points in visual space are often segregated from one another by groups of cells preferring different features. Moreover, different aspects of visual objects such as their shape, spectral composition, location in space, and motion are processed in separate, non-contiguous cortical areas (Desimone et al, 1985; Felleman and van Essen, 1991; Newsome and Pare, 1988; Ungerleider and Mishkin, 1982; Wurtz et al, 1990; Zeki, 1973; Zeki et al, 1991). Thus, a particular visual object elicits responses in a large number of spatially distributed neurons, each of which responds only to a partial aspect of the object.

This raises the intriguing question, commonly addressed as the binding problem, of how these distributed activities are reintegrated to generate unambiguous representations of objects in the brain. Such binding problems arise at very early stages of sensory processing where simple properties of visual objects are represented, such as the precise location and orientation of contours. The reason is that, even at levels as peripheral as the primary visual cortex, responses of individual feature-selective neurons are only poor descriptors of these properties.

The ambiguity results from the broad tuning of feature-sensitive neurons. The amplitudes of their responses depend on a number of different properties of a contour, such as its position relative to the center of the receptive field, its orientation relative to the preferred orientation of the neuron, and its curvature, length, and luminance contrast. Thus, in a particular cell stimuli differing along these various feature dimensions may all evoke responses of similar amplitude. This ambiguity can be resolved only by evaluating together the responses of the large numbers of different neurons that are coactivated by a particular contour. This, however, requires establishing selective relations among neurons that respond to the same contour and distinguishing these responses from those of other nearby contours. As the number of possible combinations between locations and orientations of contours is nearly infinite, a flexible binding mechanism is required for the non-ambiguous association of responses to the same contour.

Similar binding problems have to be resolved at processing stages that accomplish scene segmentation and perceptual grouping. Regardless of the sensory modality, the first step toward identifying perceptual objects consists of a grouping operation whereby the features of a particular sensory object have to be related to one another, and become segregated from features of other objects and from features of the embedding background. This requires again the establishment of highly selective relations among the responses of large populations of neurons that will often be distributed across various cortical areas. Because different objects lead to activation of different constellations of neurons whereby subsets of such populations may be the same for different objects, again, flexible binding mechanism is required that can cope with the very large number of possible combinations. Finally, binding problems arise also at the level at which perceptual objects are eventually represented.

Just as elementary features appear to be represented by a population code rather than by the responses of individual neurons, complex perceptual objects also seem to be represented by populations of neurons, each of which codes for a particular subconstellation of features. This has to be inferred from the fact that a search for individual neurons responding with high selectivity to particular perceptual objects revealed specificity only for faces and for a limited set of objects with which the animal had been familiarized extensively (Gross, Rocha-Miranda, and Bender, 1972; Baylis, Rolls, and Leonard, 1985; Desimone et al, 1984, 1985; Perret, Mistlin, and Chitty, 1987; Miyashita, 1988; Sakai and Miyashita, 1991). But even in these cases a particular face or object evokes responses in a very large number of neurons, and any particular cell can be activated by numerous, often only loosely related, patterns.

As the basic principles of cortical organization seem to be similar among sensory and motor areas, binding problems of a related kind should occur also in motor processing. Indeed, recordings from different areas of the motor cortex support the notion that specific motor patterns are represented by a population code; that is, by the graded responses of a large number of distributed neurons. The trajectories of a particular movement can be predicted correctly only if the relative contributions of large numbers of neurons are considered (Georgopoulos, 1990; Mussa-Ivaldi, Giszter, and Bizzi, 1990; Sparks, Lee, and Rohrer, 1990). As the execution of movements requires the precise association of cell assemblies representing various components of the respective movements, and as these constellations vary for different movements, a flexible binding mechanism is required here also to link together the populations of neurons that have to cooperate to generate a particular movement.

The most widely accepted proposal for the solution of binding problems in sensory processing implies that special binding units collect the responses of cells that have to be bound together by means of converging input connections. The idea is that the thresholds of these binding units are adjusted so that they respond only if the full set of the respective driving units is activated. A particular constellation of responses in the input layer would thus be signaled by the activation of the respective binding unit. To distinguish the population responses that signal the precise orientation and location of a contour, a binding unit would be required that receives its input connections from exactly the set of orientation-selective units that respond to a contour with that particular orientation and location.

This is clearly not an attractive solution. First, one could have started with the implementation of such selective units right away. Second, if coarse codes are circumvented by creating individual, sharply tuned cells, an exceedingly large number of units is required to represent with high resolution all orientations at all possible locations. Introducing binding units is thus extremely expensive in terms of hardware, because the number of required binding units scales very unfavorably with the number of different input constellations that can be bound. Despite of this, it is commonly held that the binding together of component features defining perceptual objects is achieved by such convergence onto higher-order binding units.

Such a solution to the binding problem may be exploited by simple nervous systems and is perhaps also implemented in vertebrate brains to bind frequently occurring, stereotyped constellations of features. However, it seems highly unlikely that it is used as a general mechanism because it would require too many binding units. In essence, one would require at least one binding unit for each of the nearly infinite feature constellations that characterize the vast number of distinguishable objects. Moreover, at least four or five additional units are needed per distinguishable object to bind the different response configurations that are caused by different views of the same objects.

Even if objects and their different views are represented in a more economical way by interpolation in small groups of neurons (Poggio, 1990), no single area in the visual processing stream has been identified so far that could serve as the ultimate site of convergence and that would be large enough to accommodate the still exceedingly large number of required neurons. Also, one would have to postulate a large reservoir of uncommitted cells to allow for the binding of features of new, hitherto unknown objects. These neurons would have to maintain latent input connections from all feature-selective neurons at lower processing stages. For the representation of new objects, the subsets of these connections, which are activated by the specific feature constellation of the new object, would have to be selected and consolidated instantaneously.

The equivalent of such higher-order binding units on the motor side would be command neurons, each of which would represent a particular complex motor pattern. Each of these command neurons would have to distribute its activity onto the appropriate population of neurons that produce the respective motor pattern. The problems are the same as on the sensory side. Too many binding units are required, and learning a new motor skill would demand implementation of newly committed binding units.

Yet another problem is that activity of a few command units would have to drive a vast number of cells downstream to produce a motor response, and it is difficult to see how that could be realized. The same problem is seen at the sensory side. If a particular perceptual object were indeed represented by the responses of only a few binding units, their output activity would have to be redistributed in a highly divergent way to motor systems to be able to initiate a response. A particularly delicate problem would arise if one had higher-order binding units at the sensory and command neurons on the motor side. As one can learn to associate virtually any motor response with any perceptual object, each of the sensory-binding units would have to be connected to all command neurons. This would obviously saturate the dynamic range and the integrative capacities of these neurons and render response selection impossible.

Alternative solutions have therefore been proposed. These are all based on the assumption that binding is achieved by cooperative interactions among the neurons whose responses have to be bound together. The idea is that at each level of processing, cells interact through a dense network of reciprocal, highly tuned connections, the functional architecture of which reflects the criteria according to which active cells should be grouped or bound together. Thus, once input activity becomes available and selected cells begin responding, a self-organizing process is initiated by which subsets of responses are bound together according to the joint probabilities imposed by the specific input pattern, the functional architecture of the coupling network, and the signals arriving through reentry loops from higher processing stages. The essential advantage of such a dynamic, self-organizing binding process is that individual cells can bind at different times, for example, when input constellations change, with different partners.

This greatly economizes the number of required cells. Binding units are no longer necessary, as the respective ensemble of ad hoc bound units would be the equivalent of a binding unit. Moreover, and most important, a particular cell can now be used in representations of many different feature constellations, as it can be bound in a flexible way to changing partners. This makes it possible to create with a limited set of neurons a nearly infinite number of different binding constellations. The only constraint is the dynamic range of the neurons that limits the number of inputs a cell can receive, but this problem can be overcome by iteration and parcellation (see below).

This solution to the binding problem closely resembles previously formulated concepts on sensory representations that assume that perceptual objects are represented in the brain by assemblies of interacting neurons rather than by individual, highly selective cardinal cells (Barlow, 1972; Martin, 1994). The assembly hypothesis was made explicit in Hebb's (1949) seminal book on the organization of behavior and has become considerably more elaborate and adapted to recent neurobiological evidence (Abeles, 1991; Braitenberg, 1978; Crick, 1984; Edelman, 1987, 1989; Grossberg, 1980; Hebb, 1949; Palm, 1982, 1990; Singer, 1985, 1990; von der Malsburg, 1985).

However, relatively little attention has been paid until recently to the question of how responses of neurons in a Hebbian assembly can be labeled so that they are distinguished unambiguously as belonging to the same assembly, or, in the context of our binding problem, how responses that are bound together become distinguished as being bound and can be segregated from other, often simultaneous, responses to which they should not be bound.

The simplest way to select responses for further processing is to increase their saliency by increasing their amplitude. Accordingly, most proponents of the assembly hypothesis, including Hebb, proposed that cells that have joined an assembly are distinguished because they increase their discharge rates due to reciprocal excitation and reverberation. The same strategy can be applied to label responses that should be bound together. The problem with this idea is that follower cells have to integrate over some tens of milliseconds to find out whether a feeding cell has increased its discharge rate. Thus, discharge rates have to be maintained elevated over some time to allow for effective temporal summation.

If within this integration time another assembly becomes organized, a superposition problem arises, as it becomes impossible to know which of the many simultaneous, enhanced responses belong to which assembly. This limits the number of populations that can be enhanced simultaneously without becoming confounded. Only those populations would remain segregatable that are clearly defined by a place code. But place codes are again expensive with respect to the number of required neurons, and they suffer from low combinatorial flexibility. Another disadvantage of selecting neurons solely on the basis of enhanced discharge rates is that it precludes the option to encode information about features or constellations of features in the graded responses of distributed populations of neurons because rate is no longer available as a coding space for stimulus qualities.

It was proposed, therefore, that synchronizing responses on a time scale of milliseconds is a more efficient mechanism for response selection. It also increases the saliency of responses because it allows for effective spatial summation in the population of neurons receiving convergent input from synchronized input cells. Because of certain characteristics of cortical connectivity, synchronization actually appears as a particularly effective mechanism for response selection. Many of the excitatory connections between cortical pyramidal cells exhibit a marked frequency attenuation of synaptic transmission (Thomson and West, 1993). Furthermore, any particular pyramidal cell receives input from several thousand other pyramidal cells, but each of those connections of inputs contributes only a few synapses of low efficiency. Thus, synchronization of inputs is likely to increase the saliency of responses more effectively than increasing the rate of firing.

In addition, synchronization expresses unambiguous relations among input neurons because it enhances selectively and with high temporal precision only the saliency of responses that are synchronous. Simulation studies (Softky and Koch 1993) suggest that the interval for effective summation of converging inputs is only a few milliseconds in cortical neurons. If synchronization could be achieved with a similar degree of precision, response selection would become highly specific, and different assemblies could become organized in rapid temporal succession by using a multiplexing strategy. In principle, a particular assembly could even be defined by a single barrage of synchronously emitted action potentials whereby each individual cell would have to contribute only a few discharges. Predictably, such synchronous events are very effective in eliciting responses in target populations, and because synchronous discharges of large numbers of neurons are statistically very improbable, their information content is high.

For these reasons it was theorized that binding of population responses should be achieved by synchronization (von der Malsburg 1985; von der Malsburg and Schneider, 1986; Milner, 1974). The assumption is that, during the formation of functionally coherent assemblies, the discharges of neurons undergo a specific temporal patterning so that cells participating in the encoding of related contents eventually come to discharge in synchrony. This patterning is thought to be based on a self-organizing process that is mediated by a highly selective network of reentrant connections. Thus, neurons having joined into an assembly coding for the same feature or at higher levels, for the same perceptual object, or for a particular movement trajectory, would be identifiable as members of the assembly because their responses would contain episodes during which their discharges are synchronous.

PREDICTIONS

If an assembly of cells coding for a common feature or a common perceptual object or for a particular motor act is distinguished by the temporal coherence of the responses of the constituting neurons, predictions can be derived that are accessible to experimental testing.

1. Spatially segregated neurons should exhibit synchronized response episodes if activated by a single stimulus or by stimuli that can be grouped together into a single perceptual object. This synchronization should occur with precision in the millisecond range.

2. Synchronization should be frequent among neurons within a particular cortical area, but it should also occur between cells distributed across different cortical areas if these cells respond to different features of the same perceptual object.

3. The probability that neurons synchronize their responses both within a particular area and across areas should reflect some of the Gestalt criteria used for perceptual grouping.

4. Individual cells must be able rapidly to change the partners with which they synchronize their responses if stimulus configurations change and require new associations. Thus, synchronization must occur as the result of a highly dynamic, self-organizing process, and its probabilities must depend on stimulus configurations.

5. If more than one object is present in a scene, several distinct assemblies should form. Cells belonging to the same assembly should have synchronous response episodes, but no consistent temporal relations should exist between the discharges of neurons belonging to different assemblies.

6. Synchronization should occur as the result of a self-organizing process that is based on mutual and parallel interactions among the distributed cortical cells whose responses become synchronous.

7. The connections determining synchronization probabilities should be highly specific, as the criteria according to which distributed responses are bound together reside in the functional architecture of these connections.

8. The synchronizing connections should allow for interactions at levels of processing where responses of neurons already express some feature selectivity to permit feature-specific associations. This predicts that cortico-cortical connections contribute to synchronization.

9. The synchronizing connections should be endowed with adaptive synapses allowing for use-dependent, long-term modifications of synaptic gain to permit the acquisition of new grouping criteria when new object representations are to be installed during perceptual learning.

10. These use-dependent synaptic modifications should follow a correlation rule whereby synaptic connection should strengthen if presynaptic and post-synaptic activity is often correlated, and they should weaken in case there is no correlation. This is required to enhance grouping of cells that code for features that often occur in consistent relations, as is the case for features constituting a particular object.

11. These grouping operations should occur over several processing stages, because the search for meaningful groupings has to be performed at different spatial scales and according to different feature domains. This could be achieved by distributing the grouping operations over different cortical areas, each of which processes preferentially certain aspects of the retinal input.

EXPERIMENTAL TESTING OF THE PREDICTIONS

With the exception of prediction 11, which has not been tested yet, all predictions have received experimental support, with most of the data obtained in the mammalian visual cortex. Neurons recorded simultaneously

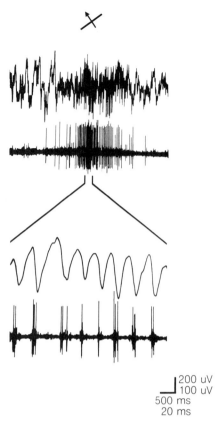

Figure 6.1 The multi unit activity (MUA) and local field potential (LFP) responses were recorded from area 17 in an adult cat to the presentation of an optimally oriented light bar moving across the receptive field. Oscilloscope records of a single trial show the response to the preferred direction of movement. In the upper two traces, at a slow time scale, the onset of the neuronal response is associated with an increase in high-frequency activity in the LFP. The lower two traces display the activity at the peak of the response at an expanded time scale. Note the presence of rhythmic oscillations in the LFP and MUA (35–45 Hz) that are correlated in phase with the peak negativity of the LFP. Upper and lower voltage scales are for the LFP and MUA, respectively. (Adapted from Gray and Singer, 1989.)

with a single electrode transiently engaged in synchronous discharges when presented with their preferred stimulus (Gray and Singer, 1987). In multiunit recordings these locally synchronous discharges often appear as clusters of spikes that follow one another at rather regular intervals of 15 to 30 msec. These sequences of synchronous rhythmic firing usually last no more than a few hundred milliseconds and may occur several times during a single passage of moving stimuli (figure 6.1). Accordingly, autocorrelograms computed from such response epochs often exhibit a periodic modulation (Gray and Singer, 1987, 1989; Eckhorn et al, 1988; Gray et al, 1990; Schwarz and Bolz, 1991; Livingstone, 1991).

This phenomenon of local response synchronization was observed with multiunit and field potential recordings in several independent studies in different areas of the visual cortex of anesthetized cats (areas 17, 18, 19, and the medial bank of the posterior suprasylvian sulcus (PMLS) (Eckhorn et al, 1988, 1992; Gray and Singer, 1989; Gray et al, 1990; Engel, König, and Singer, 1991a), in area 17 of awake cats (Raether, Gray, and Singer, 1989; Gray and Viana di Prisco, 1993), in the optic tectum of awake pigeons (Neuenschwander and Varela, 1993), and in the visual cortex of anesthetized (Livingstone, 1991) and awake behaving monkeys (Kreiter and Singer, 1992; Eckhorn et al, 1993). Similar synchronization phenomena also were observed in a variety of nonvisual structures (Singer, 1993, 1994; Singer and Gray, 1995).

Multielectrode recordings revealed that similar response synchronization can occur also among spatially segregated cell groups within the same visual area (Gray et al, 1989, 1992; Engel et al, 1990; König et al, 1993) and also among different cortical areas (Eckhorn et al, 1988; Engel, König, and Singer, 1991; Murthy and Fetz, 1992; Nelson et al, 1992a) and even across hemispheres (Engel et al, 1991a; Munk et al, 1992). Measurements in awake cats (Raether, Gray, and Singer, 1989; Gray and Viana di Prisco, 1993) and monkeys (Kreiter and Singer, 1992; Murthy and Fetz, 1992; Ahissar et al, 1992) showed that this phenomenon of response synchronization is not confined to anesthesia but is readily demonstrable in various neocortical areas (visual, auditory, somatosensory, and motor) of alert behaving animals. These single-unit data are complemented by a large body of evidence derived from field potential and electroencephalographic (EEG) recordings that all indicate that distributed groups of neurons can engage in synchronous activity (Singer, 1993; Singer and Gray, 1995).

THE DEPENDENCE OF RESPONSE SYNCHRONIZATION ON STIMULUS CONFIGURATION

As outlined above, the hypothesis of temporally coded assemblies requires that the probabilities with which distributed cells synchronize their responses should reflect some of the Gestalt criteria applied in perceptual grouping. A clear dependence of synchronization probability could be established with respect to the criteria of vicinity, continuity, and common fate (Gray et al, 1989; Engel et al, 1990).

Gray et al (1989) recorded multiunit activity from two locations in cat area 17 separated by 7 mm. The receptive fields of the cells were nonoverlapping, had nearly identical orientation preferences, and were spatially displaced along the axis of preferred orientation. This enabled stimulation of the cells with bars of the same orientation under three different conditions: two bars moving in opposite directions, two bars moving in the same direction, and one long bar moving across both fields coherently. No significant correlation was found when the cells were stimulated by oppositely moving bars. A weak correlation was present for the coherently moving bars. The long bar stimulus resulted in a robust synchronization of the activity at the two sites. This effect occurred despite the fact that the overall numbers of spikes produced by the two cells and the oscillatory patterning of the responses were similar in the three conditions.

In related experiments Engel et al (1991, 1991a) demonstrated in the cat that the synchronization of activity between cells in areas 17 and PMLS and between areas 17 in the two hemispheres has a similar dependence on the properties of the visual stimulus (figure 6.2). These findings indicate that the global properties of visual stimuli can influence the magnitude of synchronization between widely separated cells located within and between different cortical areas. Single contours but also spatially separate contours that move coherently and therefore appear as parts of a single figure are more efficient in inducing synchrony among the responding cell groups than incoherently moving contours that appear as parts of independent figures.

These results indicate clearly that synchronization probability depends not only on the spatial segregation of cells and on their feature preferences, the latter being related to the cells' position within the columnar architecture of the cortex, but also, and to a crucial extent, on the configuration of the stimuli. So far, synchronization probability appears to reflect rather well some of the Gestalt criteria for perceptual grouping. The high synchronization probability of nearby cells corresponds to the binding criterion of vicinity, the dependence on receptive field similarities agrees with the criterion of similarity, the strong synchronization observed in response to continuous stimuli obeys the criterion of continuity, and the lack of synchrony in responses to stimuli moving in opposite directions relates to the criterion of common fate.

Experiments have also been performed to test the prediction that simultaneously presented but different contours should lead to the organization of two independently synchronized assemblies of cells (Engel et al, 1991b; Kreiter, Engel, and Singer, 1992). If groups of cells with overlapping receptive fields but different orientation preferences are activated with a single moving light bar, they synchronize their response (Engel et al, 1990, 1991b). Usually, synchrony is established among all responding neurons, including those that are activated only suboptimally. This agrees with the postulate derived from the hypothesis of coarse coding that all responses of cells participating in the representation of a stimulus ought to be bound together.

However, if such a set of groups is stimulated with two independent spatially overlapping stimuli that move in different directions, the activated cells split into two independently synchronized assemblies. Cells whose feature preferences match better with stimulus 1 form one synchronously active assembly, and those matching better with stimulus 2 the other (figure 6.3). Thus, although the two stimuli now evoke graded responses in all of the recorded groups, cells representing the same stimulus remain distinguishable because their responses have synchronized response epochs while showing no consistent correlations with responses of cells activated by different stimuli.

To extract this information, a read-out mechanism is required that is capable of evaluating coincident firing at a millisecond time scale. As mentioned

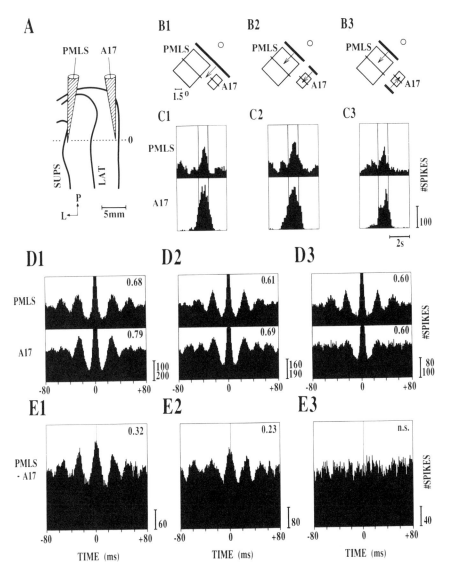

Figure 6.2 Interareal synchronization is sensitive to global stimulus features. (A) Position of the recording electrodes. A17, area 17; LAT, lateral sulcus; SUPS, suprasylvian sulcus; P, posterior; L, lateral. (B1–B3) Plots of the receptive fields of the PMLS and area 17 recording. The diagrams depict the three stimulus conditions tested. The circle indicates the visual field center. (C1–C3) Peristimulus time histograms for the three stimulus conditions. The vertical lines indicate 1-s windows for which autocorrelograms and cross-correlograms were computed. Comparison of the autocorrelograms was computed for the three stimulus paradigms. Note that the modulation amplitude of the correlograms is similar in all three cases (indicated by the number in the upper right corner). (E1–E3) Cross-correlograms computed for the three stimulus conditions. The number in the upper right corner represents the relative modulation amplitude of each correlogram. Note that the strongest correlogram modulation is obtained with the continuous stimulus. The cross-correlogram is less regular and has a lower modulation amplitude when two light bars are used as stimuli, and there is no significant modulation (NS) with two light bars moving in opposite direction. (From Engel et al, 1991a.)

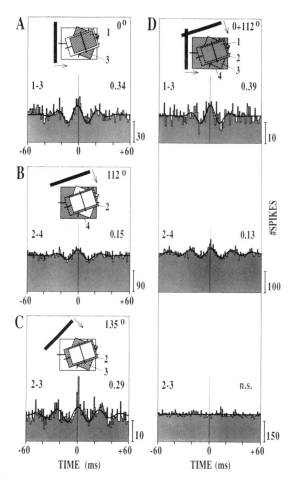

Figure 6.3 Stimulus dependence of short-range interactions. Multiunit activity was recorded from four different orientation columns of area 17 of cat visual cortex separated by 0.4 mm. The four cell groups had overlapping receptive fields and orientation preferences of 22 degrees (group 1), 112 degrees (group 2), 157 degrees (group 3), and 90 degrees (group 4), as indicated by the thick line drawn across each receptive field in A through D. The figure shows a comparison of responses to stimulation with single moving light bars of varying orientation (left) with responses to the combined presentation of two superimposed light bars (right). For each stimulus condition, the shading of the receptive fields indicates the responding cell groups. Stimulation with a single light bar yielded synchronization among all cells activated by the respective orientation. Thus, groups 1 and 3 responded synchronously to a vertically orientated zero-degree light bar (A), groups 2 and 4 to a light bar at an orientation of 112 degrees (B), and cell groups 2 and 3 to a light bar of intermediate orientation. (C) Simultaneous presentation of two stimuli with orientations of zero and 112 degrees, respectively, activated all four groups (D). However, in this case the groups segregated into two distinct assemblies, depending on which stimulus was closer to the preferred orientation of each group. Thus, responses were synchronized between groups 1 and 3, which preferred the vertical stimulus, and between 2 and 4, which preferred the stimulus oriented at 112 degrees. The two assemblies were desynchronized with respect to each other, and so there was no significant synchronization between groups 2 and 3. The cross-correlograms between groups 1 and 2, 1 and 4, and 3 and 4 were also flat (not shown). Note that the segregation cannot be explained by preferential anatomical wiring of cells with similar orientation preference because cell groups can readily be synchronized in all possible pair combinations in response to a single light bar. The correlograms are shown superimposed with their Gabor function. The number in the upper right of each correlogram indicates the relative modulation amplitude. ns = not significant. Scale bars indicate the number of spikes. (From Engel et al, 1991b).

above, recent analysis of the integrative properties of cortical pyramidal cells suggests that in these cells the window for effective temporal summation may indeed be as short as a few milliseconds (Softky and Koch, 1993).

Another important issue of these experiments is the demonstration that individual cells can actually change the partners with which they synchronize when stimulus configurations change. Cell groups that engaged in synchronous response episodes when activated with a single stimulus no longer do so when activated with two stimuli but are then synchronized with other groups. This agrees with the prediction of the assembly hypothesis that interactions among distributed cell groups should be variable and influenced by the constellation of features in the visual stimulus.

THE NATURE AND SPECIFICITY OF SYNCHRONIZING CONNECTIONS

The hypothesis requires that synchronization probability depends to a substantial extent on interactions among the neurons whose responses actually represent the features that have to be bound together. As cells in subcortical centers possess only very limited feature selectivity, one is led to postulate that cortico-cortical connections should also contribute to the synchronization process. Examination of interhemispheric response synchronization has revealed that responses of neurons in areas 17 of the two hemispheres synchronize in very much the same way as responses within the same hemisphere if evoked by coherently moving stimuli (Engel et al, 1991a). This agrees with the theory that contours extending across the midline of the visual field should be bound by the same mechanism as contours located within the same hemifield.

Sectioning the corpus callosum abolished response synchronization (Engel et al, 1991a; Munk et al, 1992). This is direct proof that cortico-cortical connections contribute to response synchronization and that synchronization with zero-phase lag can be brought about by reciprocal interactions between spatially distributed neurons despite considerable conduction delays in the coupling connections. Thus, in agreement with the predictions, the synchronization phenomena considered in the context of binding are not necessarily an indication of common input but may also occur as a result of a dynamic organization process that establishes coherent firing by reciprocal interactions and reentry (Singer and Gray, 1995).

The theory of assembly coding implies that the criteria according to which particular features are grouped together rather than others reside in the functional architecture of the assembly forming coupling connections. It is of particular interest, therefore, to study the development of the synchronizing connections, to identify the rules according to which they are selected, to establish correlations between their architecture and synchronization probabilities, and, if possible, to relate these neuronal properties to perceptual functions.

In mammals cortico-cortical connections develop mainly postnatally (Callaway and Katz, 1990; Innocenti, 1981; Luhmann, Martinez-Millan, and Singer, 1986; Price and Blakemore, 1985a) and attain their final specificity through an activity-dependent selection process (Callaway and Katz, 1990; Innocenti and Frost, 1979; Luhmann, Singer, and Martinez-Millan, 1990; Price and Blakemore, 1985b). Recently, it was found that strabismus induced in three-week-old kittens leads to a profound rearrangement of cortico-cortical connections. Normally, these connections link cortical territories regardless of whether these are dominated by the same or by different eyes. In strabismics, by contrast, the tangential intracortical connections come to link with high selectivity only territories served by the same eye (Löwel and Singer, 1992). The functional correlate of these changes in the architecture of cortico-cortical connections is a modification of synchronization probabilities. In strabismics, response synchronization no longer occurs among cell groups connected to different eyes, whereas it is normal among cell groups connected to the same eye (König et al, 1990, 1993).

These results have several implications. First, they are further support for the notion that tangential intracortical connections contribute to response synchronization. Second, they confirm the prediction that the assembly-forming connections should be susceptible to use-dependent modifications and be selected according to a correlation rule. Third, the reduced synchrony among cells driven by different eyes supports that synchronization serves as a binding mechanism. Strabismic subjects become unable to fuse signals conveyed by different eyes into coherent percepts even if the signals are made retinotopically contiguous by optical compensation of the squint angle (von Noorden, 1990). Thus, binding mechanisms appear to be abnormal or missing between cells driven from different eyes. The lack of cortico-cortical connections and the lack of response synchronization could be one of the reasons for this deficit, in addition to the loss of binocular neurons.

These correlations are compatible with the view that the architecture of cortico-cortical connections, by determining the probability of response synchronization, could set the criteria for perceptual grouping. Since this architecture is shaped by experience, it opens the possibility that some of the binding and segmentation criteria are acquired or modified by experience.

IMPAIRED RESPONSE SYNCHRONIZATION CORRELATES WITH PERCEPTUAL DISTURBANCES

Further indications for a relation between experience-dependent modifications of synchronization probabilities and functional deficits come from a study of strabismic cats who had developed amblyopia. Strabismus, when induced early in life, not only abolishes binocular fusion and stereopsis, but may also lead to amblyopia of one eye (von Noorden, 1990). This condition develops when the subjects solve the problem of double vision not by alternating use of the two eyes but by constantly suppressing the signals coming from the deviated eye. The amblyopic deficit usually consists of reduced spatial resolution and distorted and blurred perception of patterns.

A particularly characteristic phenomenon in amblyopia is crowding, the drastic impairment of the ability to discriminate and recognize figures if they are surrounded with other contours. In addition, signals conveyed by the deviating eye are less salient than those from the normal eye, as the former signals cannot be perceived as long as both eyes are open even if attention is directed to them. Identification of neuronal correlates of these deficits in animal models of amblyopia is inconclusive because the contrast sensitivity and the spatial resolution capacity of neurons in the retina and the lateral geniculate nucleus are normal.

In the visual cortex, identification of neurons with reduced spatial resolution or otherwise abnormal receptive field properties remains controversial (Crewther and Crewther, 1990; Blakemore and Vital-Durand, 1992). However, multielectrode recordings from striate cortex of cats with behaviorally verified amblyopia revealed highly significant differences in the synchronization behavior of cells driven by the normal and the amblyopic eye, respectively. Responses to single moving bars that were recorded simultaneously from spatially segregated neurons connected to the amblyopic eye were much less well synchronized with one another than the responses recorded from neuron pairs driven through the normal eye (Roelfsema et al, 1994). This difference was even more pronounced for responses elicited by gratings of different spatial frequency. For responses of cell pairs activated through the normal eye, the strength of synchronization tended to increase with increasing spatial frequency, whereas it tended to decrease further for cell pairs activated through the amblyopic eye (figure 6.4).

Apart from these highly significant differences between the synchronization behavior of cells driven through the normal eye and the amblyopic eye, no other differences were found in the commonly determined response properties of these cells. Thus, cells connected to the amblyopic eye continued to respond vigorously to gratings whose spatial frequency had been too high to be discriminated with the amblyopic eye in the preceding behavioral tests. These results suggest that disturbed temporal coordination of responses such as reduced synchrony may be one of the neuronal correlates of the amblyopic deficit. Indeed, if synchronization of responses at a millisecond time scale is used by the system to tag and identify the responses of cells that code for the same feature or contour, disturbance of this temporal patterning could be the cause for reduced spatial resolution and the crowding phenomenon. If responses evoked by nearby contours can no longer be associated unambiguously with either one contour or the other but become confounded, perceptual deficits are expected that closely resemble those characteristic for amblyopic vision.

Use-dependent modifications of synaptic connections require for their induction that postsynaptic neurons be sufficiently depolarized and hence receive enough drive from subcortical and intrinsic inputs (Artola and Singer,

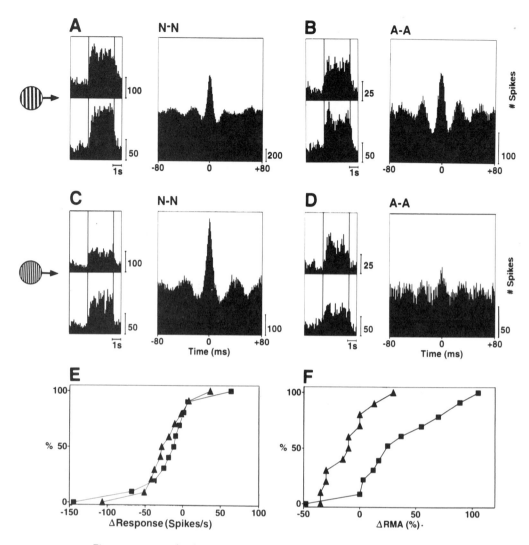

Figure 6.4 Amplitudes and synchronization of responses to gratings of different spatial frequencies recorded from cats with strabismic amblyopia. (A–D) Responses to low (A and B) and high (C and D) spatial frequency gratings, recorded simultaneously from two cell groups driven by the normal eye (N sites) (A and C) and two cell groups driven by the amblyopic eye (A sites) (B and D), respectively. The left and right pannels show the response histograms and the corresponding cross-correlograms, respectively. Note that response amplitudes decrease at the higher spatial frequency in both cases, whereas the relative modulation amplitude increases for the N-N pair but decreases for the A-A pair. (E) Cumulative distribution functions of the differences between the amplitude of responses to low and high spatial frequency gratings of optimal orientation. N sites are represented by squares ($n = 53$); A sites are represented by triangles ($n = 35$). The abscissa shows responses to high spatial frequency minus responses to low spatial frequency gratings. Note the similarity of the two distributions ($p > 0.1$). (F) Cumulative distribution functions of the differences between relative modulation amplitudes (ΔRMA of cross-correlograms obtained for responses to high and low spatial frequency gratings of N-N pairs (squares; $n = 24$) and A-A pairs (triangles; $n = 11$). The ΔRMA values (abscissa) were calculated by subtracting the relative modulation amplitude obtained with the low spatial frequency from that obtained with the high spatial frequency. The difference between the ΔRMA distributions of N-N pairs and A-A pairs is highly significant. (Roelfsema et al 1994).

1993). If, due to interocular rivalry, activity from the good eye consistently weakens responses to input from the deviating eye, appropriate experience-dependent selection of cortico-cortical connections is likely to be prevented. As a possible reason for the reduced synchronization among cells driven by the amblyopic eye, one might consider abnormalities in the network of cortico-cortical connections linking cell groups dominated by that eye. It is conceivable that the continuous suppression of signals provided from that eye impedes the experience-dependent specification of the respective intra-cortical synchronizing connections. Furthermore, reduced synchrony reduces the saliency of responses by reducing their impact on cells at higher processing levels. This is likely to account for inability to attend to signals from the amblyopic eye when both eyes are open and competing for attention.

THE RELATION BETWEEN SYNCHRONY AND OSCILLATIONS

As response synchronization on the one hand and oscillatory responses on the other are often, but not necessarily always, associated with one another, it appears appropriate to examine the relation between the phenomena more closely. The occurrence of oscillatory responses does not imply that cells discharge in synchrony. Similarly, nonoccurrence of oscillations does not exclude synchrony. Furthermore, it is useful to analyze to which extent different recording methods are appropriate for assessing synchrony and oscillatory behavior, because there are a number of difficulties with the detectability of oscillatory firing patterns in single cell recordings and with the definition of oscillations.

No inferences can of course be drawn from single cell recordings as to whether the responses of the recorded cell are synchronized with others, regardless of whether or not the cell is found to discharge in an oscillatory manner. The situation is different when multiunit recordings are obtained with a single electrode. In this case, periodically modulated autocorrelograms are always indicative not only of oscillatory firing patterns but also of response synchronization, at least among the local group of simultaneously recorded neurons. The reason is that such periodic modulations can build up only if sufficient numbers of the simultaneously recorded cells are oscillating synchronously and at a sufficiently regular rhythm. However, not observing periodically modulated autocorrelograms of multiunit recordings neither excludes that the recorded units oscillate, because nonsynchronized oscillations would not be observable, nor excludes that the recorded cells actually fire in synchrony, because they could do so in a nonperiodic way.

The same arguments are applicable to field potentials and even more so to EEG recordings. If they exhibit an oscillatory pattern, this always implies that a large number of neurons must have engaged in synchronized rhythmic activity. Otherwise the weak fields generated by activation of individual synapses and neurons would not sum to potentials recordable with macro-electrodes. But again, the reverse is not true: neither oscillatory discharge patterns nor response synchronization can be excluded if macroelectrode recordings fail to reveal oscillatory fluctuations.

Furthermore, it has to be considered that single cell recordings may not be particularly well suited for the diagnosis of oscillatory activity. This is suggested by results from the visual cortex (Gray et al, 1990) and in particular from the olfactory bulb (Freeman and Skarda, 1985). Individual discharges of single units may be precisely time locked with the oscillating field potential. This proves that these discharges participated in an oscillatory process and occurred in synchrony with those of many other cells, without, however, showing any sign of oscillatory activity in their autocorrelation function. The reasons for this apparent paradox are sampling problems and nonstationarity of the time series. If the single cell does not discharge at every cycle and if the oscillation frequency is not perfectly constant over a period of time sufficiently long to sample enough discharges for an interpretable autocorrelation function, the oscillatory rhythm to which the cell is actually locked will not be disclosable. Thus, the less active a cell and the higher and more variable the oscillation frequency, the less is it legitimate to infer from non-periodically modulated autocorrelograms that a cell is not oscillating.

This sampling problem becomes more and more accentuated as the frequency of the oscillations increases. This explains why γ-band oscillations were observed first with macroelectrodes and remain difficult to observe with microelectrodes unless one can record from several, synchronously active cells simultaneously.

Finally, some ambiguities are associated with the term "oscillations." Commonly, oscillations are associated with periodic time series such as are produced by a pendulum or a harmonic oscillator. But more irregular or even aperiodic time series are still addressed as oscillatory. Such irregular oscillations typically occur in noisy linear or nonlinear systems, and cover a large spectrum of phenotypes from slightly distorted, periodic oscillations over chaotic oscillations to nearly stochastic time series. Oscillatory phenomena in the brain are rarely of the harmonic type and, if so, only over very short time intervals. Most often, oscillatory activity in the brain is so irregular that autocorrelation functions computed over prolonged periods of time frequently fail to reveal the oscillatory nature of the underlying time series.

Evidence that in most investigated structures the phases of response synchronization tend to be associated with episodes of oscillatory activity, raises the question as to whether oscillations and synchrony are causally related. One possibility is that oscillatory activity favors the establishment of synchrony and hence is instrumental for response synchronization (König et al, 1993). In oscillatory responses the occurrence of one burst predicts with some probability the occurrence of the next. It has been argued that this predictability is a necessary prerequisite to synchronize remote cell groups with zero-phase lag, despite considerable conduction delays in the coupling connections (Engel et al, 1992). This view is supported by simulation studies showing that zero-phase lag synchronization can be achieved despite considerable conduction delays and variation of conduction times in the synchronizing connections if the coupled cell groups have a tendency to oscillate (König and Schillen, 1991; Schillen and König, 1990, 1993; Schuster and Wagner, 1990a,b).

Another feature of networks with oscillatory properties is that network elements that are not linked directly can be synchronized by intermediate oscillators (König and Schillen, 1991). This may be important, for instance, to establish relationships between remote cell groups within the same cortical area, or for cells distributed across cortical areas that process different sensory modalities. In both cases, linkages either by intermediate cortical relays or even by subcortical centers must be considered (see Llinás, this volume). These considerations suggest that oscillations, while not conveying any stimulus-specific information per se, may be instrumental for the establishment of synchrony over large distances.

It is also conceivable, however, that oscillations occur as a consequence of synchrony. Simulation studies indicate that networks with excitatory and inhibitory feedback have the tendency to converge toward states where discharges of local cell clusters become synchronous (Koch and Schuster, 1992; Deppisch et al, 1992; Sporns, Tononi, and Edelman, 1991). Once such a synchronous volley has been generated, the network is likely to engage in oscillatory activity. Because of recurrent inhibition and because of Ca^{2+}-activated K^+ conductances (Llinás, 1988, 1990) the cells that had emitted a synchronous discharge will also become simultaneously silent. On fading of these inhibitory events, firing probability will increase simultaneously for all cells and this, together with maintained excitatory input and nonlinear voltage-gated membrane conductances such as the low-threshold Ca^{2+}-channels (Llinás, 1990), favors the occurrence of the next synchronous burst, and so on. Thus, oscillations are a likely consequence of synchrony, and it actually becomes important to understand how cortical networks can be prevented from entering states of global oscillations, and if they do, how these can be terminated. These issues were addressed in a number of simulation studies (Hansel and Sompolinsky, 1992; König, Janosch, and Schillen, 1992; König and Schillen, 1990; Schillen and König, 1991, 1993; Sporns et al, 1991; von der Malsburg and Schneider, 1986).

SYNCHRONIZATION AND ATTENTION

The hypothesis that information about feature constellations is contained in the temporal relation between the discharges of distributed neurons, and in particular in their synchrony, also has some bearing on the organization of attentional mechanisms. It is obvious that synchronous activity will be more effective in driving cells at higher levels than nonorganized, asynchronous discharges. Thus, those assemblies would appear as particularly salient and hence effective in attracting attention, which makes their discharges coherent with shorter latency and higher temporal precision than others.

Conversely, responses of neurons reacting to features that cannot be grouped or bound successfully, and hence cannot be synchronized with the responses of other neurons, would have only a small chance of being relayed further and influencing shifts of selective attention. It is thus conceivable that of the many responses that occur at peripheral stages of visual processing, only a few are actually passed on toward higher levels. These would either be responses to particularly salient stimuli causing strong and simultaneous discharges in a sufficient number of neurons, or responses of cells that succeeded in being organized in sufficiently coherent assemblies. Thus, responses to appearing or disappearing targets have a good chance of being passed on even without getting organized internally because they would be synchronized by the external event.

But responses to patterns lacking temporal structure require organization through internal synchronization mechanisms to be propagated. This interpretation implies that neuronal responses that attract attention and gain control over behavior should differ from nonattended responses, not so much because they are stronger, but because they are better synchronized among each other.

Accordingly, shifting attention by top-down processes would be equivalent with biasing synchronization probability of neurons at lower levels by feedback connections from higher levels. These top-down influences could favor the emergence of coherent states in selected subpopulations of neurons, those that respond to contours of an attended object or pattern. Thus, the mechanism that allows for grouping and scene segmentation—the organization of synchrony—could also serve to manage attention. The advantage would be that nonattended signals do not have to be suppressed, which would hitherto eliminate them from competition for attention. Rather, cells could remain active and thus be rapidly recruitable into an assembly if changes of afferent activity or of feedback signals modify the balance among neurons competing for the formation of synchronous assemblies.

In a similar way, shifts of attention across different modalities could be achieved by selectively enhancing synchronization probability in particular sensory areas and not in others. This could be achieved, for example, by modulatory input from the basal forebrain or nonspecific thalamic nuclei. If these projection systems were able to modulate in synchrony the excitability of cortical neurons distributed in different areas, it would greatly enhance the probability that these neurons link selectively with each other and join into coherent activity. Such linking would be equivalent to the binding of the features represented in the respective cortical areas.

Again, this view equates grouping or binding mechanisms with attentional mechanisms. The attention-directing systems would simply have to provide a temporal frame within which distributed responses could self-organize toward coherent states through the network of selective cortico-cortical connections. In doing so, the attentional systems need not themselves produce responses in cortical neurons. It would be sufficient that they cause a synchronous modulation of their excitability.

It is conceivable that the synchronous field potential oscillations that have been observed in animals and humans during states of focused attention reflect such an attention mechanism. That these field potential oscillations are only loosely related to the discharge probability of individual neurons, are coherent across different cortical areas, are particularly pronounced when the subjects are busy with tasks requiring integration of activity across different cortical areas, and stop immediately when the binding problem is solved, as witnessed by the execution of a well-programmed motor act, is in agreement with such an interpretation (Llinás, this volume; Singer, 1993; Singer and Gray, 1995).

SYNOPSIS

In this paragraph a picture is developed in which response synchronization is used at different levels of cortical processing for feature representation, scene segmentation, perceptual grouping, and the organization of sensory representations. The essential ingredients of this model are depicted schematically in figure 6.5. The different boxes stand for some of the numerous cortical areas devoted to the processing of retinal signals. The arrows between them symbolize the possibility of a reciprocal flow of signals between areas at similar and different levels of the processing hierarchy. For a detailed description of the connectivity pattern among different visual areas, the reader is referred to Felleman and van Essen (1991) and Young (1992).

On presentation of a complex visual scene, the following sequence of events is assumed to occur. Neurons in V1 that encounter a preferred feature in their receptive field increase their activity, thus raising the probability that their discharges can be made coincident with those of other cells. At the same time, these responses are organized due to the action of the tangential connections within V1. Because of the specific architecture of these connections, neurons coactivated by the same continuous contour or by colinear contour segments tend to synchronize their activity. While this organization proceeds in V1, signals are passed on to other areas where similar organization processes are initiated. Of the many responses in V1, those that are synchronized best will be particularly effective in influencing neurons in higher areas. Therefore, response constellations that fit the grouping criteria set by the architecture of tangential connections in V1 will be passed on and processed further with greater probability than incoherent responses that also arrive from V1. Because the connections from V1 to the other areas convey already preprocessed activity, and by divergence and convergence allow for remapping of neighborhood relations, the grouping criteria in these higher areas should differ from those in V1.

Thus it is assumed, for example, that in V5 those neurons have a tendency to synchronize their responses that code for the same direction of motion.

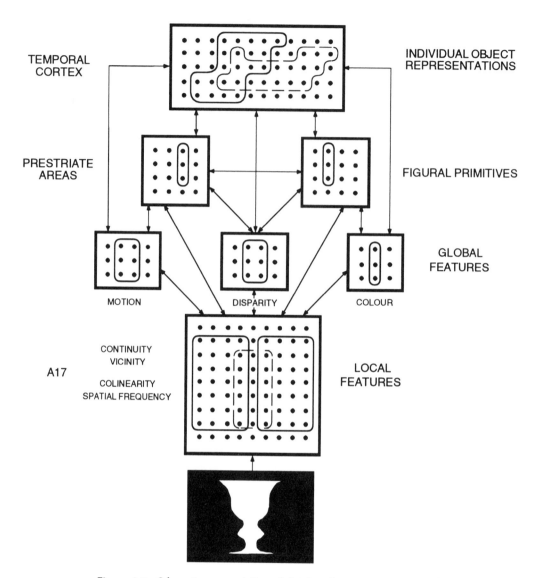

Figure 6.5 Schematic representation of distributed grouping operations during scene segmentation. The boxes represent cortical areas at different levels of processing that perform grouping operations according to increasingly complex criteria. The arrows indicate reciprocal connections among these distributed cortical areas. For details see text.

Because the neurons in V5 have large receptive fields and hence a great aperture, and are also sensitive to relative motion, this area can evaluate coherent motion both in relative and absolute terms over large distances. While the responses in V5 become organized according to the grouping criteria set by the intrinsic interactions within V5, it is assumed that they influence by back-projections the organization process in V1, adding the criterion of coherent motion to the grouping process in V1. This top-down influence is thought to bias synchronization probability among neurons in V1 toward either more or less synchrony, depending on stimulus configuration.

Responses to contour elements that are far apart and have different orientations have a low probability of becoming synchronized by local interactions within V1. However, if these contour elements move coherently, their coherence would be detected by neurons in V5, and responses to these contours would synchronize in V5 and, through back-projections, increase synchronization probability for the respective set of neurons in V1. Such top-down influences from motion-sensitive areas with large aperture could account for the observation that coherently moving line segments lead to synchronization of responses in area 17, even if the cortical representations of these line segments are much farther apart than the maximum span of the tangential intracortical connections (Gray et al, 1989).

The finding that pharmacological inactivation of cells in motion-sensitive areas reduces considerably response synchronization to coherently moving contours in V1 supports this possibility (Nelson et al, 1992b). Conversely, responses to nearby contours of similar orientation that would have a tendency to become synchronized due to the local interactions in V1 may be prevented from synchronizing by top-down influences from motion-sensitive areas if the contours move in different directions and with different speeds. Such differences in motion trajectories prevent neurons in motion-sensitive areas from synchronizing (Kreiter and Singer, 1992), and hence, activity in the back-projections would either not favor the occurrence of synchrony in V1 or even actively reduce its probability.

Similar grouping operations are assumed to occur simultaneously in numerous other prestriate areas, but according to different criteria. Thus, while one area explores similarities in color space, another may search for related textures, and yet another for similarities in retinal disparity, and so on. The results of these evaluations that can all occur in parallel are sent back to V1, where they all contribute to the continuing organization process. As a consequence, the synchronization probabilities among neurons in area 17 change, and this in turn modifies the input configurations to prestriate areas. While the distributed search for the most probable grouping constellations proceeds, areas at the top of the processing hierarchy will also be involved.

Because of the polysynaptic nature of the input, these areas will probably become active only when activity in the preceding areas has become sufficiently coherent. However, because of the high degree of parallelism in the organization of prestriate areas and the rather direct connections between prestriate and temporal areas, these processing delays should be short and not exceed a few tens of milliseconds. In the higher areas, responses should become organized according to the same general rules as at peripheral levels, given the similarity of the intrinsic organization of the different cortical areas. The grouping criteria will be much more complex at these higher levels, however, because interactions now involve neurons that represent complicated constellations of features such as figural components and higher-order geometrical shapes (Tanaka et al, 1991; Gallant, Braun, and van Essen, 1993).

These higher areas are connected to lower areas by dense back-projections, and thus it must be assumed that once coherent patterns became organized at higher levels, they influence the organization of patterns at lower levels. These processes can all occur nearly simultaneously, as the areas concerned are interconnected by oligosynaptic pathways. Thus, the process of organizing the neuronal representation of a scene consists of parallel operations that occur nearly simultaneously at different levels of the processing hierarchy and according to similar principles. But because of differences in the way in which ascending activity from V1 is mapped into different areas, the evaluation criteria differ for each area and increase in complexity as one moves away from V1. In this model, decisions required for successful perceptual grouping and scene segmentation are based on a highly distributed voting operation where each area contributes its "point of view" and where both bottom-up and top-down processes are intimately interleaved.

Each of the areas explores the feature space for which it is predisposed by its specific afferent and intrinsic connectivity, searches for coherence, and distributes the result of its computation simultaneously to all the areas to which it is connected. These messages are assumed to bias the probabilities with which neurons in the respective target areas synchronize or desynchronize their discharges.

Successful segmentation could thus be viewed at as the result of a self-organizing process that converges toward the state of maximum probability. If scenes contain little ambiguity with respect to the grouping criteria that are stored in the architecture of connections within and between areas, the organization process can be very rapid, and in extreme cases it may not even require the contribution of back-projected activity. This could even be true for complex scenes if they contain mainly familiar objects. In this case the pattern of sensory activity would match directly with the functional architecture of coupling connections that was shaped by previous learning, and the system can converge nearly instantaneously into a coherent state. Under such conditions the system would function in a way that is not too different from a multilayered feed-forward network of the Hopfield type. However, if the scene contains ambiguities allowing for several equally likely groupings, or if it is highly unfamiliar, convergence may occur only after seconds.

Such extreme processing times may actually be required for the segmentation of figures defined solely by similar disparity in Julesz patterns or for the detection of figures hidden in background textures by camouflage, as for example the well-known Dalmatian dog. In both cases it is helpful and reduces recognition time if one already knows what the figure is, a pragmatic proof of the notion that high-level representations can directly influence figure-ground segmentation by top-down biasing of peripheral grouping criteria. In case of the Dalmatian dog, for example, recognition could be speeded up either by top-down propagation if experience has already installed grouping criteria at the levels where figural attributes are bound together, or if one provided additional cues that would facilitate grouping by bottom-up processes at peripheral levels. If the contour elements constituting the dog had any of the properties in common that V1 and prestriate areas can probably evaluate and relate to one another, such as disparity, color, motion, orientation, and texture, segmentation would occur much more rapidly.

Here a pattern is perceived as soon as segmentation is completed and neurons have become organized in distinct, coherently active assemblies. In that case their output will be sufficiently coherent to allow for the propagation of signals to remote cortical areas and ultimately to effector levels. For this to occur it is not only necessary that enough cells coordinate their responses. It is also required that the spatial distribution of these coherently active cells match the receptive field properties of cells at higher levels. Just as cells in V1 are selective for particular spatiotemporal patterns of retinal input, cells in higher cortical areas are likely to be activatable only by the appropriate spatiotemporal patterns that have organized in more peripheral cortical areas. But in contrast to the retinal and thalamic activation patterns, these cortical activation patterns are no longer a direct reflection of the retinal image but are a result of a highly dynamic self-organizing process. The organization of the spatial and temporal structure of these patterns is initiated by the retinal input, but then it is extensively modified by dynamic interactions that are determined essentially by the functional architecture of connections linking cells within and between areas. The proposal is that this organization process converges toward coherent states in which responses that have to be related to one another are tagged by their synchrony.

Following the same line of reasoning, it is also possible that access to the level of processing where representations reach consciousness is gated by coherence. As proposed by Crick and Koch (1990), it is conceivable that only activation patterns (assemblies) reach the threshold of conscious awareness that are sufficiently organized, that is, coherent.

REFERENCES

Abeles M. (1991). *Corticonics*. Cambridge University Press, Cambridge.

Ahissar E, Vaadia E, Ahissar M, Bergmann H, Arieli A, Abeles M. (1992). Dependence of cortical plasticity on correlated activity of single neurons and on behavioral context. *Science* 257:1412–1415.

Artola A, Singer W. (1993). Long-term depression of excitatory synaptic transmission and its relationship to long-term potention. *Trends Neurosci* 16:480–487.

Barlow HB. (1972). Single units and cognition: A neurone doctrine for perceptual psychology. *Perception* 1:371–394.

Baylis GC, Rolls ET, Leonard CM. (1985). Selectivity between faces in the responses of a population of neurons in the cortex in the superior temporal sulcus of the monkey. *Brain Res* 342:91–102.

Blakemore C, Vital-Durand F. (1992). Different neural origins for "blur" amblyopia and strabismic amblyopia. *Ophthalmol Physiol Optom* 12:83–80.

Braitenberg V. (1978). Cell assemblies in the cerebral cortex. In: *Architectonics of the cerebral cortex. Lecture notes in biomathematics 21. Theoretical approaches in complex.* R Heim, G Palm, eds. Springer-Verlag, Berlin, 171–188.

Callaway EM, Katz LC. (1990). Emergence and refinement of clustered horizontal connections in cat striate cortex. *J Neurosci* 10:1134–1153.

Crewther DP, Crewther SG. (1990). Neural sites of strabismic amblyopia in cats: Spatial frequency deficit in primary cortical neurons. *Exp Brain Res* 79:615–622.

Crick F. (1984). Function of the thalamic reticular complex: The searchlight hypothesis. *Proc Natl Acad Sci USA* 81:4586–4590.

Crick F, Koch C. (1990). Towards a neurobiological theory of consciousness. *Semin Neurosci* 2:263–275.

Deppisch J, Bauer HU, Schillen TB, König P, Pawelzik K, Geisel T. (1992). Stochastic and oscillatory burst activities in a model of spiking neurons. In: *Artificial neural networks.* JAJ Taylor, ed. Elsevier, Amsterdam, 921–924.

Desimone R, Albright TD, Gross CG, Bruce C. (1984). Stimulus-selective properties of inferior temporal neurons in the macaque. *J Neurosci* 4:2051–2062.

Desimone R, Schein SJ, Moran J, Ungerleider LG. (1985). Contour, color and shape analysis beyond the striate cortex. *Vision Res* 24:441–452.

Eckhorn R, Bauer R, Jordan W, Brosch M, Kruse W, Munk M, Reitboeck HJ. (1988). Coherent oscillations: A mechanism for feature linking in the visual cortex? *Biol Cybernet* 60:121–130.

Eckhorn R, Bauer R, Jordan W, Brosch M, Kruse W, Munk M, Reitboeck HJ. (1992). Stimulus-specific synchronizations in cat visual cortex: Multiple microelectrode and correlation studies from several cortical areas. In: *Induced rhythms in the brain.* E Basar, TH Bullock, eds. Birkhäuser, Berlin, 47–80.

Eckhorn R, Frien A, Bauer R, Woelbern T, Kehr H. (1993). High frequency (60–90 Hz) oscillations in primary visual cortex of awake monkey. *Neuroreport* 4:243–246.

Edelman GM. (1987). *Neural Darwinism: The theory of neuronal group selection.* Basic Books, New York, 371.

Edelman GM. (1989). *The remembered present.* Basic Books, New York.

Engel AK, König P, Gray CM, Singer W. (1990). Stimulus-dependent neuronal oscillations in cat visual cortex: Inter-columnar interaction as determined by cross-correlation analysis. *Eur J Neurosci* 2:588–606.

Engel AK, König P, Kreiter A, Schillen TB, Singer W. (1992). Temporal coding in the visual cortex: New vistas on integration in the nervous system. *Trends Neurosci* 15:218–226.

Engel AK, König P, Singer W. (1991). Direct physiological evidence for scene segmentation by temporal coding. *Proc Natl Acad Sci USA* 88:9136–9140.

Engel AK, König P, Kreiter AK, Singer W. (1991a). Interhemispheric synchronization of oscillatory neuronal responses in cat visual cortex. *Science* 252:1177−1179.

Engel AK, Kreiter AK, König P, Singer W. (1991b). Synchronization of oscillatory neuronal responses between striate and extrastriate visual cortical areas of the cat. *Proc Natl Acad Sci USA* 88:6048−6052.

Felleman DJ, van Essen DC. (1991). Distributed hierarchical processing in the primate cerebral cortex. *Cerebral Cortex* 1:1−47.

Freeman WJ, Skarda CA. (1985). Spatial EEG-patterns, non-linear dynamics and perception: The neo-Sherrington view. *Brain Res Rev* 10:147−175.

Gallant JL, Braun J, van Essen DC. (1993). Selectivity for polar, hyperbolic and Cartesian gratings in macaque visual cortex. *Science* 259:100−103.

Georgopoulos AP. (1990). Neural coding of the direction of reaching and a comparison with saccadic eye movements. In: *Cold Spring Harbor symposia on quantitative biology.* Cold Spring Harbor Laboratory Press, Cold Spring Harbor, NY, 849−859.

Gray CM, Engel AK, König P, Singer W. (1990). Stimulus-dependent neuronal oscillations in cat visual cortex: Receptive field properties and feature dependence. *Eur J Neurosci* 2:607−619.

Gray CM, Engel AK, König P, Singer W. (1992). Synchronization of oscillatory neuronal responses in cat striate cortex: Temporal properties. *Vis Neurosci* 8:337−347.

Gray CM, König P, Engel AK, Singer W. (1989). Oscillatory responses in cat visual cortex exhibit inter-columnar synchronization which reflects global stimulus properties. *Nature* 338: 334−337.

Gray CM, Singer W. (1987). Stimulus-dependent neuronal oscillations in the cat visual cortex area 17. *Neurosci Lett Suppl* 22:1301P.

Gray CM, Singer W. (1989). Stimulus-specific neuronal oscillations in orientation columns of cat visual cortex. *Proc Natl Acad Sci USA* 86:1698−1702.

Gray CM, Viana di Prisco G. (1993). Properties of stimulus-dependent rhythmic activity of visual cortical neurons in the alert cat. *Soc Neurosci Abstr* 19:359.8.

Gross CG, Rocha-Miranda CE, Bender DB. (1972). Visual properties of neurons in inferotemporal cortex of the macaque. *J Neurophysiol* 35:96−111.

Grossberg S. (1980). How does a brain build a cognitive code? *Psychol Rev* 87:1−51.

Hansel D, Sompolinsky H. (1992). Synchronization and computation in a chaotic neural network. *Physiol Rev* 68:718−721.

Hebb DO. (1949). *The organization of behavior.* John Wiley & Sons, New York.

Innocenti GM. (1981). Growth and reshaping of axons in the establishment of visual callosal connections. *Science* 212:824−827.

Innocenti GM, Frost DO. (1979). Effects of visual experience on the maturation of the efferent system to the corpus callosum. *Nature* 280:231−234.

Koch C, Schuster HG. (1992). A simple network showing burst synchronization without frequency locking. *Neural Comput* 4:211−223.

König P, Engel AK, Löwel S, Singer W. (1990). Squint affects occurrence and synchronization of oscillatory responses in cat visual cortex. *Soc Neurosci Abstr* 16:523.2.

König P, Engel AK, Löwel S, Singer W. (1993). Squint affects synchronization of oscillatory responses in cat visual cortex. *Eur J Neurosci* 5:501−508.

König P, Janosch B, Schillen TB. (1992). Stimulus-dependent assembly formation of oscillatory responses. III. Learning neural computation. *Computation and Neural Systems* 4:666–681.

König P, Schillen TB. (1990). Segregation of oscillatory responses by conflicting stimuli—Desynchronizing connections in neural oscillator layers. In: *Parallel processing in neural systems and computers.* R Eckmiller, G Hartman, G Hauske, eds. Elsevier, Amsterdam, 117–120.

König P, Schillen TB. (1991). Stimulus-dependent assembly formation of oscillatory responses. I. Synchronization. *Neural Computation* 3:155–166.

Kreiter AK, Engel AK, Singer W. (1992). Stimulus-dependent synchronization of oscillatory neuronal activity in the superior temporal sulcus of the macaque monkey. *Eur Neurosci Assoc Abstr* 15:1076.

Kreiter AK, Singer W. (1992). Oscillatory neuronal responses in the visual cortex of the awake macaque monkey. *Eur J Neurosci* 4:369–375.

Livingstone MS. (1991). Visually evoked oscillations in monkey striate cortex. *Soc Neurosci Abstr* 17:73.3.

Llinás RR. (1988). The intrinsic electrophysiological properties of mammalian neurons: Insights into central nervous system function. *Science* 242:1654–1664.

Llinás RR. (1990). Intrinsic electrical properties of nerve cells and their role in network oscillation. In: *Cold Spring Harbor symposia on quantitative biology.* Cold Spring Harbor Laboratory Press, Cold Spring Harbor, NY, 933–938.

Löwel S, Singer W. (1992). Selection of intrinsic horizontal connections in the visual cortex by correlated neuronal activity. *Science* 255:209–212.

Luhmann HJ, Martinez-Millan L, Singer W. (1986). Development of horizontal intrinsic connections in cat striate cortex. *Exp Brain Res* 63:443–448.

Luhmann HJ, Singer W, Martinez-Millan L. (1990). Horizontal interactions in cat striate cortex. I. Anatomical substrate and postnatal development. *Eur J Neurosci* 2:344–357.

Martin KAC. (1994). Brief history of the "feature detector." *Cerebral Cortex* 4:1–7.

Milner PM. (1974). A model for visual shape recognition. *Psychol Rev* 81:521–535.

Miyashita Y. (1988). Neuronal correlate of visual associative long-term memory in the primate temporal cortex. *Nature* 335:817–820.

Munk MHJ, Nowak LG, Chouvet G, Nelson JI, Bullier J. (1992). The structural basis of cortical synchronization. *Eur J Neurosci Suppl* 5:21.

Murthy VN, Fetz EE. (1992). Coherent 25- to 35-Hz oscillations in the densorimotor cortex of awake behaving monkeys. *Proc Natl Acad Sci USA* 89:5670–5674.

Mussa-Ivaldi FA, Giszter SF, Bizzi E. (1990). Motor-space coding in the central nervous system. In: *Cold Spring Harbor symposia on quantitative biology.* Vol LV. Cold Spring Harbor Laboratory Press, Cold Spring Harbor, NY, 827–835.

Nelson JI, Salin PA, Munk MHJ, Arzi M, Bullier J. (1992a). Spatial and temporal coherence in cortico-cortical connections: A cross-correlation study in areas 17 and 18 in the cat. *Vis Neurosci* 9:21–38.

Nelson JI, Nowak LG, Chouvet G, Munk MHJ, Bullier J. (1992b). Synchronization between cortical neurons depends on activity in remote areas. *Soc Neurosci Abstr* 18:11.

Neuenschwander S, Varela FJ. (1993). Visually-triggered neuronal oscillations in the pigeon: An autocorrelation study of tectal activity. *Eur J Neurosci* 5:870–881.

Newsome WT, Pare EB. (1988). A selective impairment of motion perception following lesions of the middle temporal visual area (MT). *J Neurosci* 8:2201–2211.

Palm G. (1982). *Neural assemblies*. Springer-Verlag, Heidelberg.

Palm G. (1990). Cell assemblies as a guideline for brain research. *Concepts Neurosci* 1:133–147.

Perrett DI, Mistlin AJ, Chitty AJ. (1987). Visual neurones responsive to faces. *Trends Neurosci* 10:358–364.

Poggio T. (1990). A theory of how the brain might work. In: *Cold Spring Harbor symposia on quantitative biology*. Cold Spring Harbor Laboratory Press, Cold Spring Harbor, NY, 899–910.

Price DJ, Blakemore C. (1985a). The postnatal development of the association projection from visual cortical area 17 to area 18 in the cat. *J Neurosci* 5:2443–2452.

Price DJ, Blakemore C. (1985b). Regressive events in the postnatal development of association projections in the visual cortex. *Nature* 316:721–724.

Raether A, Gray CM, Singer W. (1989). Intercolumnar interactions of oscillatory neuronal responses in the visual cortex of alert cats. *Eur Neurosci Abstr* 12:72.5.

Roelfsema PR, König P, Engel AK, Sireteanu R, Singer W. (1994). Reduced neuronal synchrony: A physiological correlate of strabismic amblyopia in cat visual cortex. *Eur J Neurosci* 6:1645–1655.

Sakai K, Miyashita Y. (1991). Neural organization for the long-term memory of paired associates (see comments). *Nature* 354:152–155.

Schillen TB, König P. (1990). Coherency detection by coupled oscillatory responses—Synchronizing connections in neural oscillator layers. In: *Parallel processing in neural systems and computers*. R Eckmiller, G Hartmann, G Hauske, eds. Elsevier, Amsterdam, 139–142.

Schillen TB, König P. (1991). Stimulus-dependent assembly formation of oscillatory responses. II. Desynchronization. *Neural Comput* 3:167–178.

Schillen TB, König P. (1993). Temporal structure can solve the binding problem for multiple feature domains. In: *Computation and neural systems*. FH Eeckman, JM Bower, eds. Kluver, Norwell, 509–513.

Schuster HG, Wagner P. (1990a). A model for neuronal oscillations in the visual cortex. 2. Phase description of the feature dependent synchronization. *Biol Cybernet* 64:83–85.

Schuster HG, Wagner P. (1990b). A model for neuronal oscillations in the visual cortex. 1. Mean-field theory and derivation of the phase equations. *Biol Cybernet* 64:77–82.

Schwarz C, Bolz J. (1991). Functional specificity of the long-range horizontal connections in cat visual cortex: A cross-correlation study. *J Neurosci* 11:2995–3007.

Singer W. (1985). Activity-dependent self-organization of the mammalian visual cortex. In: *Models of the visual cortex*. D Rose, VG Dobson, eds. John Wiley & Sons, New York, 123–136.

Singer W. (1990). The formation of cooperative cell assemblies in the visual cortex. *J Exp Biol* 153:177–197.

Singer W. (1993). Synchronization of cortical activity and its putative role in information processing and learning. *Annu Rev Physiol* 55:349–374.

Singer W. (1994). Putative functions of temporal correlations in neocortical processing. In: *Large-scale neuronal theories of the brain*. C Koch, J Davis, eds. MIT Press, Cambridge, 202–237.

Singer W, Gray CM. (1995). Visual feature integration and the temporal correlation hypothesis. *Annu Rev Neurosci* 18:555–586.

Softky WR, Koch C. (1993). The highly irregular firing of cortical cells is inconsistent with temporal integration of random EPSPs. *J Neurosci* 13:334–350.

Sparks DL, Lee C, Rohrer WH. (1990). Population coding of the direction, amplitude and velocity of saccadic eye movements by neurons in the superior colliculus. In: *Cold Spring Harbor symposia on quantitative biology*. Cold Spring Harbor Laboratory Press, Cold Spring Harbor, NY, 805–811.

Sporns O, Tononi G, Edelman GM. (1991). Modeling perceptual grouping and figure-ground segregation by means of active reentrant connections. *Proc Natl Acad Sci USA* 88:129–133.

Tanaka K, Saito H, Fukada Y, Moriya M. (1991). Coding visual images of objects in the inferotemporal cortex of the macaque monkey. *J Neurophysiol* 66:170–189.

Thomson AM, West DC. (1993). Fluctuations in pyramid-pyramid excitatory postsynaptic potentials modified by presynaptic firing pattern and postsynaptic membrane potential using paired intracellular recordings in rat neocortex. *Neuroscience* 54:329–346.

Ungerleider LG, Mishkin M. (1982). Two cortical visual systems. In: *Analysis of visual behavior*. DJ Ingle, ed. MIT Press, Cambridge, 564–586.

von der Malsburg C. (1985). Nervous structures with dynamical links. *Ber Bunsenges Phys Chem* 89:703–710.

von der Malsburg C, Schneider W. (1986). A neural cocktail-party processor. *Biol Cybernet* 54:29–40.

von Noorden GK. (1990). *Binocular vision and ocular motility. Theory and management of strabismus*. CV Mosby, St. Louis.

Wurtz RH, Yamasaki DS, Duffy DJ, Roy JP. (1990). Functional specialization for visual motion processing in primate cerebral cortex. In: *Cold Spring Harbor symposia on quantitative biology*. Cold Spring Harbor Laboratory Press, Cold Spring Harbor, NY, 717–727.

Young MP. (1992). Objective analysis of the topological organization of the primate cortical visual system. *Nature* 358:152–155.

Zeki SM. (1973). Colour coding in the rhesus monkey prestriate cortex. *Brain Res* 53:422–427.

Zeki S, Watson JDG, Lueck CJ, Friston KJ, Kennard C, Frackowiak RSJ. (1991). A direct demonstration of functional specialization in human visual cortex. *J Neurosci* 11:641–649.

7 The Binding Problem of Neural Networks

C. von der Malsburg

The life of a person or animal is a succession of scenes: arrangements of animate and inanimate objects and their trajectories in time. The survival depends in large part on an animal's skill in exploiting the regularities in scenes to its advantage. No two scenes in a lifetime are alike in detail, and their regularity never has the form of a literal repetition of sensory patterns. Therefore, relevant structure cannot be formulated directly on a primary sensory level. Rather, it is necessary for the brain to formulate abstract patterns, or schemata, that relate indirectly to concrete sensory or motor patterns by complex computations. The great flexibility of even the humblest animal in dealing with its environment shows that the relevant regularities are general. The brain's architecture must capture the style of these regularities, must provide a framework for making the right distinctions and identifications, and must provide for the organizational mechanisms to create appropriate representations and action patterns as well as for learning.

COGNITIVE ARCHITECTURE

The set of basic structures and mechanisms that enable the brain to extract and process the regularities behind sensory and motor patterns may be called its cognitive architecture. Four basic issues span much of the issue (figure 7.1):

1. The brain is a physical system. Its states can be interpreted as representations of scenes. What are the relevant physical quantities and how are they to be interpreted? *What is the data structure of short-term memory?*

2. Under the influence of sensory information and of stored information (i.e., the data referred to under issue 3), the contents of short-term memory are organized. *What is the mechanism of short-term memory organization?*

3. Activity in the brain leaves behind physical traces that can be interpreted as representing knowledge, experience, patterns, rules, procedures, skills, and memories. What is the nature of those traces and how are they to be interpreted? *What is the data structure of long-term memory?*

4. Depending on the state, that is, the contents of short-term memory, the contents of long-term memory are modified to store information that may be

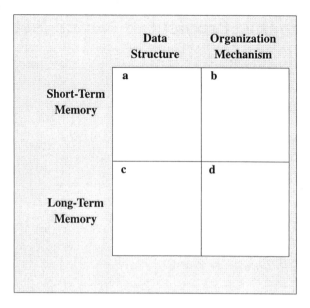

	Data Structure	Organization Mechanism
Short-Term Memory	a	b
Long-Term Memory	c	d

Figure 7.1 Cognitive architecture. Two fundamental questions must be addressed to understand the relationship between brain and mind: how are physical states of the brain to be interpreted as representing mental states (in computer terms, what is the brain's data structure)? and what are the mechanisms by which brain states are organized? Both questions require answers on at least two time scales: that of short-term memory, representing the present scene, and that of long-term memory, representing our knowledge and experience. These questions can be conveniently arranged as a 2 × 2 matrix. The letters a through d in the four boxes refer to the issues discussed in the text.

useful at a later time. What is the nature of this process? *What is the mechanism of long-term memory organization?*

These questions asked about the computer would not make much sense. Each particular program has its own data structures and algorithms that have to be interpreted one by one. There are general answers to those general questions, but they refer to a trivial level and are not very interesting. However, we have reason to believe that answers concerning the brain will be much more interesting.

The brain's architecture is the result of phylogenetic development. Phylogeny could not afford to pay attention to very specific situations, at least not for animals that are able to adapt flexibly to new environments. Consequently, it had to formulate structure on a principled, architectonic level, specifying application-oriented structures only on a general level and letting the individual adapt its nervous system to its particular needs.

CLASSIC NEURAL NETWORKS AS COGNITIVE ARCHITECTURE

The baseline from which to start is the conceptual framework currently discussed under the name of neural networks. This framework is the fruit of decades of conceptual development, and its main points are well grounded in neuroscience. Here is how it deals with the four architectural issues:

1. The physical variables relevant to short-term memory are neural firing rates. Each neuron can be interpreted as an elementary symbol. The meaning of that symbol can be investigated by recording from the neuron in the active brain and finding the precise context that activates it. Typical symbolic meanings of neurons are a blue light bar moving with orientation o over position x of retina, or muscle y twitched, and grandmother. The symbol is alive and part of the actual perceived scene when the corresponding neuron is active.

2. Activity states of neurons are organized with the help of excitatory and inhibitory signals exchanged between neurons and received from sensory cells. The system is regulated such as to converge toward stationary states. These last a fraction of a second, a time scale tuned to the typical progression of events in real life situations.

3. The physical quantities constituting long-term memory are synaptic strengths. If the customary definition is stretched a bit, one can interpret a synapse as an elementary rule: the excitatory connection from neuron j to neuron i, reading, when j is on, the probability that neuron i should also be on is to be raised by an amount related to the strength T_{ij} of the synapse between them.

4. Long-term memory is reorganized with the help of mechanisms of synaptic plasticity. One of these mechanisms is Hebbian plasticity, according to which the (excitatory) connection between two neurons is strengthened when both neurons are active at the same time. The effect of this rule is to increase the likelihood of those activity states that occurred in the past. Other plasticity rules implement supervised learning and use external information on the desirability of the present activity state, or partial information on which state should have been activated.

This set of concepts dominates current thinking about the function of the brain and has much to recommend it. It structures our thinking about the brain and raises relevant issues. It is in line with much of the experimental evidence about the nervous system and suggests further experiments in a fruitful way. Most important, it constitutes a vision that encourages us to formulate and attack the issue of cognitive architecture.

However, problems exist with classic neural networks as a candidate for cognitive architecture (Fodor and Pylyshyn, 1988). Although the formation of specific functional structures by learning from examples has been demonstrated, these demonstrations are restricted to small problem spaces and are successful only if the input patterns are encoded already in a way that is adapted to the problem at hand. (Neural networks have inherited these constraints from the more general framework of statistical estimation.) Thus, the technology of forming functional structures is still too much a matter of construction rather than self-organization. With their limitations, neural network structures can serve only as small subsystems in a larger system, the construction of which is a matter of construction and not of autonomous learning.

Another closely related difficulty with classic neural networks (again, taken as a technological tool) is their lack of power to generalize. Thus, the greater goals of representing natural scenes or of organizing the behavior of a complex organism seem totally out of reach of neural network-based theorizing. The dynamic link architecture is an attempt to solve a fundamental problem with neural networks, binding, and may thus help to overcome some of their difficulties.

THE BINDING ISSUE

Imagine a neural network for the inspection of a visual scene as mediated by its image on the retina. The network is internally structured such that it can derive four propositions and represent them by output neurons. Two of them recognize objects: a triangle (neuron *triangle*) or a square (*square*), both generalizing position. The other two indicate the position of objects: in the upper half (*top*) or the lower half (*bottom*) of the retina, both generalizing the nature of the object. When shown single objects, the network responds adequately, with (*triangle, top*) or (*square, bottom*). A problem arises, however, when two objects are presented simultaneously. If the output reads (*triangle, square, top, bottom*) it is not clear whether the triangle or the square is in the upper position. This is the binding problem: the neural data structure does not provide for a means of binding the proposition *top* to the proposition *triangle*, or *bottom* to *square*, if that is the correct description. In a typographical system this could easily be done by rearranging symbols and adding brackets: [(*triangle, top*), (*square, bottom*)]. The problem with neural networks is that they provide neither for the equivalent of brackets nor for the rearrangement of symbols.

This example, due to Frank Rosenblatt, uncovers a fundamental problem with the classic neural network version of a cognitive architecture. The problem refers to issue 1, the data structure of short-term memory. Neural networks have no flexible means of constructing higher-level symbols by combining more elementary symbols [(in the example, the composite symbol (*triangle, top*) out of *triangle* and *top*)]. The difficulty is that simply coactivating the elementary symbols leads to binding ambiguity when more than one composite symbol is to be expressed. This weakness can have grave consequences. If it were vital for the organism to trigger some action in response to a triangle, but only if it was in an upper position, the scene representation given above would not be sufficient. The reaction would have to be tied to the coincidence of activity in cells *triangle* and *top*, which, however, would also occur if the triangle was at the bottom and a square was at the top. The animal therefore would respond to a so-called false conjunction.

It pays to analyze the origin of the binding problem in this example. The correspondence between object type and position is explicit on the retinal level. Its loss on the way to the output of the circuit is due to the generalization that is taking place within the circuit: the triangle and square cells perform generalization regarding position, the top and bottom cells perform generalization regarding object type. (In this sense, the circuit has its own "what" and "where" systems, in analogy to the response types discussed for the temporal and parietal pathways of primate cortex.)

Remaining in the classic neural network framework for a moment, the hole can be stopped by introducing combination-coding cells, a neuron that stands for the combination (*triangle, top*), for instance. This solution, however, is problematic on more than one account. Our nervous system cannot afford to contain combination-coding neurons to represent all possible bindings, combinatorics quickly leading to astronomical numbers. It also cannot be imagined that evolution has found a way of endowing our brain at birth with a complement of neurons that is affordable in size and yet covers all combinations that can ever play a role in our life. What remains is the potential of creating new combination-coding neurons by learning whenever they turn out to be important.

This is the route taken by most current neural network models. The idea runs like this. A feature combination that is to be represented by a neuron first has to be recognized as being important, and for that it has to be picked from all the other combinations that are present in scenes actually occurring. This is achieved with the help of scene statistics: if the combination (*top, triangle*) occurs more often than other combinations, then it must be important and is to be represented by a new neuron.

This approach runs into a serious problem. The number of possible feature combinations in a scene is very large, growing exponentially with the number of features in a sensory modality. To estimate frequencies of occurrence with statistical significance, the necessary number of scenes would be much larger than the animal experiences in its lifetime. For this quantitative reason the statistical estimation approach to the learning of combination-coding neurons works only in very small model systems. This problem creates a barrier to the scaling up of model systems that has to be broken before the dream of systems that learn from a natural environment can become real and before we can claim to understand the brain.

This learning time problem for the formation of combination-coding cells is due to the absence of a flexible, dynamic binding mechanism in classic neural networks. Such a mechanism could obviate the need for most of these cells, and it could also be extremely useful for identifying important combinations to be represented by neurons should the need arise. In the example above, the relevant binding information is still explicitly present at the retinal level—it only has to be handed down and represented at the output despite the generalizations taking place in the circuit. If that could be achieved somehow, learning could be speeded up tremendously because the significant bindings would be made to stand out in individual scenes. In short, classic neural networks present us with the paradoxical situation that binding is possible with combination-coding cells, but combination-coding cells are not easily available without binding.

Conventional symbol systems all have flexible means of expressing binding and hierarchical composition of higher-level symbols from more elementary symbols. For that they mostly employ spatial or temporal arrangements of subsymbols. However, these solutions to the binding problem cannot serve as models here. The brain poses the added difficulty that its data structure should not only express binding but must also be structured by general mechanisms of self-organization.

Binding addresses very deep issues concerning the brain and the mind. When the physical structure of the brain is examined, one finds molecules, cells, and connections. When we examine the mind by introspection or with the help of psychophysics, we encounter entities that integrate large amounts of detail into global patterns, imaginations, and decisions. It is very likely that these two faces of the coin can be united in a view according to which the detail is identified with the activity of individual neurons, and the global aspects are identified with coherent dynamic patterns on the array of all neurons. Realization of this view requires a vision of how the collective dynamics of detail-encoding individual neurons can be integrated into higher-level mental entities. The classic neural network architecture tries instead to fold the mental entities back onto the single cell level.

DYNAMIC LINK ARCHITECTURE

The cells of the central nervous system are extremely complex. Classic neural networks are based on a simple caricature of this complexity. Perhaps this caricature leaves out essential traits, already known or yet to be discovered. They dynamic link architecture (von der Malsburg, 1981) modifies neural networks in five essential ways:

1. Rapid neural signal fluctuations are considered an essential aspect of neural activity, not as inessential noise.

2. Dynamic links are introduced as a new set of variables in the form of rapidly modifiable synaptic weights.

3. Synaptic and neural activity processes are interpreted in a novel way as data structures for short-term memory, issue 1 of the cognitive architecture.

4. A more complex organization mechanism for short-term memory is introduced (2).

5. The process of long-term synaptic plasticity (4) takes on a somewhat more refined form.

Several mathematical formulations have been attempted for these ideas (von der Malsburg, 1988; Bienenstock and von der Malsburg, 1987; Konen,

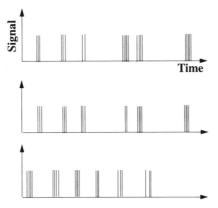

Figure 7.2 Temporal binding. Neurons can dynamically express grouping into composite structures by synchronizing their activity. In the figure, the middle neuron is bound to the upper neuron and not to the lower. If the middle neuron stood for a position and the other two for objects, the position would in the present situation apply to the upper object, not the lower. At another time, the lower neuron's object might be in that same position, expressed by spike synchrony between the middle and bottom neurons.

Maurer, and von der Malsburg, 1994), but it would be premature to give preference to any one of them. Consequently, I will define the architecture here as a conceptual rather than as a mathematical structure.

Correlations

Neurons in the brain are taken to be elementary symbols, just as in the neural network architecture. The signals of neurons are evaluated under two aspects. One of them is the rate or mean frequency of firing, and is interpreted as the intensity with which the elementary symbol is presently active. The other aspect refers to fine temporal signal structure, which is evaluated in terms of correlations among sets of cells. If, during a time interval, the signals on a set of neurons are found to be significantly correlated, the set is interpreted as being bound during that interval (figure 7.2).

There is experimental evidence for the existence in the nervous system of temporal signal structure of appropriate nature to encode binding by temporal synchrony. It has even been observed that signal correlations between cells occur and disappear when the features to which the cells respond are integrated into one figure or are part of distinct figures (e.g., two vertical light bars moving horizontally as one long bar or moving independent of each other). For a review of some of the experimental evidence see Engel et al (1992) and Singer, this volume.

The simplest case involves just two neurons and their binary correlation. It is to be borne in mind, however, that correlations involving just two neurons cannot play a central role in the brain. Binary correlations are too easily drowned in the noise of accidental coincidences. Therefore, more important correlations will be those involving larger numbers of neurons. A few events, each involving simultaneous spikes on fifty neurons, can easily be recognized as being statistically significant. A variety of possible temporal signal structures could serve as a basis for correlation patterns, with irregular spike trains at one end of a spectrum and regular oscillatory signals (Engel et al, 1992) at the other. In the latter case, correlations between two signals express themselves as agreement in frequency and phase.

This interpretation is to be applied on a hierarchy of several time scales. An event at a coarser time scale is composed of a rapid succession of short events. The hierarchy is limited below by the precision with which relative timing of signals can be reproduced in the central nervous system. This may be somewhat above one millisecond.

The hierarchy of time scales corresponds to a hierarchy of complexity. Speaking about the visual system, on the finest scale neurons may be bound together that are activated from the same point on a retina and that refer to different submodalities such as shape, color, motion, or stereo depth. On a higher level of the binding hierarchy, neurons in the same neighborhood within a figure are correlated with somewhat less temporal precision. Binding on this level has been invoked to bind together the elements of shape primitives, or geons (Hummel and Biederman, 1992). On a next higher level, cells anywhere within the same figure are synchronized. If, for instance, two colored letters are seen side by side, the spatial resolution of color-sensitive neurons may not be good enough to distinguish between the positions of the two letters. Without a binding mechanism, this would lead to ambiguity as to which color goes with which letter. The corresponding "conjunction error" is actually observed when subjects are not given sufficient viewing time (Treisman, 1985). With temporal binding, the signals of all those neurons that are activated from the same retinal point are correlated in time, disambiguating the situation. This would also solve the binding problem in the triangle-and-square example.

On a still higher level of the hierarchy, entire objects are bound to form the representation of a whole scene or sentence or complex argument. It has been argued that the phase relations of oscillatory firing can be employed to implement reasoning in neural networks (Shastri and Ajjanagadde, 1993).

The lower end of the binding hierarchy is not accessible to our own introspection. At scales larger than, say, 0.5 second our brain is able to observe and remember the actual sequence of events. They are experienced as the coherent chunks of structure that appear in flashes of attention. On coarser time scales, events are to a large part staged by eye and body movements and by real external events. On these scales the phenomenon of binding by simultaneous activity has always been taken for granted. It is also implicit in the usual way of driving neural networks as a sequence of stimulus-response events: simultaneously active input units are thereby bound as part of the same stimulus. The dynamic link architecture simply continues the hierarchy to finer temporal scales and thereby to events that are created by the network itself rather than the input.

On the scale of a few milliseconds, signal correlations may actually not be restricted to precise synchrony, and the spikes that form an event may be slightly scattered in time. It is necessary, however, that the actual sequence be reproducible and that the circuitry be in place to distinguish the temporal patterns.

One could go to the extreme and imagine a system that started out entirely composed of low-level sensory and motor neurons and that built up all higher-level entities as connectivity and correlation patterns. Objects would then be represented in a natural way as arrays of their initially given sensory elements, the same way that the tea mug in front of me is constituted entirely by its atoms and does not contain any high-level units to correspond to its subpatterns, its parts, or its entirety. This view in its extreme form is certainly not realized in the brain. The bandwidth of neural signals in our nervous system is too low to permit the build-up of very deep correlation hierarchies. For this reason, intermediate levels in symbol hierarchies have to be represented to a large extent by new units that are to be recruited along the way, temporal correlations stepping in to represent those combinations that are not (yet) represented by cells.

It has been claimed repeatedly that the observation of combination-coding neurons in a brain is evidence for a solution to the binding problem without temporal coding. This argument misses the point. The binding problem arises only when the combination-coding neurons in the brain cannot disambiguate the situation.

Neurophysiologists have traditionally considered random aspects of cellular responses to test stimuli as a nuisance, and they averaged them out by adding responses over many identical stimulations. Also, modeling studies of neural activity in the brain tended to ignore fine temporal signal structure (and, *a fortiori*, their correlations) with the following argument. The number of synapses converging onto a neuron is very large. Under the assumption that the signals carried by them are statistically independent, their temporal structure will average out, resulting in a temporally smooth summed input signal to the neuron. Correspondingly, the output of the neuron will vary smoothly, and this would be true for all neurons. Any temporal signal structure would thus quickly disappear. According to this argument it seems to be a self-consistent view to expect neural signals to vary smoothly in time. However, this view does not stand up to fact. As any recording shows, cortical neural signals do have a very pronounced stochastic structure, and nervous tissue is evidently designed to create and preserve it. The assumption of statistical independence of signals therefore must be faulty, and strong signal correlations must be present in the brain.

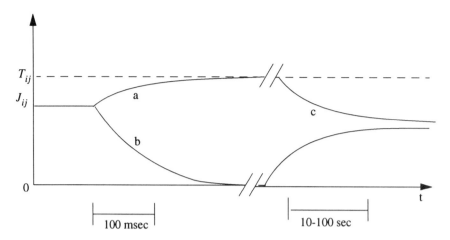

Figure 7.3 Dynamic links. The synaptic weight J_{ij} between neurons j and i can vary on a fast time scale. (a) If the neurons i and j fire synchronously, the dynamic weight J_{ij} is rapidly increased from a resting value to the maximum value set by the permanent synaptic strength. (b) If both neurons are active but fire asynchronously, the synaptic weight is rapidly decreased to zero. This dynamic switching can take place within small fractions of a second. (c) When there is no more activity in one or both of the neurons, the dynamic weight slowly falls back to the resting value, with the time constant of short-term memory.

Rapid Synaptic Modification

The temporal bandwidth of neural signals is severely limited, and it is not possible within short periods of time to express complicated multilevel binding structures in terms of signal correlations. If it is necessary to do so, longer periods of time have to be invested to process the many disambiguations sequentially. If it has been observed that two neurons are actually not bound in the present scene, that observation can conveniently be stored in short-term memory by temporarily switching off any connections that may exist between them and to common target cells.

This observation leads to the hypothesis of rapid synaptic modification (figure 7.3). Synapses are characterized by two quantities, T and J, where T is the conventional permanent synaptic weight, which may be slowly modified by mechanisms of plasticity (see below). The momentarily effective strength of a synapse is J. This quantity can vary on a rapid time scale between zero and a maximum determined by T. When J is zero, the synapse does not transmit signals. At rest, J takes on an intermediate value between zero and its maximum. When the two connected cells become active in a correlated fashion, J is regulated upward, to its maximum if the correlation is sufficiently strong. When the two cells are both active but in an uncorrelated fashion, J is regulated downward, to zero in the extreme case. Forceful activity events can modify synapses in a small fraction of a second, perhaps a few milliseconds. When there is no further activity in the two cells connected by a synapse,

J slowly returns to its resting value, with the time constant of short-term memory.

Although experimental evidence exists for rapid synaptic modification (Zucker, 1989), the precise mode of control postulated in dynamic link architecture remains to be demonstrated in experiments. The effective synaptic weights of whole fields of synapses can be reset to their resting values by central command signals.

The two central hypotheses of dynamic link architecture, binding by signal correlations and short-term synaptic modification, amount to a massive increase in the number of dynamic variables, to a much richer structure and to a profound reinterpretation of neural dynamics as part of the cognitive architecture. Signal correlations are the glue by which high-level symbols can be formed from lower-level ones to suit the needs of individual scenes and the constellation of objects and patterns in them. If, as done above, synaptic connections are interpreted as elementary rules, then by dynamically switching synapses, the system can decide which of the rules are actually applicable in a given situation, switching off those that are not consistent with the situation and with each other. To manage all this rich structure, more sophisticated mechanisms of organization have to be considered (to deal with issues 2 and 4 of the cognitive architecture).

State Organization

In the classic neural network architecture, the only variables on the psychological time scale are neural signals. These are organized by the exchange of excitation and inhibition, regulated to create attractor states that are quasistable over fractions of a second. In the dynamic link architecture, signal dynamics are modified to create signals that fluctuate on several time scales. This raises a number of issues, especially questions of how functionally appropriate correlations are created and how correlations are used by the brain in a meaningful way.

Some of the signal correlations are already implicit in the sensory signals and express the causal relations in the external world. More correlations are created, however, in the neural circuits themselves: the existence of excitatory connections between two neurons raises the probability for one of them to fire in correlation with the other. The essence of this is that the signal correlations come to express the patterns of connections in the circuit, that is, the underlying causal structure of the nervous system itself, just as afferent signal correlations express the causal structure in the external world. The "fast enabling links" (Hummel and Biederman, 1992), for instance, are connections within the visual system that encode those relations of features that are indicative of binding within a geon.

How are signal correlations evaluated in the brain? According to what we know about the structure of the nervous system, signal correlations play a very important role in neural dynamics. The excitatory effect of afferent spikes can pile up and fire a cell only if they coincide with a precision comparable to the membrane time constant. Thus, neurons are coincidence detectors and are superbly sensitive to signal correlations. Now, if coincidence-detecting neurons were the only means of evaluating correlation, one would not be much better off than classic neural networks, and the brain would still need a combination coding cell for each binding pattern. Fortunately, that is not so. A correlation pattern can selectively activate receiving circuits of appropriate structure. In the simplest case this is possible if the circuit that receives the pattern is isomorphic to the circuit that created it, in the sense that subsets of coupled cells in one circuit are connected to subsets of coupled cells in the other. This principle was extensively exploited for the invariant recognition of visual patterns (Konen, Maurer, and von der Malsburg, 1994).

Whereas in classic neural networks neurons do not pay attention to fine signal structure, in the dynamic link architecture the incoming signals have to be correlated in time. This leads to a much more differentiated dynamics, and a given set of neurons can now support a large number of activity patterns that differ only in their fine temporal structure. This principle is also implicit in Abeles' (1991) synfire chains. These are chains of sets ("pools") of neurons, each one connected nearly all-to-all with the next pool. A synfire chain can be traversed by an activity process in which all the cells in a pool fire simultaneously and thus succeed in firing the cells in the next pool simultaneously. Each neuron can participate in many synfire chains and even several times in the same chain. Synfire chains are proposed as the basic building blocks of a compositional cognitive system (Bienenstock, 1994).

Signal correlations are also evaluated by synapses, by modifying their dynamic weight. The interaction between signal correlations and synaptic dynamics has the form of a positive feedback loop. A strong synapse helps to create a correlation in the two cells connected, and the correlation strengthens that synapse. This feedback loop is the basis for a system of rapid network self-organization. A given network creates a signal process that is characterized by correlations shaped by the connectivity structure in the network. These signal correlations act back on the network and modify its structure by rapid synaptic modification. This leads to a run-away situation that comes to a halt when a network is reached in which the signal structure and the connectivity structure are consistent with each other. These specific structures are called connectivity patterns. Presumably (von der Malsburg, 1981), connectivity patterns are sparse, that is, have relatively few active connections per node; and the active connections are maximally cooperative, that is, for each pair of neurons in the pattern, different direct and indirect connections help each other to link those neurons.

Scene Representation

The reality we perceive is first and foremost the reality of the states of our mind. It is for us an issue of central importance to find out how the physical states of our brain can come to represent that rich world. This is exactly the architectural issue 1: how can activity states or processes in our brain act as physical symbols to represent the mental objects that we see and experience? I will argue that the dynamic link architecture is a major step toward solving that issue due to its property of compositionality (see Bienenstock and Geman, this volume), which distinguishes it from classic neural network theory.

Our inner experience can be described as a continuous sequence of scenes. Voluminous tomes have been written to describe scenes from an introspective point of view (an extreme example is the work of E. Husserl). Briefly, a scene is a short, real or imagined sequence of events that are simultaneously and explicitly accessible, and usually contain a description of ourselves as part of the scene. Scenes can be decomposed into separate objects, their trajectories, and their relationships. Mental scene descriptions are constructed (issue 2) from sensory data and from stored knowledge (issue 3). We must at the very least understand how scenes can be composed from simpler entities and descriptors, how they can be decomposed, and how new patterns can be referred back to known, old patterns.

Presumably, our mental system is composed of relatively fixed elementary patterns that can be dynamically linked to form more complex descriptors. To take an example, my tea mug is described in terms of shape aspects (elongated, upright form, cylindrical body, handle), shape elements (curvature of surface, flared rim, bend of the handle), surface markings (flower decor, shiny reflections), its material, its position relative to me and the table as reference surface, its function as a container of liquid and source of vapor, its role in the potential action of grasping and drinking, and, if I care to elicit them, many more aspects.

The dynamic link architecture affords the infrastructure required for scene representation. Complex (sensory) patterns can be segmented in a meaningful way into subpatterns that correspond to separate objects or functional components of the scene. This is done by temporally correlating signals within a segment and decorrelating signals between elements in different segments. During the process of segmentation, experience on likely groupings of elements, stored in the form of permanent connections, can be brought to bear (Hummel and Biederman, 1992). Segmentation in the context of the dynamic link architecture has been described by a number of authors (von der Malsburg and Buhmann, 1992).

Whereas the formation of segments is possible with the help of very simple signal patterns in the form of blocks uniting all elements within a segment in an undifferentiated correlation, the description of the internal structure of an object requires detailed correlation patterns that amount to intricate arrays of pointers that attach descriptors to their referents. This attachment is achieved with the help of binary signal correlations between descriptors and referents.

A paradigm of object representation and the attachment of descriptors was studied in the context of visual object recognition (von der Malsburg, 1988;

Konen, Maurer, and von der Malsburg, 1994). The two-dimensional visual aspect of an object is constructed by linking neural elements in the form of a two-dimensional array. Individual elements represent wavelet components (roughly, oriented edges on various levels of resolution) of the gray-level distribution on the retina. Such elements are found as receptive fields of single neurons in primary visual cortex. A collection of such visual aspects is stored as models in some part of the brain ("model domain") as networks of permanent connections. An element can take part in many such networks. In a concrete situation all the links belonging to one aspect are dynamically activated and all others are deactivated. This is possible without creating confusion (Bienenstock and von der Malsburg, 1987). When a new aspect of an object appears in the primary visual cortex (and is naturally represented as a two-dimensionally linked array of wavelet elements), it can be recognized with the help of a dynamic process in which an appropriate aspect model is activated and its parts are linked to the new visual aspect, attaching corresponding elements to each other (Konen, Maurer, and von der Malsburg, 1994). An appropriate model is one that is loosely isomorphic to the new aspect in containing the same element types in the same two-dimensional arrangement. Object recognition that is invariant to position, size, and orientation and that is robust with respect to lighting, background, partial occlusion, deformation, and rotation in depth, and that can reliably distinguish between hundreds of objects (human faces) has been demonstrated in this style. Part of this work is described and reviewed by Lades et al (1993). In this way, a scene is interpreted and built up by the activation and interlinking of structural descriptions, attaching them to each other as suggested by structural relations of partial isomorphy. As this interlinking is represented with the help of temporal signal structure and correlations, these physical symbols for mental entities are processes rather than static structures.

It is often necessary for the brain to process temporally structured input patterns, especially in the auditory modality. These temporal patterns are in danger of colliding with the temporal processing required by the dynamic link architecture. This conflict is resolved with the help of peripheral circuits that detect temporal patterns in the sensory input and represent them with the help of slowly varying signals on specialized neurons, thus freeing the temporal domain on central levels from the interference by external patterns.

Learning

The amount of genetic information to structure the brain is limited, and especially for humans, genes cannot address the living environment of the individual in a very specific way. The brain therefore has to build up autonomously or absorb much of the required structure. The vision motivating the field of neural computing is to understand and imitate this ability. To date this goal is distant, and all neural model systems still rely heavily on very specific initial connectivity structure. The dynamic link architecture may bring the vision within reach, by solving a fundamental difficulty of neural learning.

So far I have discussed the organization (issue 2) of the active state of the system (issue 1), making use of the constraints implicit in the permanent connectivity parameters T, which constitute the long-term memory (issue 3). An important modifaction is also introduced with respect to modification of the long-term memory (issue 4). The mechanisms for modifying synaptic connections in classic neural networks architecture, Hebbian plasticity, reinforcement learning, and supervised learning, are all plagued by the difficulty that the significant and meaningful connections that have to be modified are easily drowned among the many meaningless connections that correspond to accidental patterns active in a given state. As discussed above, this leads to bad scaling behavior of neural networks. Efficient learning requires mechanisms to single out those connections in a situation that are essential and significant, and distinguish them from those arising from accidental coexistence.

The dynamic link architecture offers a potent mechanism to do that. If, in a given state, two cells are active, and between them is neither a direct nor a short indirect connection, then the activity on these cells will indicate this fact by not being correlated. A plasticity mechanism that is sensitive to the fine signal correlations, called refined plasticity, easily picks up this fact and keeps them apart, neither creating a direct connection between them nor helping to create a hidden unit to represent a pattern that includes them. The power of this effect was demonstrated by Konen and von der Malsburg (1993).

Expressed in more general terms, the activity and connectivity patterns created in the dynamic link architecture constitute differentiated structure in a given state that goes way beyond merely expressing which cells are active in the state (as does the classic neural network architecture), making evident the way in which these cells are connected according to the knowledge already implicit in the network. This information is to a large extent ignored in the classic architecture. In the dynamic link architecture it is used to keep those connections from growing for which there is not at least indirect evidence of functional significance in the form of indirect connections linking the same end points.

Another way of seeing how the dynamic link architecture improves the learning situation is this. A given state of the neural network is broken down into a quick succession of microstates, each of which activates only a small subset of the cells in the state. Plasticity is restricted to act only within microstates. In this way the plasticity mechanism is saved from the need to scale to states with many active cells. The burden falls on the dynamic mechanism to break the network's state into microstates in a significant way.

REFERENCES

Abeles M. (1991). *Corticonics: Neuronal circuits of the cerebral cortex*. Cambridge University Press, Cambridge.

Bienenstock E. (1994). *A model of neocortex*. Technical report. Division of Applied Mathematics, Brown University, Providence, RI.

Bienenstock E, von der Malsburg C. (1987). A neural network for invariant pattern recognition. *Europhys Lett* 4:121–126.

Engel AK, König P, Kreiter AK, Schillen TB, Singer W. (1992). Temporal coding in the visual cortex: New vistas on integration in the nervous system. *Trends Neurosci* 15:218–226.

Fodor J, Pylyshyn ZW. (1988). Connectionism and cognitive archtecture: A critical analysis. *Cognition* 28:3–71.

Hummel JE, Biederman I. (1992). Dynamic binding in a neural network for shape recognition. *Psychol Rev* 99:480–517.

Konen W, Maurer T, von der Malsburg C. (1994). A fast dynamic link matching algorithm for invariant pattern recognition. *Neural Networks* 7:1019–1030.

Konen W, von der Malsburg C. (1993). Learning to generalize from single examples in the dynamic link architecture. *Neural Computation* 5:719–735.

Lades M, Vorbrüggen JC, Buhmann J, Lange J, von der Malsburg C, Würtz RP, Konen W. (1993). Distortion invariant object recognition in the dynamic link architecture. *IEEE Trans Comput* 42:300–311.

Shastri L, Ajjanagadde V. (1993). From simple associations to systematic reasoning: A connectionist representation of rules, variables and dynamic bindings. *Behav Brain Sci* 16:417–494.

Treisman A. (1985). Preattentive processing in vision. *Comput Vision Graphics Image Processing* 31:156–177.

von der Malsburg C. (1981). *The correlation theory of brain function*. Internal report 81-2. Max-Planck-Institut für Biophysikalische Chemie, Göttingen, Germany. Reprinted (1994). In: *Models of neural networks*. K Schulten, HJ van Hemmen, eds. Springer-Verlag, Berlin.

von der Malsburg C. (1988). Pattern recognition by labeled graph matching. *Neural Networks* 1:141–148.

von der Malsburg C, Buhmann J. (1992). Sensory segmentation with coupled neural oscillators. *Biol Cybernet* 67:233–242.

Zucker RS. (1989). Short-term synaptic plasticity. *Annu Rev Neurosci* 12:13–31.

8 Recognition and Representation of Visual Objects in Primates: Psychophysics and Physiology

N. K. Logothetis and D. L. Sheinberg

THE PROBLEM OF RECOGNITION

The ability to recognize objects is a remarkable accomplishment of biological systems. Familiar objects can be readily recognized based on their shape, color, or texture. Even when partially occluded, an object's identity can be deduced based on contextual information. Furthermore, visually similar members of object classes can become easily disciminable by repeated exposure, as when a geologist learns to recognize rock formations or an ornithologist learns to discriminate species of birds.

Reliable artificial recognition systems have proved to be surprisingly difficult to achieve. A major obstacle in this endeavor is that we know very little about what actually constitutes an object. Components of objects are not clearly labeled as belonging to one object or another. Indeed, there is nothing special about individual objects in the way they are presented to the visual system. The shape of an object, or its characteristic regions, are almost never visually primitive constructions, determined by a predictable combination of primary cues. Any given two-dimensional image can be parsed into an arbitrary set of objects, each of which can be decomposed recursively into smaller objects. Moreover, what we consider to be an object depends on the visual input, yet it is also determined by the task at hand.

The neural representation of objects is a mystery even when considering simple geometrical objects, such as a cube, a cone, or a cylinder, seen in isolation. A key question concerning the perception of three-dimensional objects is the spatial reference frame used by the brain to represent them. The rapidity of the recognition process could be explained by the visual system's ability to transform stored models of three-dimensional familiar objects quickly, or by its ability to specify the relationship among viewpoint-invariant features or volumetric primitives that can be used to accomplish a structural description of an image. Alternatively, viewpoint-invariant recognition could be realized by a system endowed with the ability to perform an interpolation between a set of stored two-dimensional templates created for each experienced viewpoint.

LEVELS OF RECOGNITION

In attempting to determine a possible reference system for object representation it is useful to consider first the different taxonomic levels of abstraction at which object recognition can occur. Objects are usually recognized first at the basic level (Rosch et al, 1976). This level refers to the initial classification of individual visual entities, such as a piano or a tree. When detailed distinctions among objects of the same category are required, for instance, when discriminating different kinds of trees, recognition is said to occur at the subordinate level. Subordinate categories share a great number of object attributes with other subordinate categories, and have to a large extent similar shape (Rosch et al, 1976; Rosch, 1975; Jolicouer, Gluck, and Kosslyn, 1984).

Atypical exemplars of basic-level categories can be occasionally classified faster at the subordinate than at the basic level (Jolicouer, Gluck, and Kosslyn, 1984). For example, the image of a penguin is more likely to be initially identified as penguin before it is determined to be a bird. Since the notion of basic level was defined for entire categories based on the degree of inclusiveness of perceptual and functional attributes (Rosch et al, 1976), the term entry point level was coined (Jolicouer et al, 1984) to denote the abstraction level at which stored information can be accessed fastest, regardless of the taxonomic level. Of interest, clinical studies indicate that recognition at different categorization levels may involve different neural circuitry (Damasio, 1990; Tranel, Damasio, and Damasio, 1988).

SPATIAL REFERENCE FRAMES FOR OBJECT RECOGNITION

To explain how visual objects may be represented, two basic reference frames for recognition have been proposed. Object-centered representations imply the existence of a complete three-dimensional description of an object (Ullman, 1989), or of a structural description of the image specifying the relationships among viewpoint-invariant volumetric primitives (Marr, 1982; Biederman, 1987). A prediction of object-centered representations is that recognition performance (in terms of error rate) is independent of viewpoint, provided that the information necessary to access the correct model is present in the image; in other words, as long as the image is not the result of an accidental alignment of the eye and the object, where information about an object's structure is entirely lost (Biederman, 1987). For example, imagine an ice cream cone seen from below. If the axis of gaze is aligned with the axis of the cone (a rare event indeed), the ice cream cone's profile will simply be a circle.

Viewer-centered representations model three-dimensional objects as a set of two-dimensional views, or templates, and recognition consists of matching image features against the views in this set. Viewpoint-invariance in systems based on viewer-centered representations may therefore rely on object familiarity, and performance may be progressively worse for views that are far from those experienced previously.

N. K. Logothetis and D. L. Sheinberg

When tested against human behavior, verification of the predicted performance of object-centered representations appears to depend on the object classification level. Whereas humans can recognize familiar objects or objects of the entry point level in a viewpoint-independent fashion (Biederman, 1987), they fail to do so at the subordinate level, at which fine, shape-based discriminations are required for identifying an individual entity (Rock and DiVita, 1987; Rock, DiVita, and Barbeito, 1981; Tarr and Pinker, 1989, 1990; Bülthoff and Edelman, 1992; Edelman and Bülthoff, 1992; Logothetis et al, 1994).

Viewer-centered representations, on the other hand, can explain human recognition performance at any taxonomic level, but they often are considered implausible because of the amount of memory required to store all views that a three-dimensional object can generate when viewed from different distances and orientations. Yet, recent theoretical work indicated that a viewer-centered representation system may accomplish viewpoint invariance relying on a small number of two-dimensional views. For example, under conditions of orthographic projection, all possible views of an object can be expressed simply as the linear combination of as few as three distinct two-dimensional views, given that the same features remain visible in all three views (Ullman and Basri, 1991). The model of linear combinations of views, however, relies only on geometrical features, and fails to predict human behavior for recognizing objects at the subordinate levels (Edelman and Bulthoff, 1992; Logothetis et al, 1994).

Alternatively, generalization could be accomplished by nonlinear interpolation among stored orthographic or perspective views that can be determined on the basic of geometric features or material properties of the object. Indeed, a simple network can achieve viewpoint invariance by interpolating among a small number of stored views (Poggio and Edelman, 1990). Computationally, such a network uses a small set of sparse data corresponding to an object's training views to synthesize an approximation to a multivariate function representing the object. The approximation technique, which is known by the name of generalized radial basis functions (GRBFs), is mathematically equivalent to a multilayer network (Poggio and Girosi, 1990). A special case of such a network is that of the radial basis functions (RBFs), which can be conceived of as hidden-layer units, the activity of which is a radial function of the disparity between a novel view and a template stored in the unit's memory. Such an interpolation-based network makes psychophysical predictions (Poggio, 1990) that are supported by human psychophysical work (Rock and DiVita, 1987; Rock, DiVita, and Barbeito, 1981), and can be tested directly against the recognition performance of monkeys.

OBJECT RECOGNITION IN PRIMATES: PSYCHOPHYSICAL DATA

Recently, we began to explore the nature of object representation in the primate. To this end, we set out first to examine how nonhuman primates achieve viewpoint invariance for previously unfamiliar objects. Monkeys can clearly recognize faces and facial expressions, as well as a variety of other objects in their natural environment. Moreover, they do so despite differences in the retinal projections of objects seen at different orientations, sizes, and positions. Is their performance in acquiring viewpoint invariance, however, consistent with a viewer-centered representation of objects? If so, is view invariance achieved by interpolating among a small number of views learned and stored through frequent exposure?

In the behavioral experiments, monkeys were trained to recognize novel objects from a given viewpoint and subsequently were tested for their ability to generalize recognition for rotated views of the objects. The stimuli, examples of which are shown in figure 8.1, were similar to those used by Edelman and Bülthoff (1992) in human psychophysical experiments or a variety of other two- or three-dimensional patterns, including commonplace objects, scenes, and body parts.

One view was arbitrarily designated as the zero view for each object. The viewpoint coordinates of the observer with respect to the object were defined as the longitude and the latitude of the eye on an imaginary sphere centered on the object (figure 8.2). We used a right-handed coordinate system for the object transformations.

The monkeys were trained to recognize objects regardless of position or orientation. They were first allowed to inspect an object, the target, presented from a given viewpoint, and subsequently were tested for recognizing views of the object from different viewpoints. Objects were presented sequentially, with the target views dispersed among a large number of other objects, the distractors. Two levers were attached to the front panel of the monkey's chair, and reinforcement was contingent on pressing the right lever each time the target was presented. Pressing the left lever was required on presentation of a distractor. Correct responses were rewarded with fruit juice.

Initially, the animals were trained to recognize the target's zero view among a large set of distractors, and subsequently were trained to recognize additional target views resulting from progressively larger rotations around one axis. After a monkey learned to recognize a given object from any viewpoint in the range of ± 90 degrees, the procedure was repeated with a new object.

Figure 8.3 illustrates the sequence of events in a single observation period of a typical experiment. Successful fixation was followed by the learning phase in which the target was inspected from one or two viewpoints, called the training views. To provide the monkey with three-dimensional structure information, the target was presented as a motion sequence of 10 adjacent, Gouraud-shaded views, 2 degrees apart, centered around the zero view. The learning phase was followed by a short fixation period, after which the testing phase started. Each testing phase consisted of up to 10 trials. The beginning of a trial was indicated by a low-pitched tone, immediately followed by the presentation of the test stimulus—a shaded, static view of either the target or a distractor.

N. K. Logothetis and D. L. Sheinberg

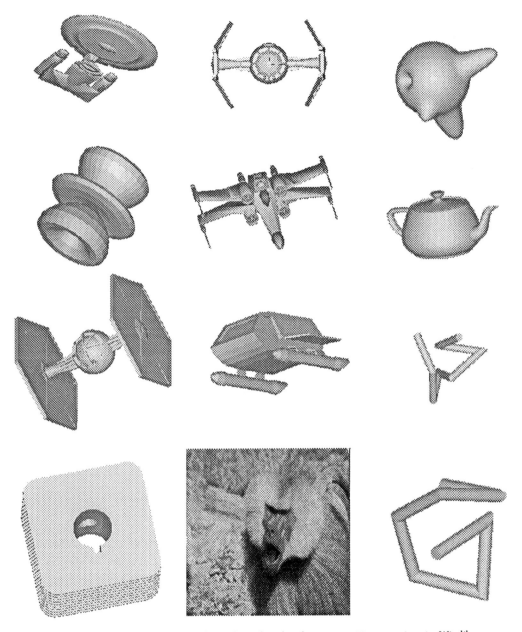

Figure 8.1 Examples of stimuli used in the object recognition experiments. Wirelike, amoeboid, and common-type objects were created mathematically and rendered by a computer. Pictures of various natural objects such as hands and faces were digitized using a camera and frame grabber.

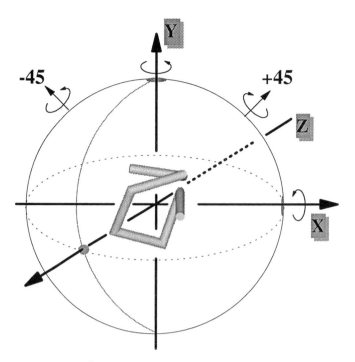

Figure 8.2 The viewing sphere. Images depicting the various views of the objects tested were achieved by mathematically calculating the appearance of the object after undergoing an arbitrary rotation. Recognition was tested for views generated by rotations around the vertical (y), horizontal (x), and the two oblique (± 45-degree) axes lying in the fronto-parallal plane. Thus, rotations around the x, y, and z axes resulted in vertical, horizontal, and diagonal rotations in the plane, respectively. Any arbitrary view of the object could be achieved by the appropriate combination of rotations around the three axes.

View-Specific Recognition Performance

The perception of three-dimensional novel objects was found to be a function of the object's retinal projection at the time of the recognition encounter. Recognition became increasingly difficult for the monkeys as the stimulus was rotated away from its familiar view. The generalization field for novel wire-like and spheroidal objects extended to about ± 40 degrees around an experienced viewpoint. However, when the animals were trained with as few as three views of the object, spaced 120 degrees apart, they could often interpolate recognition for all views resulting from rotations around the same axis.

Figure 8.4 shows the average performance of two monkeys tested for the recognition of two different stimuli, one wire and one spheroidal amoebalike object. For each of the target shapes, distractors of the same object class were generated using identical mathematical constraints (i.e., the same moment of inertia, variability in segment orientation, and identical segment length for the wires, and the same number of protrusions and range of protrusion sizes

N. K. Logothetis and D. L. Sheinberg

Recognition Task

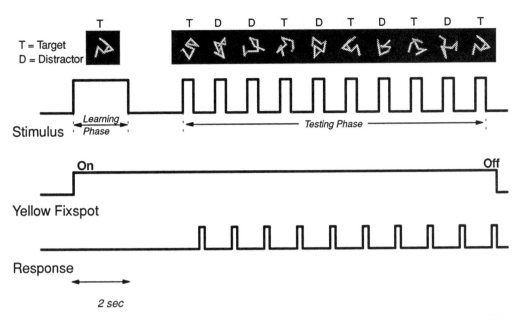

Figure 8.3 The recognition task. An observation period consisted of a learning phase, within which the target object was presented oscillating ± 10 degrees around a fixed axis, and a set of test trials during which the subjects were presented with up to 10 single, static views of either the target or the distractors. Training and testing, as well as individual test trials, were separated by brief blank periods. Subjects were required to maintain fixation throughout the entire observation period, as indicated by the persistence of the fixspot. They responded by pressing one of two levers, right for the target and left for the distractors. Feedback was not given under testing conditions.

for the spheroids). There was, therefore, a high degree of visual similarity between the targets and distractors.

For both test stimuli, numerous target views generated from rotations around the vertical axis, and at least 60 distractor objects, were used during testing. Figures 8.4a and 8.4c show the average experimental hit rate for the wire object and the amoeba object, respectively, plotted as a function of rotation angle. The monkeys could correctly identify the views of the target around the trained, zero view, but their performance dropped significantly for disparities larger than about ± 45 degrees. Performance below chance level is probably the result of the large number of distractors used within a session, which limited learning of specific distractors. Therefore an object that was not clearly perceived as a target view was readily classified as distractor. Figures 8.4b and 8.4d show the false alarm rates for the two sets of stimuli.

The view-specific performance also was also observed for object rotations around axes other than the vertical (figure 8.5). For both the wires (figure 8.5a) and the amoebas (figure 8.5b), the monkeys' ability to identify the target

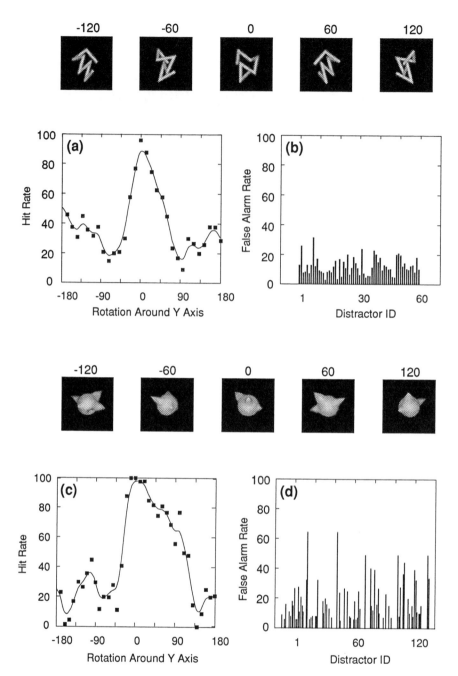

Figure 8.4 Recognition performance as a function of rotation in depth for two target objects. The abscissa of (a) and (c) show the rotation angle and the ordinate the hit rate. The small rectangles represent recognition performance for 12-degree increments around the horizontal meridian. When the object is rotated more than about 30 to 40 degrees away from the preferred view performance falls below 50%. Plots (b) and (d) show false alarm rates for the 60 different distractor objects used during testing.

N. K. Logothetis and D. L. Sheinberg

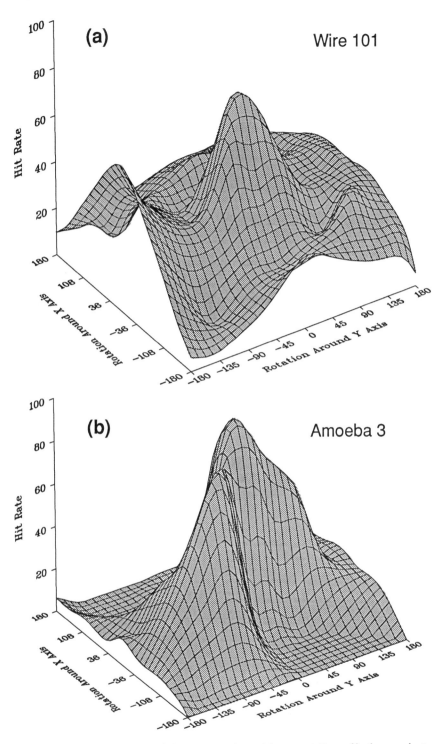

Figure 8.5 Performance around the viewing sphere. Arbitrary rotations of both a novel wire object (**a**) and an amoebalike object (**b**) away from the zero view impaired recognition of the target.

object correctly was severely impaired when the target was rotated more than approximately 45 degrees from the zero view.

Interpolating Between Familiar Views

The ability of the monkeys to generalize recognition to novel views was also examined after training the animals with two successively presented views of the target 75, 120, and 160 degrees apart. Each monkey was initially trained to identify 2 views of an object among 60 distractor objects of the same class. Training was considered complete when the monkey's hit rate for the two target views was consistently above 95% and the false alarm rate remained below 10%. Interpolation was complete (>95%) for training views 75 degrees apart. Error rate increased for views 120 degrees apart where the monkey could no longer interpolate recognition.

The psychophysical performance of the animals seems to be consistent with the idea that view-based approximation modules synthesized during training may indeed be one of several algorithms the primate visual system uses for object recognition. Training the monkey with one single view results in a bell-shaped generalization field for both the wire and the amoeba objects. Moreover, the ability of the monkey to interpolate between two familiar views depends on their distance from each other, a finding difficult to reconcile with a recognition system based on linear interpolation (Ullman and Basri, 1991), but directly predicted by a system relying on nonlinear approximation (Poggio and Girosi, 1990). Sets of neurons that are tuned broadly to individual object views may represent the neural substrate of such approximation modules.

Pseudomirror-Symmetry Effects

For some objects the monkeys' behavioral pattern deviated from the typical view-dependent performance, in that they could also recognize the target from views resulting from approximately 180-degree rotations of the training view (figure 8.6; see also figure 8.5a). As can be seen, performance drops for views farther than 30 degrees but it resumes as the unfamiliar views of the target approach the 180-degree view of the target. This behavior was specific to those wirelike objects for which the zero- and 180-degree views appeared as mirror-symmetrical images of each other, due to minimal self-occlusion. We call such views pseudomirror-symmetrical. In this respect, the improvement in performance parallels the reflectional invariance observed in human psychophysical experiments (Biederman and Cooper, 1991).

Such reflectional invariance may also partly explain the observation that information about bilateral symmetry simplifies the task of three-dimensional recognition by reducing the number of views required to achieve object constancy (Vetter, Poggio, and Bülthoff, 1994). It was not surprising that

N. K. Logothetis and D. L. Sheinberg

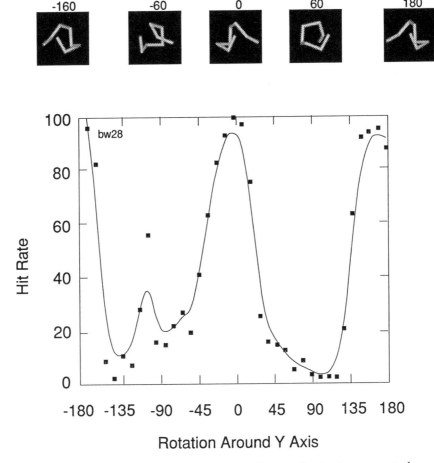

Figure 8.6 Responses to pseudomirror-symmetrical images showing improvement of recognition performance for views generated by 180-degree rotations of wirelike objects. This type of performance was specific to wirelike objects that possessed zero- and 180-degree views resembling mirror-symmetrical, two-dimensional images due to accidental lack of self-occlusion. Conventions are as in figure 8.4.

performance around the 180-degree view of an object did not improve for any of the self-occluding, spheroidal objects used in these experiments.

It is worth noting that in our studies, the recognition of pseudomirror-views improved for rotations around any of the four tested rotation axes. At first this might appear surprising, since most of the mirror symmetry that humans experience is around the vertical axis. In fact, rotations of faces around the horizontal axis usually have a robust effect on human performance, whereas they have no significant effect on the performance of the monkey (Bruce, 1982). The difference might be attributed to the development of laterality in humans, or simply to the fact that monkeys often look at each other from an upside-down attitude. Of interest, children up to 10 years old, who may still have incompletely developed laterality, can remember faces presented upside down almost as well as they do those presented upright (Carey and Diamond, 1977).

View-Invariant Recognition Performance

Although we obtained clear evidence for view-dependent recognition for the novel wire and amoebalike objects, these results should not be taken to mean that all, or even most, of the monkeys' recognition performance is affected by viewpoint. Given adequate experience with the novel objects, the monkeys could achieve, with remarkable consistency, perfect recognition performance for all target rotations. It is telling, however, that this view-independent performance seemed to emerge only after an initial period of viewpoint dependence. These observations are much more consistent with a model of object recognition based on interpolation between experienced views rather than internal manipulation of a three-dimensional structural model.

In addition, to complement the results of the subordinate-level testing conditions, we also examined the monkeys' generalization performance in more basic-level tasks. The term basic-level is used here simply to denote that the objects were largely different in shape from the distractors.

For these experiments, two monkeys were each trained on a single view of a novel object, the starship *Enterprise*. In the testing phase, distractors were selected from a set of 120 objects, including geometrical constructs, wire, spheroidals, plane models, and fractal objects. Under these testing conditions, hit rates for the target object were almost perfect ($> 95\%$) for all rotation angles, whereas false alarm rates were below 5% for each of the distractor objects. Thus, when the animals were tested for basic-level classifications, performance was viewpoint invariant even in the absence of extensive training.

Discussion

The first demonstration of strong viewpoint dependence in the recognition of novel three-dimensional objects in humans was by Rock and collaborators (Rock, DiVita, and Barbeito, 1981; Rock and DiVita, 1987). These investigators examined the ability of subjects to recognize smoothly curved, wirelike objects experienced from one viewpoint, when presented from a novel viewpoint. They found that humans are unable to recognize views corresponding to object rotations as small as 30 to 40 degrees around a given axis. This result was obtained even though their stimuli provided the subjects with full three-dimensional information. Furthermore, subsequent investigations showed that subjects could not even imagine what a wirelike object looks like when rotated, despite instructions for visualizing the object from another viewpoint (Rock, Wheeler, and Tudor, 1989). Similar results were obtained in later experiments with computer-rendered, wirelike objects presented stereoscopically or as flat images (Bulthoff and Edelman, 1992).

Our data provide evidence of similar view dependency of recognition in monkeys. All tested monkeys were unable to recognize novel objects when presented among similar distractors and rotated more than approximately 40 degrees from a familiar view. These results are hard to reconcile with theories postulating object-centered representations. Such theories predict uniform performance across different object views, provided that three-dimensional information is available to the subject at the time of the first encounter. Thus, one essential issue is whether information about the object's structure was available to the monkeys during the learning phase of these experiments.

For one, the objects were computer rendered with appropriate shading (Gouraud-shaded views) and were presented in slow oscillatory motion. The kinetic depth effect (motion parallax) produced by such motion yields vivid and accurate perception of the three-dimensional structure of an object or surface (Braunstein, 1968; Rogers and Graham, 1979). Experiments on monkeys show that nonhuman primates, too, possess the ability to see such structure from motion in random-dot kinematograms (Siegel and Andersen, 1988). In addition, the wire objects were visible in their entirety since, unlike most opaque natural objects in the environment, regions in front do not substantially occlude regions in back. Thus, during the learning phase of each observation period, information about the three-dimensional structure of the target was available to the monkeys by virtue of shading, the kinetic depth effect, and minimal self-occlusion.

The strongly view-dependent performance at the subordinate level of recognition was not specific to the wirelike objects. Similar performance was observed within an entirely different object class whose members had extensive surface and occlusion like many objects in daily life. Thus, it appears that monkeys, just like human subjects, show rotational invariance in basic-level tasks, but they fail to generalize recognition at the subordinate level when identification of individual entities relies on fine, shape-based discriminations. Of interest, training with a limited number of views was sufficient for all the animals tested to achieve view-independent performance. Hence, view invariance based on familiarity does not require the storage of a formidable number of object views.

Could the view-dependent behavior be a result of the monkeys' failing to understand the task? The monkeys could indeed recognize a two-dimensional pattern as such, without necessarily perceiving it as a view of an object. Correct performance around the familiar view could then be simply explained as the animals' inability to discriminate adjacent views. Several lines of arguments refute such an interpretation, however.

First, the animals easily generalized recognition to all novel views of common objects. Second, when the wirelike objects had prominent characteristics, such as very sharp or very wide angles, closures, or other pronounced combinations of features, the animals were able to perform in a view-invariant fashion. Evidently the visual system will use any information available to identify an object. A representation can be built based on a detailed description of shape as well as on only some characteristic features of an object, including nongeometrical properties such as color and texture. There is no reason to expect that either humans or monkeys will rely on subordinate shape discriminations when the objects can be clearly identified otherwise. Third, when more than one view of the target was presented in the training phase, the animals successfully interpolated between the trained views, often with 100% performance. Interpolation between views was not merely matching to the trained views and their generalization gradient, since performance for the views between the samples was at least two times better than that expected from the conjunction of the bell-shaped performance curves. Finally, the monkeys' ability to recognize pseudomirror views of the familiar views also represents a form of generalization.

It is worth noting that recognition based entirely on fine shape discriminations, such as those described here, is not uncommon in daily life. Face identification is a striking example of subordinate-level recognition. Despite the great structural similarity among individual faces, it is easy for both humans and monkeys to recognition faces. We are certainly able to recognize mountains and cloud formations, as well as humanmade objects such as modern sculptures and different types of cars. Many of these objects are recognized based on their shape, and most of them cannot necessarily be structurally decomposed in simpler parts. Moreover, even theories suggesting that recognition involves the indexing of a limited number of volumetric components (Biederman, 1987) and the detection of their relationships have to face the problem of learning those components that cannot be further decomposed.

OBJECT RECOGNITION IN PRIMATES: NEUROPHYSIOLOGICAL DATA

Inferotemporal Cortex

The inferior temporal area (IT) is composed of the large region of cortex extending from just anterior to the inferior occipital sulcus to just posterior to the temporal pole, and from the fundus of the superior temporal sulcus to the fundus of the occipitotemporal sulcus. Neuropsychological reports in humans and lesion studies in monkeys have consistently found that damage to this area can lead to severe impairments in form perception. After unilateral temporal lobectomy for the relief of epilepsy, humans revealed significant deficits in remembering complex shapes (Milner, 1968, 1980). Lesion studies in monkeys showed that damage to IT spares low-level visual tasks, such as orientation discrimination, but disrupts pattern perception and recognition (Iwai and Mishkin, 1969; Gross, 1973; Dean, 1976).

In the earliest single unit studies in IT, Gross and collaborators (1967, 1969) reported that cells in this area have large receptive fields that almost always include the fovea, and that most of these cells are selective for stimulus attributes such as size, color, orientation, and direction of movement (Gross, Rocha-Miranda, and Bender, 1972). The authors also described a few cells that responded best to complex shapes, such as hands, trees, and faces, providing the first potential evidence for the existence of object-specific cells in the brain. Subsequent studies failed to support the notion that individual objects are specifically represented by individual cells in IT, and instead indicated that certain feature classes appear to be coded by these neurons.

The selectivity of IT neurons to shape was studied by presenting various natural or humanmade objects (Desimone et al, 1984; Tanaka et al, 1991), or by presenting a set of parametric shape descriptors, such as the Fourier descriptors (Schwartz et al, 1983). The IT cells showed stimulus selectivity for complex patterns such as fractals, brushes, and faces (Desimone et al, 1984; Miyashita, 1988; Tanaka et al, 1991). Cell selectivity also was maintained over changes in stimulus size, contrast, color, or orientation (Gross and Mishkin, 1977), although absolute levels of firing can be affected by changing stimulus size (Schwartz et al, 1983).

Shape is clearly a prevailing stimulus feature in IT cortex. The IT neurons respond in a selective manner to the shape of various natural or humanmade objects (Desimone et al, 1984), parametric shape descriptors (Schwartz et al, 1983), and two-dimensional functions that can be made to synthesize any visual pattern to a required degree of accuracy (Richmond et al, 1987). Pattern-tuned neurons maintain their selectivity even when the stimuli are defined by visual cues other than luminance or color contrast, such as motion or texture differences (Sáry, Vogels, and Orban, 1993). The shape selectivity of IT neurons is also maintained over changes in stimulus position and size (Gross and Mishkin, 1977). Although such changes usually alter the absolute firing rate of the neurons (Schwartz et al, 1983), the relative preference for a particular stimulus is maintained; to this extent IT neurons exhibit size and position invariance.

The most striking class of highly selective cells in IT are those responding to the sight of faces (Bruce, Desimone, and Gross, 1981; Perrett, Rolls, and Caan, 1982; Hasselmo, Rolls, and Baylis, 1986; Yamane et al, 1987). Face neurons have been recorded in both adult and infant monkeys (Rodman, Scalaidhe, and Gross, 1993). They are usually deep in the lower bank and fundus of the superior temporal sulcus (STS), and in the polysensory area located dorsal to IT cortex in the fundus and upper bank of the STS (Desimone et al, 1984; Perrett, Rolls, and Caan, 1982). Most face-selective neurons are 2 to 10 times more sensitive to faces than to other complex patterns, simple geometrical stimuli, or real three-dimensional objects (Perrett, Rolls, and Caan, 1979, 1982). Presenting different views or parts of a face in isolation revealed that the neurons may respond selectively to face views (Desimone et al, 1984; Perrett et al, 1985), features, or subsets of features (Perrett, Mistlin, and Chitty, 1989; Young and Yamane, 1992). Thus, they have properties reminiscent of an RBF network. Is such view-selectivity specific to faces? Could one expect to find neurons in this area that are tuned to views (or parts thereof) of nonsensical objects that the monkey learns to recognize?

To address these questions, we recorded from neurons in IT cortex while monkeys performed the experimental paradigm described above. Specifically, we asked whether IT cells respond selectively to novel objects that the monkey learns to recognize, and whether or not those cells that might be selective show view-dependent activity.

View Selectivity of IT Neurons for Three-Dimensional Objects

We examined the activity of over 700 IT neurons in two macaques during either a simple fixation task or the recognition task. Figure 8.7 shows the recording sites as estimated from the stereotaxic coordinates. Since the animals are being used in additional experiments on object recognition, no histological reconstructions are currently available.

Isolated units were tested with a variety of simple or complex patterns while the animal was involved in a fixation task. The animal was trained to maintain fixation within a 1 × 1-degree window. The activity of the cells that

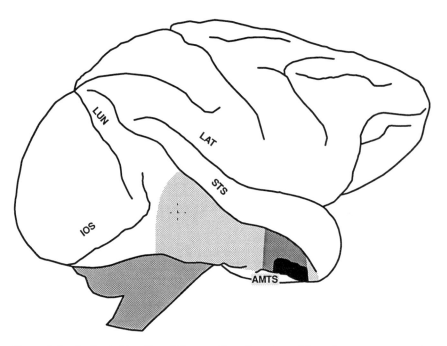

Figure 8.7 Anatomical location of the recording site estimated from the stereotaxic coordinates. Lateral view of a macaque brain. Labeled are the lunate sulcus (LUN), the inferior occipital sulcus (IOS), the lateral fissure, the superior temporal sulcus (STS), and the anterior medial temporal sulcus (AMTS). The dashed cross represents the Horsley-Clarke zero. The anteroposterior and mediolateral extent of the primary recording site were from 14 to 21 mm anterior and 16 to 24 mm lateral. We concentrated our recordings in the dorsal lip, dorsal bank, and fundus of the AMTS.

N. K. Logothetis and D. L. Sheinberg

responded to either the wire or the amoebalike objects were examined further while the animal performed the recognition task.

We found a number of units that showed a remarkable selectivity for individual views of wire and amoebalike objects that the monkey had learned to recognize. An example of highly selective neuron is shown in figure 8.8. The responses of this cell were studied for 30 different views of a wire object that the monkey learned. For this cell, the monkey's psychophysical performance was above 95% for all the views of this object. However, the cell was highly selective for views located around −72 degrees. Its activity decreased considerably with even a 12-degree deviation from the preferred view. The view 180 degrees away from the preferred view did elicit firing of the neuron, albeit weaker. Figure 8.8b shows the responses of the same cell for 15 wire-like and nonwire distractor objects. As can be seen in the figures, none of these objects elicited any significant response from the neuron.

Figure 8.9 shows an example of a similar cell from another monkey. Again, having been exposed to this wire over the course of many sessions, the monkey had learned to identify it perfectly, independent of viewpoint. The cell, however, was highly selective for views of the wire centered around the zero view (figure 8.9a). Of the 70 distractors presented, not one made the cell fire more than 35% as fast as the zero view of the target (figure 8.9b).

In addition, many cells showed a tuning that appeared more closely coupled to the animal's behavioral performance (figure 8.10). As seen in figure 8.10a, the monkey's ability to recognize the target was strongly viewpoint dependent. For object rotations of more than ±30 degrees around the y axis, the monkey consistently misclassified the target as a distractor. Figure 8.10c illustrates that a strikingly similar pattern was found in the cell's response to the same object. The monkey never responded positively to one of the 60 distractors (figure 8.10b), and the cell showed no selectivity for any of the distractor objects (figure 8.10d).

These observations provide strong evidence that the activity of these neurons is not simply a reflection of arousal, attention, or a sensation of familiarity, but rather relates to the object's characteristic features or views. To date, 71 (9%) of the 773 analyzed cells showed view-selective responses similar to those illustrated in figure 8.10. The majority of the rest of the neurons were visually active when plotted with other simple or complex stimuli, including faces. A small percentage of neurons, although often firing with a rate of between 5 and 20 Hz, could not be driven by any of the stimuli used in these experiments.

Dissociation of Cell and Monkey Response

As shown in figures 8.8 and 8.10, even when the animal could recognize a target from all tested viewpoints, some cells were still selective to only a small number of target views. This dissociation between performance and cell activity also was observed for targets for which the monkey did not show

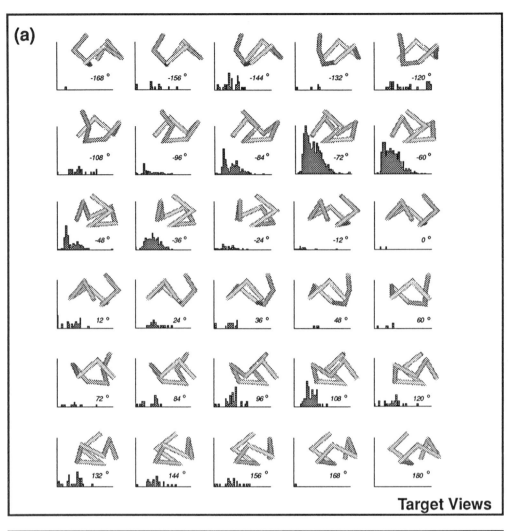

Target Views

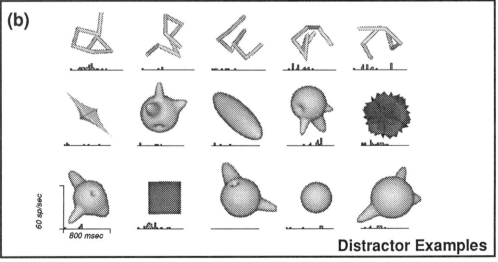

60 sp/sec

800 msec

Distractor Examples

viewpoint-invariant recognition. Figure 8.11 gives an example of a cell that is tuned to one of two target views that the monkey could recognize. The monkey could properly identify the wire if presented in either the zero view or a view approximately 180 degrees away from the zero view (figure 8.11a). However, as seen in figure 8.11b, the cell was selective only for the zero view. The thick line in figure 8.11b indicates a hypothetical tuning curve for some other cell. Note that its peak is outside of the region in which the animal can recognize the target. Such selectivity is, of course, theoretically possible; and if these cells were simply passive filters, one might imagine that they might actually be encountered. This does not appear to be the case, though. We have never found a cell that was selective for particular views of an object that the animal systematically failed to recognize.

Pseudomirror-Symmetric and Viewpoint-Invariant Cells

Of the view-selective cells, a small number (5 of 71) responded strongly for a particular view and its pseudomirror-symmetrical view. An example of neuron responding to pseudomirror-symmetrical views is shown in figure 8.12. This cell was most responsive for a set of views around 100 degrees, however, it also gave a large response for a set of views around the −80-degree view of the target. The monkey's performance was 100% for almost all the tested views. The high performance is the result of giving feedback to the animal for several views of the object. Neither of the neuron's preferred views, however, represents the view that the monkey was shown in the training period.

A few cells (8 of 773) also responded to wirelike objects presented from any viewpoint, thereby showing view-invariant response characteristics. For these cells, the monkey had been exposed to the wires repeatedly and had achieved viewpoint-invariant behavioral performance as well.

Discussion

Cells selective for specific patterns or object views are clearly not rare throughout the inferotemporal cortex. View selectivity for face-selective inferotemporal neurons has been reported previously (Desimone et al, 1984). Cells were sensitive to the orientation of the head in depth. Some were maximally sensitive to the front view of a face, and their response fell off as

Figure 8.8 Example of a view-selective cell. The abscissa of each small plot represents time. and the ordinate is the mean spike rate. Angles refer to the corresponding view of the target. Performance of the monkey was above 95% for all views of the targets (not shown). (a) This cell was highly selective for views located around −72 degrees. Activity decreased considerably with even a 12-degree deviation from the preferred view. Note the improved response for the view 180 degrees away from the preferred view. (b) None of the distractor objects, including other wires, elicited any notable response from the cell.

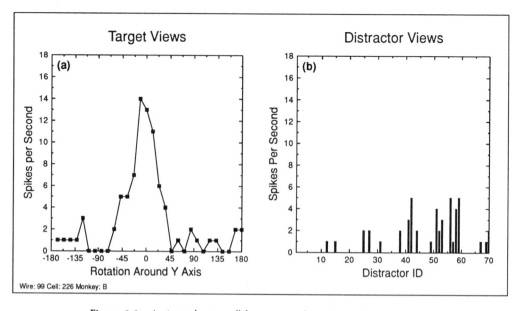

Figure 8.9 A view-selective cell from a second monkey. (a) This cell was selective for views located around the zero view of the target. Cell activity was reduced almost to zero as the target was rotated approximately 45 degrees. (b) Of the 70 distractor wires tested, none made the cell fire even 35% as vigorously as the preferred view of the target. Behavioral performance for this wire was perfect.

the head was rotated into the profile view; others were sensitive to the profile view with no reaction to the front view of the face. In this example the cells' activity fell to half of its maximum when the face was rotated about 30 to 40 degrees, which is in close agreement with the data presented here using the wire or amoebalike objects.

A detailed investigation of these type of cells revealed a total of five cell types in the superior temporal sulcus, each maximally responsive to one view of the head (Perrett et al, 1985). The five types of cells were separately tuned for full face, profile, back of the head, head up, and head down. Most of these neurons were 2 to 10 times more sensitive to faces than to simple geometrical stimuli or three-dimensional objects (Perrett, Rolls, and Caan, 1979, 1982).

Recent studies showed that such selectivity appears early in the development of the visual system. Rodman, Scalaidhe, and Gross (1993) found cells in the IT cortex of infant monkeys that had responses selective for shape, faces, geometrical patterns, and color. So it seems that at least some of the neurons that are selective to highly complex patterns are available to the recognition system even at the earliest developmental stages of the visual system.

We found neurons that responded selectively to novel visual objects that the monkey learned to recognize during the experiments. None of these objects had any prior meaning to the animal, and none of them resembled anything familiar in the monkey's environment. Thus it appears that neurons

N. K. Logothetis and D. L. Sheinberg

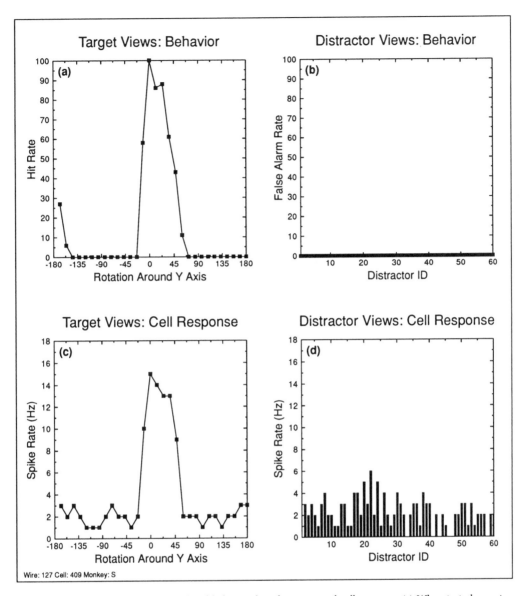

Figure 8.10 Correlated behavioral performance and cell response (a) When tested on wire 127, the monkey was able to recognize only those rotations centered around the zero view. (b) No false alarms were made for any of the 60 distractors, indicating that the monkey was very conservative about which images he classified as the target. (c) The response of an IT cell (c409) during the recognition task shows a remarkably similar response pattern to the behavioral data. (d) Cell responses to each of the 60 distractor objects.

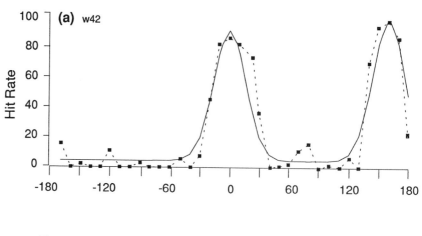

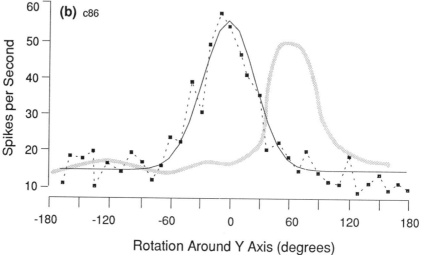

Figure 8.11 Dissociation of cell and monkey responses. (a) Behavior data for this wire shows that the monkey could recognize both the zero view and the 180-degree view of the target. (b) The neuron responded vigorously to only the zero view, even though the monkey reponded correctly to both it and 180-degree view. The thick gray line depicts a hypothetical tuning curve for a cell that is tuned to view of the wire which the monkey did not recognize. Interestingly, no cell like this has ever been found. All selective cells were selective for views of objects that the monkey could recognize.

in this area can develop a complex receptive field organization as a result of extensive training in the discrimination and recognition of objects.

The monkeys were trained with different types of objects, such as the wirelike, spheroidal, and basic objects shown in figure 8.1. Of interest, the frequency of encountering neurons selective to a particular object type seemed to be related to the animal's familiarity with the object class. In one of the monkeys, the wirelike objects, which were used extensively during the psychophysical experiments, were much more likely to elicit cell responses (71 selective cells) than, for example, spheroidal objects (10 selective cells),

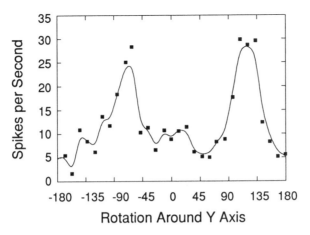

Figure 8.12 Cell responses for pseudomirror-symmetrical views. The monkey was trained on one view, at zero degrees and subsequently tested at 10-degree intervals around one axis. Note that at the time these data were collected, the recognition performance for the monkey for this object was above 90% for all views around the y axis. The graph depicts spike rate of a single neuron as a function of rotation angle. This particular cell was most selective for a set of views around 100 degrees, however, it also gave a large response for the set of views around the view at −80 degrees.

which were used to a much lesser extent. The converse was observed in another animal that was extensively trained with the amoeba objects. Most selective neurons responded best to one view of the object, and their response decreased as the object was rotated away from the preferred view. Plotting the cell responses as a function of rotation angle revealed systematic view-tuning curves similar to those obtained from striate neurons tested with lines rotated in the frontal plane.

CONCLUSIONS

From these observations, we can draw a number of preliminary conclusions. First, even when complete information about the structure of a novel object is available, recognition at the subordinate level depends on the object's attitude. Second, it seems that a memory-based, viewer-centered recognition system provides a plausible mechanism for object constancy. Both theoretical work and the results of experiments described here suggest that only a small number of object views have to be stored to achieve the perceptual invariance that biological visual systems exhibit in everyday life.

In addition, our physiological data revealed a small population of neurons in inferior temporal cortex that respond selectively to individual members of the object classes tested. The response of some neurons was a function of the object's view, although some of the view-selective neurons responded equally well to mirror-symmetrical views. Finally, for all objects used in the combined psychophysical-electrophysiological experiments, tuning was observed only for views that the monkey could recognize. Several neurons were also found that responded to the sight of unfamiliar or distractor objects. Such cells, however, gave nonspecific responses to a variety of other patterns presented while the monkey performed a simple fixation task.

ACKNOWLEDEGMENTS

The authors wish to thank J. Pauls for his contribution to this work. Portions of this chapter have appeared in Logothetis et al (1994) and Logothetis and Pauls (1995). Nikos K. Logothetis was supported by grants from the National Institutes of Health (NIH 1R01EY10089-01), the Office of Naval Research (N00014-93-1-0290), and a McKnight Endowment Fund for Neuroscience; David L. Sheinberg was supported by the National Institutes of Health (NRSA 1F32FY06624).

REFERENCES

Biederman I. (1987). Recognition-by-components: A theory of human image understanding. *Psychol Rev* 94:115–147.

Biederman I, Cooper E. (1991). Evidence for complete translational and reflectional invariance in visual object priming. *Perception* 20:585–593.

Braunstein M. (1968). Motion and texture as sources of slant information. *J Exp Psychol* 78:247–253.

Bruce C. (1982). Face recognition by monkeys: Absence of an inversion effect. *Neuropsychologia* 20:515–521.

Bruce C, Desimone R, Gross C. (1981). Visual properties of neurons in a polysensory area in superior temporal sulcus of the macaque. *J Neurophysiol* 46:369–384.

Bülthoff H, Edelman S. (1992). Psychophysical support for a two-dimensional view interpolation theory of object recognition. *Proc Natl Acad Sci USA* 89:60–64.

Carey S, Diamond R. (1977). From piecemeal to configuration representation of faces. *Science* 195:312–313.

Damasio A. (1990). Category-related recogntion defects as a clue to the neural substrates of knowledge. *Trends Neurosci* 13:95–99.

Dean P. (1976). Effects of inferotemporal lesions on the behavior of monkeys. *Psychol Bull* 83:41–71.

Desimone R, Albright T, Gross C, Bruce C. (1984). Stimulus-selective properties of inferior temporal neurons in the macaque. *J Neurosci* 4:2051–2062.

Edelman S, Bülthoff H. (1992). Orientation dependence in the recognition of familiar and novel views of 3D objects. *Vision Res* 32:2385–2400.

Gross C. (1973). Visual functions of the inferotemporal cortex. In: *Handbook of sensory physiology*. R Jung, ed. Springer-Verlag, Berlin, 451–482.

Gross C, Bender D, Rocha-Miranda C. (1969). Visual receptive fields of neurons in inferotemporal cortex of the monkey. *Science* 166:1303–1306.

Gross C, Mishkin M. (1977). The neural basis of stimulus equivalence across retinal translation. In: *Lateralization in the nervous system*. S Harnad, R Doty, J Jaynes, L Goldstein, G Krauthamer, eds.) Academic Press, New York, 109–122.

Gross C, Rocha-Miranda C, Bender D. (1972). Visual properties of neurons in inferotemporal cortex of the macaque. *J Neurophysiol* 35:96−111.

Gross C, Schiller P, Wells C, Gerstein G. (1967). Single-unit activity in temporal association cortex of the monkey. *J Neurophysiol* 30:833−843.

Hasselmo M, Rolls E, Baylis G. (1986). Object-centered encoding of faces by neurons in the cortex in the superior temporal sulcus of the monkey. *Soc Neurosci Abstr* 12:1369.

Iwai E, Mishkin M. (1969). Further evidence on the locus of the visual area in the temporal lobe of the monkey. *Exp Neurol* 25:585−594.

Jolicouer P, Gluck M, Kosslyn S. (1984). Pictures and names: Making the connection. *Cogn Psychol* 16:243−275.

Logothetis N, Pauls J. (1995). Psychophysical and physiological evidence for viewer-centered representations in the primate. *Cerebral Cortex* 5:270−288.

Logothetis N, Pauls J, Bülthoff H, Poggio T. (1994). View-dependent object recognition in the primate. *Curr Biol* 4:401−414.

Marr D. (1982). *Vision*. WH Freeman, San Francisco.

Milner B. (1968). Visual recognition and recall after right temporal-lobe exicision in man. *Neuropsychologia* 6:191−209.

Milner B. (1980). Complementary functional specialization of the human cerebral hemispheres. In: *Nerve cells, transmitters and behaviour*. R Levy-Montalcini, ed. Pontificiae Academiae Scientiarium Scripta Varia, Vatican City, 601−625.

Miyashita Y. (1988). Neuronal correlate of visual associative long-term memory in the primate temporal cortex. *Nature* 335:817−820.

Perrett D, Mistlin A, Chitty A. (1989). Visual neurones responsive to faces. *Trends Neurosci* 10:358−364.

Perrett D, Rolls E, Caan W. (1979). Temporal lobe cells of the monkey with visual responses selective for faces. *Neurosci Lett Suppl* S3:S358.

Perrett D, Rolls E, Caan W. (1982). Visual neurones responsive to faces in the monkey temporal cortex. *Exp Brain Res* 47:329−342.

Perrett D, Smith P, Potter D, Mistlin A, Head A, Milner A, Jeeves M. (1985). Visual cells in the temporal cortex sensitive to face view and gaze direction. *Proc R Soc Lond* [Biol] 223:293−317.

Poggio T. (1990). A theory of how the brain might work. *Cold Spring Harbor Symp Quant Biol* 55:899−910.

Poggio T, Edelman S. (1990). A network that learns to recognize three-dimensional objects. *Nature* 343:263−266.

Poggio T, Girosi F. (1990). Regularization algorithms for learning that are equivalent to multilayer networks. *Science* 247:978−982.

Richmond B, Optican L, Podell M, Spitzer H. (1987). Temporal encoding of two-dimensional patterns by single units in primate inferior temporal cortex. I. Response characteristics. *J Neurophysiol* 57:132−146.

Rock I, DiVita J. (1987). A case of viewer-centered object perception. *Cogn Psychol* 19:280−293.

Rock I, DiVita J, Barbeito R. (1981). The effect on form perception of change of orientation in the third dimension. *J Exp Psychol* 7:719−732.

Rock I, Wheeler D, Tudor L. (1989). Can we imagine how objects look from other viewpoints? *Cogn Psychol* 21:185–210.

Rodman H, Scalaidhe S, Gross C. (1993). Response properties of neurons in temporal cortical visual areas of infant monkeys. *J Neurophysiol* 70:1115–1136.

Rogers B, Graham M. (1979). Motion parallax as an independant cue for depth perception. *Percept Psychophysics* 8:125–134.

Rosch E. (1975). Cognitive representations of semantic categories. *J Exp Psychol* [Gen] 104:192–233.

Rosch E, Mervis C, Gray W, Johnson D, Boyes-Braem P. (1976). Basic objects in natural categories. *Cogn Psychol* 8:382–439.

Sáry G, Vogels R, Orban G. (1993). Cue-invariant shape selectivity of macaque inferior temporal neurons. *Science* 260:995–997.

Schwartz E, Desimone R, Albright T, Gross C. (1983). Shape recognition and inferior temporal neuron. *Proc Natl Acad Sci USA* 80:5776–5778.

Siegel R, Andersen R. (1988). Perception of three-dimensional structure from motion in monkey and man. *Nature* 331:259–261.

Tanaka K, Saito HA, Fukada Y, Moriya M. (1991). Coding visual images of objects in the inferotemporal cortex of the macaque monkey. *J Neurophysiol* 66:170–189.

Tarr M, Pinker S. (1989). Mental rotation and orientation-dependence in shape recognition. *Cogn Psychol* 21:233–282.

Tarr M, Pinker S. (1990). When does human object recognition use a viewer-centered reference frame? *Psychol Sci* 1:253–256.

Tranel D, Damasio A, Damasio H. (1988). Intact recognition of facial expression, gender, and age in patients with impaired recognition of face identity. *Neurology* 38:690–696.

Ullman S. (1989). Aligning pictorial descriptions: An approach to object recognition. *Cognition* 32:193–254.

Ullman S, Basri R. (1991). Recognition by linear combinations of models. *IEEE Trans Pattern Anal Mach Intell* 13:992–1005.

Vetter T, Poggio T, Bülthoff H. (1994). The importance of symmetry and virtual views in three-dimensional object recognition. *Curr Biol* 4:18–23.

Yamane S, Kaji S, Kawano K, Hamada T. (1987). Responses of single neurons in the inferotemopral cortex of the awake monkey performing human face discrimination task. *Neurosci Res* S5:S114.

Young M, Yamane S. (1992). An analysis at the population level of the processing of faces in the inferotemporal cortex. In: *Brain mechanisms of perception and memory: From neuron to behaviour*. L Squire, T Ono, M Fukuda, D Perrett, eds. Oxford University Press, New York, 47–71.

9 Olfactory Perception and Memory

H. Eichenbaum

Olfaction is thought of, if at all, as the odd sensory modality. It is the sense whose properties are commonly believed to be very different from those of vision, touch, audition, and even taste. This view is not without good justification, because olfaction is different than the other sensory modalities both in perceptual properties and in how sensory processing is organized within the brain. However, one of the major points of this chapter is that the oddities are confined to early, modality-specific stages of odor processing. By contrast, at supramodal levels of information processing where sensory information merges in the temporal and prefrontal areas, olfactory pathways are remarkably similar to those of the conventional sensory systems. Indeed, based on this observation, Nauta (1972) once characterized the olfactory system as providing a "flow diagram for telencephalic processing in the mammalian brain."

A PRELIMINARY OUTLINE OF THE OLFACTORY SYSTEM AND ITS CENTRAL PROJECTIONS

A schematic diagram of the olfactory system and its interconnections with other parts of the brain in rats and humans is provided in figure 9.1. The anatomy of the olfactory system is remarkable in its simplicity compared with that of other sensory systems in that it is composed of three main structures: the olfactory epithelium, the olfactory bulb, and the piriform cortex. Also present are an additional, parallel olfactory pathway by way of the accessory olfactory bulb that is concerned with pheromone-elicited, species-specific behaviors (Keverne, 1987), and a pathway for interhemispheric olfactory interactions by way of the anterior olfactory nucleus; these systems are not considered here.

The olfactory epithelium (not pictured) involves a large sheet of receptor cells lining the nasal turbinates through which odors pass during inhalation. The unmyelinated axons of these receptors project through the cribiform plate above the nasal cavity and enter at the superficial layer of the olfactory bulb where they terminate on distal dendrites of the principal neurons, the

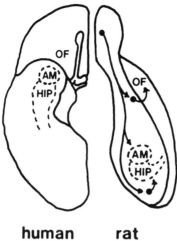

human   rat

Figure 9.1 Ventral views of the human (left) and rodent (right) brains show the main targets of the higher olfactory pathways. OF = orbitofrontal cortex; AM = amygdala; HIP = hippocampus.

mitral and tufted cells. These connections occur in glomeruli that include complex and bidirectional interactions among the receptors, principal cells, and interneurons (Shepherd, 1972). Projections of the mitral and tufted cells course in the lateral olfactory tract with somewhat different distributions along the piriform cortex along the broad surface of the base of the brain. The axons of these cells reach as far as the entorhinal cortex, which is contiguous with the piriform cortex at the caudal end of the ventral surface of the brain. Processing within the olfactory system per se is completed at this stage, except to note that major sources of nonsensory input to the olfactory bulb involve centrifugal pathways from the piriform cortex by way of the nucleus basalis and indirectly from the hippocampus to interneurons in the bulb (Macrides, Eichenbaum, and Forbes, 1982).

Processed olfactory information is directed into structures of the temporal and prefrontal areas through three main pathways. These are a dual pathway to the orbital prefrontal cortex, one direct from cells of the piriform cortex, and an indirect projection from deep piriform (endopiriform) cells to the central segment of the mediodorsal thalamic nucleus and then to the orbital prefrontal area (Price et al, 1991). In addition, the olfactory bulb and piriform cortex project to the amygdala and then to the hypothalamus. Finally, both the olfactory bulb and piriform cortex project to the entorhinal area, including very heavy projections to the lateral entorhinal area. The pathways between the olfactory system and these three the temporal and prefrontal supramodal processing stages constitute what Nauta referred to as the olfactory-telencephalic flow diagram for the sensory processing reaching limbic structures, recognizing that the conventional sensory pathways culminate in parallel routes to these areas.

ODDITIES OF OLFACTORY PERCEPTUAL PROCESSING

Some have attributed the unusual characteristics of olfaction to its early appearance in evolution. For example, one long-standing explanation for the absence of an olfactory thalamocortical relay is simply that the evolution of the thalamocortical route of sensory processing postdated the development of olfactory systems. Several other oddities of the olfactory system have invoked the same accounting, but the phylogenetic explanation does not shed light on why olfactory perception is so different. An alternative approach taken here is to combine unique properties of olfactory stimuli with unusual aspects of the olfactory anatomy and physiology, suggesting some fundamental principles of sensory processing that might better account for observed differences in perceptual properties across sensory modalities.

To this end, the following are some of the unusual characteristics of olfaction:

1. Failure to identify odor primitives or dimensions

2. No systematic topography

3. No thalamocortical pathway

4. Continuous receptor turnover

5. Lifetime plasticity in the olfactory bulb

6. Poor odor-identification capacity

7. Powerful odor memories

8. No merging of odor representations with those of other modalities prior to the supramodal convergence areas (except with taste)

I will dwell mostly on the first three, attempting to draw a connection between the biggest problem in understanding olfactory perception and some striking aspects of olfactory circuitry, and then stretch my speculations even further to suggest associations between other oddities of olfactory experience and properties of the olfactory pathways.

Dimensions of Odor Perception

Perhaps the best-known oddity of olfaction is our failure to identify odor primitives, or dimensions of odor quality. This failure does not reflect the absence of attempts to do so or lack of proposals for odor categorizations. Serious attempts to classify odors date back to Linnaeus in 1756 and include schemes of 4 to 44 odor classes described by distinct primitive qualities (Engen, 1982). Despite these many attempts, none has resulted in a consensus about dimensions that can be varied or measured systematically across odor stimuli.

Whereas no serious consideration has been given to the possibility that odor primitives do not exist, one possible explanation for this failure may be the opposite—that there are simply too many. Among the multiplicity of chemical factors that have been suggested to be operating at the receptors are stereochemical specificities; force, weight, and vibration of molecules; chemical reactions between receptor sites or enzymes and odors; and interface dynamics of odors adsorbed into the receptor. One possibility is that many or all of these proposals are correct and, furthermore, that every odor molecule involves a combination of several of these properties operating and interacting simultaneously. Unfortunately, this makes it very unlikely that we will ever find molecules that are primarily characterized by a single primitive, or that we can account for the perceptual consequences of interactions among many molecular factors in a straightforward experimental analysis.

The futility of attempts to develop an odor-categorization scheme is illustrated by an effort that was based on the phenomenon of cross-adaptation. Odor receptors rapidly adapt to stimulation such that exposure to an odor for a brief period raises the threshold for detecting it. In addition, adaptation to one odor often raises the perceptual threshold for others; this is the phenomenon of cross-adaptation. Assuming that the basis of perceptual adaptation is the blocking of specific receptors for an odor molecule, cross-adaptation may be based on shared properties of the adapted and cross-adapted odors that block the same receptors. Exploiting this phenomenon, assessment of cross-adaptations among a list of odors should yield a pattern of diminished sensitivities that reveal the common receptor primitives for those odors.

This rationale was promising in guiding a straightforward experimental design to deduce primitive adaptation elements from the pattern of cross-adaptations, but the results of its application have proved frustrating. The degree to which odors cross-adapt seems to bear no relation to perceptual similarities of odors. Even the same pair of odors does not cross-adapt equally when presented in opposite order (Cain & Engen, 1969). The basic question left open by the failure to find odor primitives is whether there are just too many dimensions, involving too many different nonlinear or nonmontonic functional effects, to permit any foreseeable quantitative analysis.

Topographical Mapping

In addition to the major problem of identifying olfactory perceptual features, the anatomy of olfaction is odd in that it lacks the usual systematic topographical mapping and involves a pathway lacking a thalamocortical circuit. To some investigators the first of these characterizations is outdated; much excitement was generated when the application of several anatomical mapping techniques revealed the beginnings of a topographical system. These techniques showed that individual odors excite specific areas of the olfactory epithelium, that there are specific, albeit complex, mappings of projections from the epithelium to the olfactory bulb, and that different odors also excite specific patches of glomeruli in the olfactory bulb (Shepherd, 1991). This organization of odor representation prompted some to conclude that olfaction does have a topographical map after all. However, no systematic relationship exists between perceived similarities or differences in odor quality and the loci of activation for odors. In addition, whereas an organization of some aspect of activation is present at the level of the nasal epithelium, and it is transmitted to the input layer of the olfactory bulb, we have no evidence that this organization involves a systematic mapping of sensory features onto structure beyond that level.

Thalamocortical Pathways

Virtually every sensory pathway other than olfaction involves a serial set of connections that bring information from the sensory ganglion to a thalamic nucleus and then (reciprocally) to an area of cortex. Some view recent descriptions of the projection from deep cells in the piriform cortex to the mediodorsal nucleus and then to a part of the prefrontal area as evidence of an olfactory thalamocortical circuit, albeit one that comes after a stage of early cortical processing. However, such an interpretation is unsettling because it relegates the piriform cortex to the position in the circuit analogous to that of a brain stem ganglion, and because it leaves the olfactory prefrontal cortex with a dual role as a primary sensory area in addition to its traditional position as the highest of association areas (Eichenbaum, Eckmann, and Shedlack, 1980; Eichenbaum, Clegg, and Feeley, 1983).

I suggest that the failure to find odor primitives and the peculiarities of olfactory topography and pathways are all closely related, and different forms of coding may exist at levels before and after the olfactory bulb. At the input stage, it is probably safe to assume that the transduction process involves the detection of some aspect of odor chemical properties. However, these properties may differ from those of other modalities in that the dimensions are both numerous, as noted above, and nonmonotonic, such that graded changes in the dimension do not produce continuous graded changes in receptor activation. These two distinctions of olfaction are strikingly unlike properties of visual and auditory perception, where stimuli can be readily qualified by primitive dimensions (color and frequency, respectively) and responses are monotonic to stimulus amplitude (brightness and loudness, respectively). Somatosensation has a more complex yet still a short list of dimensions, all of which exhibit monotonic coding. Even taste can be simplified to four primitive chemical categories and responses are monotonic to concentration.

My suggestion is that the primitive chemical properties of olfactory receptors give rise to the organizational patterns observed in the olfactory epithelium only as far as the input layer to the olfactory bulb. Beyond this stage I suggest the olfactory coding process behaves as if there were no olfactory dimensions. This notion is based on a comparison between the nature of the information processed in olfactory bulb and cortex versus that at high levels of processing in other sensory systems. Within early stages of the visual, auditory, and somatosensory systems it is precisely the relevant and mono-tonically coded dimensions, and relations among them, that are mapped so systematically. Thus, for example, in the visual system, early cortical pro-cessing stages detect specific features such as contrast, color, depth, and movement separately, and the representations of these features are systemati-cally organized.

But what about the highest levels of processing where combinations of these simpler features form perceptual objects? In the visual system, for exam-ple, this processing occurs in the inferotemporal area where there is an enor-mous convergence of inputs about visual features, and at this stage of visual processing, no topography has been identified. Instead, there is at best a clustering of cells involved in encoding particular stimuli (Perret, Mistlin, and Chitty, 1987). Attempting to draw a connection between the infero-temporal cortex and olfactory bulb and cortex, in both the dimensions of sensory processing are numerous and complexly related, and topographic mapping is not observed. Accordingly, I suggest that the role of the piriform cortex in olfaction is analogous to the role of inferotemporal cortex in vision.

But what then is the nature of the representation supported in these non-topographic areas? Haberly (1985; Ketchum and Haberly, 1991) also com-pared the visual and olfactory systems, concluding from anatomical data that the piriform cortex and the inferotemporal cortex involve organizations of distributed representation through extensive horizontal connections. Further-more, they argued that the prevalence of reexcitatory pyramidal collaterals, using fast oscillatory cycles, may support storage and recognition mecha-nisms that form the basis of a content-addressable memory. Thus, the nature of representation in primary sensory projection areas of the visual and other systems, and that characterizing the piriform cortex and association cortex of other sensory systems, are proposed to be fundamentally different. Represen-tation at early stages of conventional sensory systems involves a mapping of primitive sensory dimensions and their combinations. By contrast, representa-tion in piriform cortex in the conventional sensory association area involves the learning of stimulus categories, supported within a distributed network that can be characterized as a content-addressable, random-access memory (Eichenbaum, 1993; Haberly, 1985).

Two other points about thalamic connections are consistent with this proposal. First, the observation that the projection from the primary olfactory area (the olfactory bulb) to piriform cortex involves no thalamic pathway parallels the fact that the projections from the primary visual areas to infero-temporal cortex have no requisite thalamic relay. Second, it seems to me that the olfactory pathway to the mediodorsal thalamus and prefrontal area occurs too late to serve as the primary olfactory thalamocortical route; furthermore, this olfactory pathway strongly parallels the visual thalamo-prefrontal path originating in the inferotemporal cortex (Leonard, 1972). Of course, this accounting of olfactory processing is highly speculative and almost inconse-quential, since there is no direct way to test such a simplification of the evolution of sensory circuitries. However, my notions may have some use-fulness, as they suggest that the search for odor primitives is not likely to succeed and should be abandoned in favor of more emphasis on categorization mechanisms by distributed olfactory cortical networks (Bower, 1991; Granger et al, 1991). In addition, analyses of sensory processing by cell assemblies in the relatively simple olfactory cortex may offer insights into coding at higher levels in other sensory systems (Ketchum and Haberly, 1991; Bower, 1991; Lynch, 1986).

Receptor Turnover and Plasticity in the Olfactory Bulb

Moving on in my list of oddities of olfaction, the next pair of observations may also be connected to each other, and they may be related to the above proposals about odor coding. Unlike other sensory systems, a continuous turnover of receptor cells occurs in the olfactory sensorium (Farbman, 1992). This fact raises the question of how odor perception remains relatively constant over life, even though the receptors that support in keep being renewed. An observation that might be related to receptor turnover is that the olfactory bulb remains surprisingly plastic beyond its full development such that injury or odor deprivation can result in reorganization in the bulb well into adulthood (Farbman, 1992; Leon, Wilson, and Guthrie, 1991). My suggestion is that the unusual plasticity of the olfactory bulb compensates for the receptor turnover in the following way. As receptor cells are gradually renewed, remaining cells support a continuity of perception while the circuitry of the bulb "trains" the connections of the new cells to identify odors correctly. The random-access memory organization of the bulb thus permits a continuous accommodation for the turnover of inputs.

Olfactory Identification and Memory

Finally, getting to issues of odor identification and memory, I have two superficially contradictory observations. First, in the absence of other contextual cues, such as the sight of an odorous object, olfactory identification is very poor. Thus, humans often misidentify highly familiar odors when required to do so using only olfactory cues. In our own work, we found that normal subjects often mistake the odors of lemon and orange when only olfactory cues are provided. Such common anecdotal observations have been confirmed by systematic investigations (Engen, 1982).

Standing in stark contrast to these findings is the often-cited observation that odor memories can be exceedingly powerful. Virtually everyone can relate an experience in which an unanticipated stench evoked memories about a city experienced in their youth, or a fragrant perfume brought forth strong memories associated with a long-forgotten romance. Accounts of this type typically reveal that the evoked memories include an entire period of one's life or various aspects of the environment surrounding the time associated with the odor. Combining these observations about odor identification and memory, perhaps odors have the capacity to evoke memories of the context in which they were acquired even though they are poor cues in evoking specific verbal labels.

Multimodal Convergence

The characterization of olfactory memory just given may be related to the last of the oddities of olfaction on my list: unlike other sensory modalities, odor processing does not converge with that of other senses until the final common paths into the entorhinal cortex, amygdala, and prefrontal area. By contrast, vision, audition, and somatosensation merge in temporal and parietal association areas of the neocortex well before these ultimate convergence sites. Indeed, the common processing of conventional sensory modalities includes a convergence in the verbal areas of the neocortex, but these areas are not accessed directly by the olfactory system.

I suggest the reason why we perform so poorly in verbal labeling of odors is precisely because the verbal neocortical connection is absent. Conversely, perhaps odors are such good cues for evoking contextual memories because they have a more immediate access to the prefrontal and limbic convergence sites where contexts are formed. Following on these musings about the odd facts of olfactory perception and circuitry, the next sections will attempt to provide more solid evidence regarding the lessons olfaction may carry for one of these higher stages of sensory processing.

ODOR MEMORY AND OLFACTORY-HIPPOCAMPAL PROCESSING

The other half of this chapter concerns the higher-order processing of odor representations, particularly those accomplished by the hippocampus. In 1947 Brodal crushed the long-standing view that the hippocampus was a part of the olfactory brain, or rhinencephalon, showing that it has myriad connections with many brain areas. Since then it has become abundantly clear that the hippocampus processes information from many input sources (Deacon et al, 1983; Eichenbaum, Stewart, and Morris, 1990). Nevertheless, converging data from neuroanatomical, physiological, and behavioral studies indicate that the olfactory system projects heavily onto and has especially immediate access to the hippocampal system. This suggests that the olfactory-hippocampal pathway may be particularly useful for explorations of sensory-limbic interactions leading to the higher-order coding of perceptual information. The intimate anatomical associations between the olfactory and hippocampal systems are paralleled by the strong influence of olfactory processing over the physiological activity in the hippocampus both at the level of rhythmic electroencephalograph (EEG) activity and at the level of neuronal firing patterns, and by the critical role played by the hippocampal system in odor-guided learning and memory. In the spirit of a "renaissance of the rhinencephalon," I will argue that olfaction is a particularly advantageous model system for studies of sensory processing by the hippocampus.

Coherent Sensory-Limbic Activity

A pronounced rhythm dominates both EEG and unit activity throughout the nonprimate mammalian limbic system during exploratory activity, including that associated with learning. This pattern of electrical activity is known as theta rhythm because it lies mainly within the theta band (actual range 5–12 Hz). Hippocampal theta is initiated by activity in the pontine reticular formation (Vertes, 1981), and the pacemaker for its rhythm appears to be in the medial septum (Gray, 1971; Winson, 1978). The theta rhythm coincides with a cycle of neuronal excitability (Rudell, Fox, and Ranck, 1980), suggesting that hippocampal processing may occur in discrete processing periods akin to clock cycles in digital computers. Historically, concern has been expressed about the significance of theta rhythm across species, because earlier work failed to identify prominent slow wave activity in primates. However, a recent study revealed a clear pattern of 7- to 9-Hz rhythmic activity in the monkey hippocampus; this EEG pattern has the same laminar profile, sensitivity to pharmacological manipulation, and correlation with movement as the theta activity described in nonprimates (Stewart and Fox, 1990).

Hippocampal theta is pronounced during behaviors associated with spontaneous investigatory behavior (Vanderwolf et al, 1975), suggesting its appearance reflects hippocampal information processing. For example, Macrides et al (1982) explored the degree to which the occurrence and cyclic aspects of theta rhythm relate to specific events in learning by training rats in an odor-discrimination task. The animals were required to repeat a behavioral sequence that effectively separated a relatively high-frequency theta component (peak 7–9 Hz) associated with locomotory approach movements from a lower-frequency theta component (peak 6–8 Hz) that occurred reliably during odor sampling. Rats typically investigated an odor cue with a bout of three to five sniffs synchronized to the continuing theta rhythm (figures 9.2A and 9.2B). Furthermore, the phase relationship of sniff cycles and theta rhythm varied with the dominant sniff frequency such that sniff bouts held a preferred latency relationship with the continuing theta; sniff cycles tended to lead theta by about 140 msec (or about one cycle at 7 Hz). The reliability of this relationship varied with training such that synchronization was maximum just before the animal reached accurate performance in the discrimination and just after a reversal of odor valences ensued. These findings suggest that the sensory and motor phenomena associated with acquisition of relevant stimuli are engaged with the internal cycle of hippocampal processing during the analysis of cues critical to discriminative performance.

Taking these coherent patterns to the cellular level, we examined the firing patterns of CA1 pyramidal cells in rats performing different types of odor-discrimination tasks. In each task we identified a population of cells that fired selectively when rats sampled the odors and prepared to make their behavioral response (Eichenbaum et al, 1986; Otto and Eichenbaum, 1992b; Wiener, Paul, and Eichenbaum, 1989). Moreover, the activity of the cells was typically time locked to the continuing sniffing and hippocampal theta

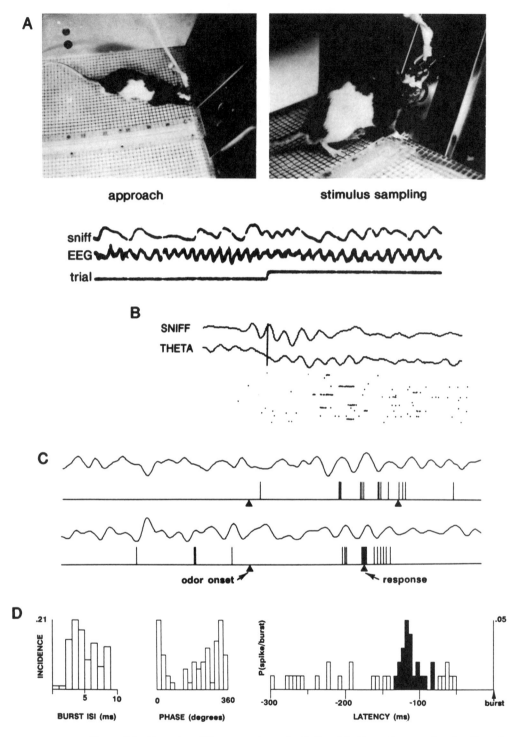

Figure 9.2 Examples of hippocampal neural activity related to performance in odor discrimination. (A) Photographs of a rat approaching (left) and sniffing at (right) the odor stimulus port. Note synchronization of the inhalation cycle and theta rhythm beginning at trial onset. (B) Sniffing, hippocampal theta, and CA1 unit activity (raster display) time locked to the peak of the first sniff after odor onset. (C) Theta rhythm and unit spike activity during odor sampling on two example trials. The observed pattern of multiple spike bursts paced and phase locked to theta is called theta bursting. (D) Averaging across all trials, histograms show, respectively, periodicity of spikes in bursts, burst position in relation to theta phase, and latency of spike activity preceding each burst. (From Eichenbaum et al, 1992.)

rhythm (figures 9.2B and 9.2C). At an even more detailed level of characterization, the synchronized activity of CA1 neurons involved bursts of action potentials sharply time locked to the continuing theta rhythm.

Several investigators exploited the observation of the bursting patterns of hippocampal cells associated with theta activity to develop paradigms for studying basic phenomena of synaptic plasticity in the hippocampus. Their results indicate that hippocampal long-term potentiation (LTP) is induced preferentially by electrical stimulation that is based on three separate but related patterns of afferent activation. The LTP in CA1 is preferentially induced by high-frequency bursts of stimulation (4 pulses at 100 Hz) repeated at 5 to 10 Hz (Larson, Wong, and Lynch, 1986), and can be induced by a single burst if another burst (Larson and Lynch, 1986) or single pulse (Rose and Dunwiddie, 1986) precedes that burst by 130 to 200 msec (i.e., at latencies that parallel frequencies of 5–7 Hz). Finally, patterned stimulation is most effective in inducing LTP in dentate gyrus when delivered at the peak of dentate theta rhythm (Pavlides et al, 1988). Together, these data suggest that brief episodes of high-frequency stimulation, when applied in the appropriate temporal relationship to prior activity and to continuing theta rhythm, can reliably enhance synaptic efficacy in a brain area critical to the formation of certain types of memory.

Our examination of the firing patterns of putative hippocampal CA1 pyramidal cells (Ranck, 1973) in rats engaged in learning hippocampal-dependent spatial and olfactory tasks revealed that all three of these characteristics of patterned stimulation, together optimal for hippocampal LTP induction, occur simultaneously and selectively during episodes of mnemonic processing (Otto et al, 1991a). We confirmed that CA1 pyramidal cells discharge in high-frequency bursts, phase locked to the positive peak of the dentate theta rhythm (figures 9.2C and 9.2D). Furthermore, these bursts were preceded by neural activity preferentially at intervals corresponding to the theta rhythm. Of importance, these patterns emerged only during significant behavioral events associated with likely periods of stimulus analysis, selection, or storage in during odor-discrimination performance. Thus the optimum conditions for inducing hippocampal LTP indeed are present when animals actively engage hippocampal processing for putative mnemonic functions.

Coherent activity associated with theta bursting appears to pervade the hippocampal cell population. Furthermore, our initial observations suggest that subsets of hippocampal cells achieve near-synchronous activity related to particular phases of theta rhythm. Evidence for this possibility came from a study in which long-term recordings were made in behaving rats using a 24-channel, printed-circuit microelectrode (Kuperstein, Eichenbaum, and VanDeMark, 1986; figure 9.3). We were able to record and isolate the activity of up to 14 cells simultaneously across an area of less than 1 mm in these rats as they performed various behaviors, including sleeping and exploratory activity (figure 9.3A). The firing of most cells was strongly related to the theta rhythm, although all cells did not have the same preferred phase (figure 9.3B).

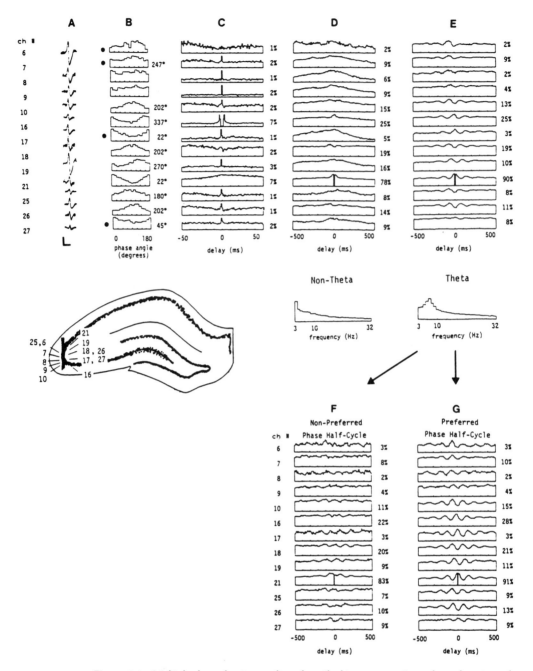

Figure 9.3 Multiple-channel unit recordings from the hippocampus. Inset shows locations of recording sites in the CA3 area of the hippocampus. (A) Unit waveforms at each site. (B) Normalized firing rate relative to theta phase recorded in the dentate gyrus. (C) Fine time resolution cross-correlation of firing synchronized to target channel 16. (D and E) Coarse time resolution cross-correlation of firing synchronized to target channel 21 during theta and nontheta states, respectively, as defined by power spectra below each column. (F and G) Coarse time resolution cross-correlation of firing synchronized to target channel 21 during preferred and nonpreferred firing theta half-cycles for the target cell.

To examine the coherent activity of the cell population, we performed numerous pairwise cross-correlations on the frequency of spikes using different cells as targets to which the activity of all other cells were correlated. Analyses focused at high temporal resolution indicated a considerable degree of coactivation of hippocampal neurons across the population (figure 9.3C). In addition, at lower temporal resolution aimed at revealing patterns associated with theta rhythm, in one of these analyses the activity of a large fraction of the cells was coherent around the theta rhythm. These patterns were most pronounced when the sample of unit activity was restricted to period of intense theta (figures 9.3D and 9.3E). When further selections were performed, such that the activity of all cells was compared for the phase of theta in which the target cell preferred to fire, coherence was even stronger (figures 9.3F and 9.3G). Moreover, during such periods of firing, distinct coherent patterns were observed for subsets of cells firing together associated with different phases of continuing theta rhythm. Thus, for example, figure 9.3G indicates that the cell in channel 17 fired coherently with the target cell in channel 21, but cells in channels 6, 7, 8, 9, 10, 18, 25, and 26 fired at a different phase coherently, whereas channels 16 and 19 may represent yet another coherent grouping. Perhaps these distinct cell ensembles reflect the coherent populations Singer predicted might encode the binding of specific perceptual wholes (this volume).

Hippocampal Coding of Sensory Information

We attempted to understand the nature of odor coding in hippocampal neurons as revealed from two lines of research. These experiments involved complementary neuropsychological characterizations of the consequences of damage to the hippocampal system, and observations on the functional correlates of hippocampal neural activity in animals performing odor learning and memory tasks (Eichenbaum, Otto, and Cohen, 1992; Eichenbaum and Otto, 1993).

The first set of studies consisted of neuropsychological assessments of odor learning in animals with damage to the hippocampal system. They were focused on the effects of transection of the fornix, the fiber bundle that supports connections between the hippocampus and subcortical structures including the septum. Notably, fornix lesions eliminate hippocampal theta rhythm, which is normally generated by pacer cells in the septum and transmitted to the hippocampus by way of the fornix. The studies revealed that this and other forms of damage to the hippocampal system do not produce anosmia, but do result in a pattern of odor learning and memory impairment that suggests ways in which odor and other sensory information are processed by the hippocampus.

Our investigations were guided by findings on human amnesia indicating that this syndrome involves a selective deficit in declarative memory, the memory for everyday facts and events that can be brought to conscious recollection and are subject to verbal or other explicit means of expression (Cohen and Eichenbaum, 1993). By contrast, procedural memory is intact even in dense amnesics. Procedural memory is characterized as the non-conscious acquisition of a bias or adaptation that is typically revealed only by implicit measures of performance. These characterizations of impaired and spared memory capacities in amnesia present a formidable challenge for the study of declarative memory in animals. However, other more detailed descriptions gave us the opportunity to develop objective definitions of declarative memory that could be applied equally well to animals and humans.

Cohen (1984) offered descriptions that could be helpful toward this goal. He suggested that "...a declarative code permits the ability to *compare and contrast* information from different processes or processing systems; and it enables the ability to *make inferences* from and generalizations across facts derived from multiple processing sources. Such a common declarative code thereby provides the basis for access to facts acquired during the course of experiences and for conscious recollection of the learning experiences themselves" (p. 97, italics added). Conversely, procedural learning was characterized as the acquisition of particular skills, adaptations, and biases and that such "procedural knowledge is tied to and expressible only through activation of the particular processing structures or procedures engaged by the learning tasks" (p. 96).

We exploited two distinctions revealed in these characterizations during our development of assessments of declarative and procedural memory that may be applicable to animal studies. First, declarative memory is distinguished by its role in comparing and contrasting items in memory; procedural memory involves the facilitation of particular routines for which no such comparisons are executed. Second, declarative memory is distinguished by its capacity to support inferential use of memories in novel situations; procedural memory supports only alterations in performance that can be characterized as rerunning more smoothly the neural processes in which they were acquired.

We extended these distinctions to make contact with the literature of hippocampal function in animals, resulting in a proposal for the representational mechanisms that might underlie declarative memory. Based on this general aspect of hippocampal-dependent memory, our hypothesis is that the hippocampal system supports a relational representation of items in memory, and that the individual representations for those items are hippocampal independent (Eichenbaum, Otto, and Cohen, 1992). Furthermore, we suggested that a critical property of the hippocampal-dependent memory system is its representational flexibility, a quality that permits inferential use of memories in novel situations. Conversely, according to our view, hippocampal-independent memories are isolated in that they are encoded only within the brain modules in which perceptual or motor processing is engaged during learning. These individual representations are inflexible in that they can be revealed only through reactivation of modules within the restrictive range of stimuli and situations in which the original learning occurred. One might expect such individual representations to support the acquisition of general procedures that are performed consistently across training trials; individual representations should also support the acquisition of specific information that does not require comparison and consequent relational representation.

Our investigations on the role of the hippocampal system in declarative memory exploited rats' excellent learning and memory capacities in odor-discrimination learning (Eichenbaum, Fagan, and Cohen, 1986; Eichenbaum et al, 1988; Eichenbaum, Mathews, and Cohen, 1989). The learning ability of intact rats versus rats with fornix transection was evaluated in variations of the odor-discrimination learning paradigm, assessing the capacity for relational representation by manipulating the demand for comparison and representation of relations among identical odor cues (Eichenbaum et al, 1988). In a simultaneous discrimination task, two odor cues were presented at the same time and in close spatial juxtaposition; the discriminative response required selecting between equivalent left and right choices. Under these training conditions, rats with fornix lesions were severely and persistently impaired on a series of different odor-discrimination problems (figure 9.4). Alternatively, in a successive discrimination task, odors were presented separately across trials, hindering comparison among items, and the response required only completing or discontinuing the stimulus-sampling behavior, thus eliminating the response choice. In striking contrast to the first results, under these training conditions, rats with fornix lesions were superior to normal rats in acquiring the same series of discrimination problems that they had failed to learn under other task demands (Eichenbaum, Fagan, and Cohen, 1986; Otto et al, 1991b; Staubli, Ivy, and Lynch, 1984).

More recently, we examined the performance of animals with hippocampal system damage in an odor-guided, delayed, nonmatch to sample task (Otto and Eichenbaum, 1992a) that is similar in memory demands to the object-cued task used successfully in studies of the hippocampal system in primates. In this task odor cues were presented sequentially, just as in the successive discrimination task, but the availability of reward was contingent on the relationship between previous and current items; the appropriate response to the odor on a particular trial was rewarded only if it was different from (i.e., a nonmatch with) that on the previous trial. Under these training conditions rats with lesions of the entorhinal and perirhinal cortex were impaired on odor memory when the delays between odor repetitions were sufficiently long. Our interpretation of these findings is that severe impairment, transient impairment, or even facilitation may be observed under different task demands, even with the identical stimulus materials. Moreover, the differences in performance by rats with hippocampal system damage can be related to the demand for stimulus and response comparison.

To assess the capacity for representational flexibility in normal rats and rats with hippocampal system damage, we pursued a follow-up experiment based on the simultaneous discrimination task (Eichenbaum, Mathews, and Cohen, 1989). Our investigation exploited a surprising finding in the results

ODOR DISCRIMINATION

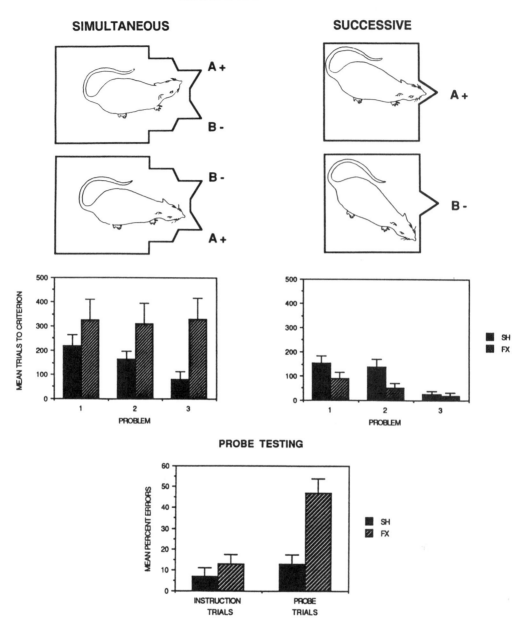

Figure 9.4 Performance of sham-operated (SH) rats and rats with lesions of the fornix (FX) on simultaneous and successive odor-discrimination learning and probe trials. Top panels illustrate the format for presentation of odors (labeled A and B) on different trials. Middle panels show learning scores for three sequentially presented discrimination problems in both formats. Bottom panel shows performance during probe trials on two successfully acquired simultaneous discrimination problems; repetitions of the instruction trials involved pairings of odors identical to that during training, but probe trials involved mispairings of rewarded and nonrewarded odors from different problems. (From Eichenbaum et al, 1988, 1989.)

from that training condition; although rats were generally impaired on this task, they succeeded in learning some of the discrimination problems at least as rapidly as normal animals. To understand why they occasionally succeeded, and to explore the nature of memory representation when they did succeed, we trained yoked pairs of normal and rats with fornix lesions on a series of simultaneous odor-discrimination problems until the rat with the fornix lesion in each pair had acquired two problems within the normal range of scores. Then we assessed the flexibility of their representations by challenging them with probe trials composed of familiar odors mispaired in combinations not previously experienced.

According to our notion of relational representation, normal animals encode all the odor stimuli presented both within and across trials using an organized scheme that would support comparisons among odors not previously experienced together. Conversely, we postulated that the representation of rats with hippocampal system damage would not support recognition of the separate elements within each compound. To test these predictions, we intermixed within a series of trials on two different instruction problems occasional probe trials composed of a mispaired rewarded odor from one problem and the nonrewarded odor from the other. Both normal rats and rats with fornix lesions continued to perform well on the trials composed of the odor pairings used on instruction trials, and normal rats performed accurately on the probe trials (figure 9.4, bottom). By contrast, rats with fornix lesions performed at chance levels on the probe trials when they were introduced, as if presented with novel stimuli.

A further analysis focusing on the response latencies of animals performing the simultaneous discrimination provided additional evidence that the nature of learned odor representations was abnormal in rats with hippocampal system damage; this analysis also provided insight into how they succeeded in learning some simultaneous discrimination problems. We determined that each rat with a fornix lesion had a quantitatively shorter average response latency than each normal rat, even though all rats performed consistently at high accuracy and showed the speed-accuracy tradeoff typical of reaction time measures. Furthermore, rats with fornix lesions also had an abnormal pattern of reaction times (figure 9.5). Each normal rat had a bimodal distribution of response latencies, and each of the two modes was associated with one of the positions where the rewarded odor was presented and response executed. This pattern of reaction times suggests that the rat consistently approached and sampled one odor port first, then either performed a nose-poke there, or approached and sampled the other odor port. By contrast, rats with fornix lesions had unimodal distribution of response latencies, and the pattern of their response latencies was the same regardless of odor and response positions.

Our interpretation of these results was that rats with hippocampal system damage sample the entire stimulus compound at once, requiring less time to complete the trial. On just those problems where different left-right

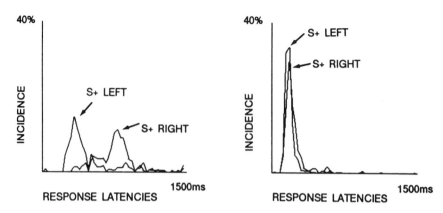

Figure 9.5 Response latencies (reactions times) for an example sham-operated rat (SH75) and an example rat with a fornix lesion (FX74) in simultaneous odor discrimination. Data are separated for trials on which the rewarded (S+) odor and the correct response was on the left or right stimulus port. (From Eichenbaum et al, 1989.)

combinations of the odors were distinguishable, they succeeded in learning an individual association for each odor compound and the appropriate response. Indeed, this account of representational strategies suggests that their performance was inflexible on our probe tests because novel mispairings of odors were perceived as unfamiliar odor compounds.

To support further the view that the hippocampus is involved in encoding stimulus relationships, and to understand how such information is encoded by the hippocampus, we recorded from hippocampal cells in rats performing in the same odor-discrimination tasks employed in our lesion experiments (Eichenbaum et al, 1986; Otto and Eichenbaum, 1992b; Wiener, Paul, and Eichenbaum, 1989). In each task we found cells that fired time locked to nearly every significant behavioral event. For example, some cells fired as the animal approached the area where odor stimuli were sampled, others fired selectively during odor sampling or response generation, and yet others fired during reward retrieval. In each task we focused our analyses on a subset of cells that fired selectively when rats sampled the odors and prepared to make the behavioral response.

Some of these cells were activated throughout the stimulus-sampling period on all types of trials, beginning to fire at onset of the cues and ceasing to fire abruptly at onset of the response. Other cells were much more selective; they increased firing dependent on the conjunction or combination of several odors presented either in different spatial configurations or temporal sequences. In simultaneous discrimination, these cells fired maximally only during sampling of a specific left-right configuration of a particular pair of odors (figure 9.6A). In successive odor discrimination, these cells fired maximally only during sampling of the rewarded odor preceded by the

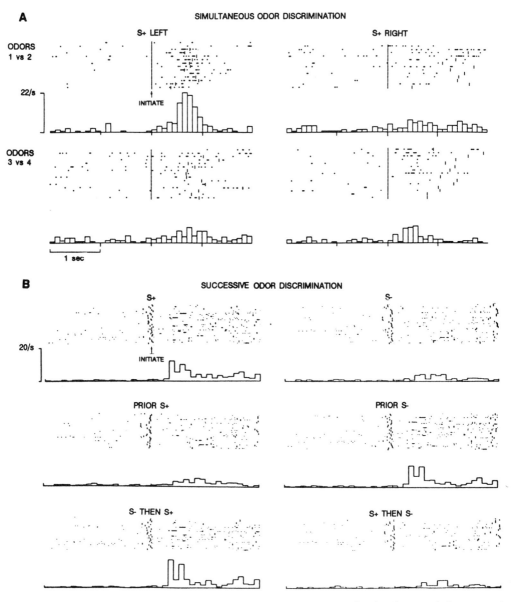

Figure 9.6 Raster displays and cumulative histograms of spikes from single hippocampal neurons activated during stimulus sampling during performance of different versions of the odor-discrimination task. In the simultaneous odor discrimination, unit activity is time locked to the trial initiation and onset of odor presentation. (From Wiener et al, 1989.) The unit response is greatest on trials when the stimulus configuration was odor 1 on the left and odor 2 on the right. In the successive discrimination, unit activity is time locked to the peak of the first inhalation after odor presentation. (From Eichenbaum et al, 1986.) Note unit activity time locked to odor onset. The unit response is larger when the current stimulus is S+ rather than S−, and when the stimulus on the immediately prior trial was S− rather than S+, and maximal on when there is an S− trial followed by an S+ trial.

nonrewarded odor on the previous trial; that is, their firing was dependent on the sequence of odor presentations (figure 9.6B). Thus, the activity of a subset of hippocampal output neurons reflects the relevant stimulus relations in each variant of the odor-discrimination paradigm, even in variants of the task in which the hippocampal system is not required for performance.

Finally, we more recently recorded from hippocampal output neurons while rats performed our odor-guided, delayed, nonmatch to sample task. In this task, some cells fired selectively on trials in which the odor cue was a non-match and others fired only when the cue was a match; these responses occurred consistently regardless of the odors involved across trials. Thus, unit activity reflected the outcome of the comparison process, the relationship between two odor cues abstracted from the items on which the comparison was based.

HIPPOCAMPAL REPRESENTATION AND THE BINDING PROBLEM

Several other chapters of this volume discuss the so-called binding problem. The problem, as it applies to early levels of sensory processing, refers to how stimulus elements that overlap or are separated throughout the sensory landscape are sorted and combine to form perceptually distinct complex stimuli (see by Ramachandron, Singer, and Logothetis, this volume). I suggest that a similar problem must be solved at the level of the hippocampal system, although at this higher stage of processing the binding problem is distinguished from that of lower levels in two ways.

First, the landscape includes information from all sensory modalities. Indeed, the afferents to the hippocampal system may be better conceived as functionally rather than perceptually defined inputs. By this characterization I mean that the cortical areas that project to the hippocampal system contain multimodal information that defines the meaning of a stimulus according to functional designations of cortical modules. Nevertheless, for the purposes of this discussion, it is simpler to think of inputs to the hippocampal system as perceptually distinct elements that are the products of sensory binding processes that occur at earlier cortical levels. Second, the kind of binding I suggest occurs in the hippocampal system is much more "conceptual" than "perceptual." It is, nevertheless, a real issue in binding such that the question I am asking is how perceptually distinct items are bound by association in memory.

Our recent data on this issue with regard to odor memory come from studies on the effects of hippocampal system damage on the learning of paired associates; that is, the learning of arbitrary associations between perceptually distinct stimuli. Our studies involving the development of a paradigm for paired associate learning in rats demonstrated a striking dissociation between the kind of binding functions performed by the hippocampus versus those that might be mediated by the surrounding parahippocampal region (Bunsey and Eichenbaum, 1993a, b).

The paired associate task typically used for humans involves studying a list of arbitrarily paired words followed by testing in which the subject is cued with the first item of each pair and must recall the second item. We designed an analogous task using odor stimuli and a recognition format that required rats to distinguish appropriate odor pairings from a large number of foils. Animals were trained to sample a stimulus sequence consisting of two odors separated by a period when airflow was reversed to prevent stimulus blending (figure 9.7a). When the stimulus sequence was one of four arbitrarily assigned paired associates, approaching a water port was rewarded; no reward was given for water port responses to either of two types of foils (figure 9.7b). One type of foil involved odors taken from different paired associates and recombined to form 48 different mispairings. Distinguishing mispairings from paired associates thus required learning the arbitrarily assigned relations among items. The other type of foil involved 64 different nonrelational sequences that included 1 of 4 odors that was never associated with reward. Distinguishing nonrelational pairings from paired associates did not require relational processing because these sequences could be identified by single never-rewarded items.

Both sham-operated rats and rats with parahippocampal area lesions rapidly learned to distinguish nonrelational pairs from paired associates (figure 9.7c). In addition, normal rats gradually learned to distinguish paired associates from odor mispairings. By contrast, rats with parahippocampal lesions could not learn to distinguish paired associates from mispairings, even when given nearly twice as many training trials as normal rats. Examination of the pattern of increments in performance during learning also indicated qualitative differences in performance on the two types of foils. Both groups rapidly acquired appropriate responses to the nonrelational sequences, and normal rats incrementally learned to distinguish mispairs from paired associates. Rats with parahippocampal lesions, by contrast, remained near chance levels of performance with respect to mispairs throughout testing. Taken together, these observations indicate a specific deficit in learning the appropriate stimulus relationships after parahippocampal lesions.

In a subsequent study we evaluated the role of the hippocampus itself in paired associate learning using the same task. In this study, selective neurotoxic lesions of the hippocampus significantly affected the learning. However, in contrast to the severe impairment seen after parahippocampal region lesions, hippocampal lesions resulted in a facilitation of the learning (figure 9.7d). This combination of findings indicates that the parahippocampal region and the hippocampus play important but different and likely interactive roles in paired associate learning. One possible explanation is that stimuli involved in a paired associate could be represented in two fundamentally different ways, one subserved by the hippocampus and another mediated by the parahippocampal region. First, the two stimuli could be represented as a unitized structures (Schacter, 1985) or configural cues (Sutherland and Rudy, 1989). This kind of representation is often made when stimuli are presented

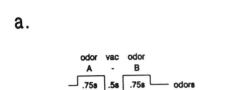

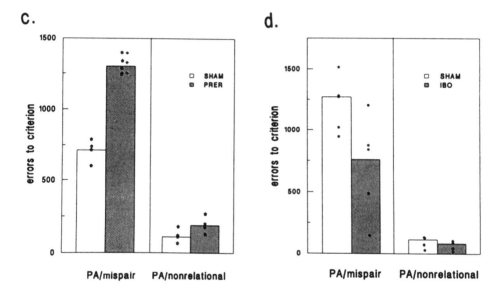

Figure 9.7 The odor-guided paired associate task. (From Bunsey and Eichenbaum, 1993a, b.) (a) The format of odor presentations. As the rat held its nose in the sniff port, odor A was presented for 0.75 second, followed by a blank interval when the air flow direction was reversed, followed by presentation of odor B. A correct response to the water port during or just after odor B presentation resulted in a water reward. (b) The list of four odor-paired associates presented in either order (with letters representing different odors), mispairs composed of the same eight odors, and nonrelational odor sequences that involved one of four other odors. (c) Performance of sham-operated rats and rats with lesions of that parahippocampal region (PRER) in distinguishing paired associates from mispairs (PA/mispair) and paired associates from nonrelational sequences (PA/nonrelational). (d) Performance of sham-operated rats and rats with selective neurotoxic lesions of hippocampus (IBO) in distinguishing paired associates from mispairs (PA/mispair) and paired associates from nonrelational sequences (PA/nonrelational).

simultaneously, such as when elements of a scene are combined to form a single compound cue. Unitized structures can also be formed when stimuli are presented successively, such as in the case of verbal idioms (e.g., "sour grapes," "small potatoes"; Schacter, 1985).

Recent evidence from both human amnesia and studies of animals with hippocampal damage (Eichenbaum et al, 1991) indicate that such learning may be accomplished in some circumstances even after damage to the hippocampus, but that this learning is rigid, or hyperspecific, in that memory for the elements of such unitized structures cannot be expressed in amnesic humans or animals with hippocampal damage. The representation of unitized structures of this type may be mediated by the parahippocampal region and, in the present case, can mediate the representation of odor pairs by compressing them as unitized or configural cues (Eichenbaum, Otto, and Cohen, 1994).

The second form of representation that could support paired associate learning involves encoding stimulus elements as perceptually distinct items organized within a network of memories in terms of assigned pairwise relations. Such a representation differs from learning unitized structures in that relational representation maintains the compositionality of the items; that is, encoding items both as perceptually distinct objects and as parts of larger scale scenes and events that capture the relevant relations between them. Such a representation also supports the expression of memories for odor elements and novel applications of knowledge about the relationships between them. The acquisition of such relational representations is proposed to be dependent on the hippocampus.

In normal paired associate learning, it is suggested that the hippocampus "wins" a competition between the representational strategies mediated by the hippocampus and parahippocampal regions and, consequently, odors are stored separately in terms of their pairing relationships. In rats with hippocampal damage, processing by the parahippocampal region and its connections with cortical areas remains intact, supporting performance based on the conceptual compression of perceptual distinct items and the storage of such unitized odor-pair representations. Indeed, our data indicate this form of representation is associated with abnormally rapid acquisition of this particular variant of the task. By contrast, after damage to the parahippocampal region neither the unitized nor the relational form of representation is intact. The ability of the parahippocampal region to make unitized representations is directly eliminated, and this lesion disconnects the hippocampus with cortical inputs carrying the odor information, also effectively preventing the hippocampus from mediating a relational representation of odor pairings. Continuing research is aimed at distinguishing these forms of representation through tests for flexible expression of paired associate memories, akin to our approach with discrimination learning described above. Relevant preliminary data are now at hand, coming from novel behavioral paradigms that exploit natural situations in which rats use their memory flexibly. Bunsey and

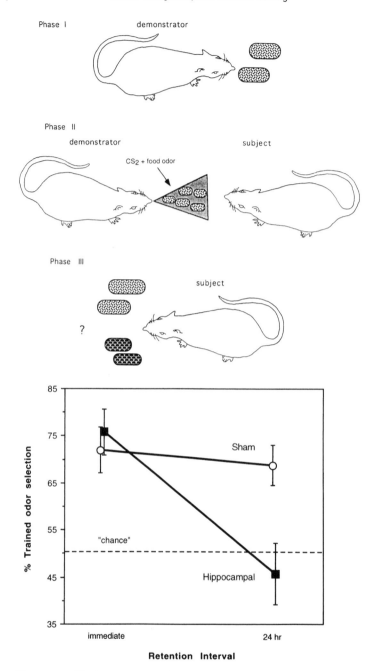

Figure 9.8 The hippocampus and memory for social transmission of food preferences. In this task a demonstrator rat is given a distinctively scented food (Phase I), and then presented to an experimental subject for a brief period of social interaction. During this experience subjects associate two odors carried on the demonstrator's breath, the distinctive food odor and carbon disulfide (CS_2), a natural constituent of rats' breath (Galef, 1990; Phase II). To test memory for the food odor-CS_2 association, subjects are presented with the same food or another distinctively scented food, either immediately or after a 24-hr delay (Phase III). Normal rats subsequently show a strong selection preference for the trained food odor in both tests. Similar to the pattern of impairment in human amnesics, rats with selective hippocampal damage show intact short-term memory, but completely forget the association within 24 hours.

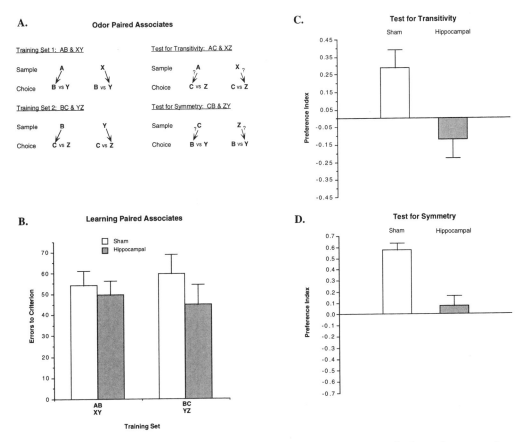

Figure 9.9 The hippocampus, odor paired associate learning, and inferential responses from memory. (A) Paired associate training and probe tests. Each training and testing trial consisted of two phases. In the sample phase, the subject was presented with a cup containing a scented mixture of sand and ground rat chow with a buried reward. In the choice phase, two scented choices were presented. Both choice items involved odors that were different from the sample odor, and which of them was correct depended on the identity of the sample odor. Initially subjects were trained on two sets of paired associates with overlapping elements. Then two types of probes were presented to test for flexible access to these memory representations. In the probe for transitivity, subjects were presented with trials comprising a sample odor from set 1 and unbaited choice odors from set 2. Transitivity was indexed by preferential digging in the choice cup associated only indirectly with the sample. In the test for symmetry trials on set 2 were re-presented, but now the sample and choice items were reversed, i.e., the former sample items were now the choices and vice versa. (B) Hippocampal lesions did not block the acquisition of odor paired associates. (C) Controls showed strong transitivity across the sets with a preference index corresponding approximately to 2:1 digging in favor of choice items indirectly associated with the presented sample (see panel A). By contrast, rats with hippocampal damage were severely impaired in that they showed no evidence of transitivity. (D) Controls had a preference index corresponding approximately to 3:1 choices in the direction of the symmetrical association (see panel A). By contrast, rats with hippocampal damage again were severely impaired, showing no significant capacity for symmetry.

Eichenbaum (1995) showed that selective hippocampal cell loss does not affect acquisition but blocks long-term expression of a naturally acquired association between odors (figure 9.8). A central component of their experimental paradigm was that learning involved mere exposure to stimulus pairings in a social situation, whereas memory was expressed in a quite a different situation to guide food selection. In addition, Bunsey and Eichenbaum (1996) used a more formal testing paradigm that exploited rats' natural foraging behavior to examine flexible expression of learned stimulus associations. As observed in our earlier studies and consistent with previous reports of intact acquisition of stimulus-stimulus associations in animals with hippocampal damage (Cho and Kesner, 1995; Murray, Gaffan, and Mishkin, 1993), rats with selective hippocampal cell loss successfully acquired sets of paired associates. However, the same rats failed when challenged to identify indirect relations between the items, specifically *transitive* relations between never-paired items that shared a common association and *symmetrical* relations for stimulus pairings presented in reversed order (figure 9.9). These findings strongly support my suggestion that the hippocampus itself is critical for the establishment of a relational representation.

In closing, a clear picture emerges from this evidence on different forms of binding of perceptual elements by components of the hippocampal system. In the parahippocampal region perceptual elements may be bound by a conceptual fusion or compression into a single configural representation. This can involve multimodal elements that occur simultaneously or even in sequence, but they are bound into a single composite encoding. By contrast, it appears the job of the hippocampus is to prevent the representational compression when perceptual elements and their relations may need to be recognized separately at a later time. In this situation the hippocampus presumably plays its role by preventing the representational compression and instead organizing a set of separate cortical representations according to their relevant relationships among the items. In this way representations are bound only by the memory network in which they reside. These complementary forms of "binding" in memory can substantially affect the nature of memory representation and subsequent memory performance.

ACKNOWLEDGMENTS

This work was supported by NIA grant AG09973, NIMH grant MH52090, and ONR grant N00014-94-1-0131.

REFERENCES

Bower JM. (1991). Piriform cortex and olfactory object recognition. In: *Olfaction: A model system for computational neuroscience.* JL Davis, H Eichenbaum, eds. MIT Press, Cambridge, 265–286.

Bunsey M, Eichenbaum H. (1993a). Paired associate learning in rats: Critical involvement of the parahippocampal region. *Behav Neurosci* 107:740–747.

Bunsey M, Eichenbaum H. (1993b). Selective hippocampal lesions facilitate performance in a paired associate task in rats. *Soc Neurosci Abstr* 19:358.

Bunsey M, Eichenbaum H. (1995). Selective damage to the hippocampal region blocks long term retention of a natural and nonspatial stimulus-stimulus association. *Hippocampus* 5:546–556.

Bunsey M, Eichenbaum H. (1996). Conservation of hippocampal memory function in rats and humans. *Nature* 379:255–257.

Cain WS, Engen T. (1969). Olfactory adaptation and the scaling of odor intensity. In: *Olfaction and taste* III. C Pfaffman, ed. Rockefeller University Press, New York.

Cho YH, Kesner RP. (1995). Relational object association learning in rats with hippocampal lesions. *Behav Brain Res* 67:91–98.

Cohen NJ. (1984). Preserved learning capacity in amnesia: Evidence for multiple memory systems. In: *The neuropsychology of memory*. N Butters, LR Squire, eds. Guilford Press, New York, 83–103.

Cohen NJ, Eichenbaum H. (1993). *Memory, amnesia, and the hippocampal system*. MIT Press, Cambridge.

Deacon TW, Eichenbaum H, Rosenberg P, Eckman KW. (1983). Afferent connections of the perirhinal cortex in the rat. *J Comp Neurol* 220:168–190.

Eichenbaum H. (1993). Thinking about brain cell assemblies. *Science* 261:993–994.

Eichenbaum H, Clegg RA, Feeley A. (1983). A re-examination of functional subdivisions of the rodent prefrontal cortex. *Exp Neurol* 79:434–451.

Eichenbaum H, Cohen NJ, Otto T, Wible C. (1991). A snapshot without the album. *Brain Res Rev* 16:209–215.

Eichenbaum H, Eckmann KW, Shedlack KJ. (1980). Thalamocortical mechanisms in odor guided behavior. I. The effects of lesions on the mediodorsal nucleus and frontal cortex on olfactory discrimination in the rat. *Brain Behav Evol* 17:255–275.

Eichenbaum H, Fagan A, Cohen NJ. (1986). Normal olfactory discrimination learning set and facilitation of reversal learning after combined and separate lesions of the fornix and amygdala in rats: Implications for preserved learning in amnesia. *J Neurosci* 6:1876–1884.

Eichenbaum H, Fagan A, Mathews P, Cohen NJ. (1988). Hippocampal system dysfunction and odor discrimination learning in rats: Impairment or facilitation depending on representational demands. *Behav Neurosci* 102:3531–3542.

Eichenbaum H, Kuperstein M, Fagan A, Nagode J. (1986). Cue-sampling and goal-approach correlates of hippocampal unit activity in rats performing an odor discrimination task. *J Neurosci* 7:716–732.

Eichenbaum H, Mathews P, Cohen NJ. (1989). Further studies of hippocampal representation during odor discrimination learning. *Behav Neurosci* 103:1207–1216.

Eichenbaum H, Otto T. (1993). Where perception meets memory: Functional coding in the hippocampus. In: *Brain mechanisms of perception and memory: From neuron to behavior*. T Ono, LR Squire, RE Raicle, D Perrett, M Fukuda, eds. Oxford University Press, New York, 301–329.

Eichenbaum H, Otto T, Cohen NJ. (1992). The hippocampus—What does it do? *Behav Neural Biol* 57:2–36.

Eichenbaum H, Otto T, Cohen NJ. (1994). Two functional components of the hippocampal memory system. *Brain Behav Sci* 17:449–518.

Eichenbaum H, Stewart C, Morris RGM. (1990). Hippocampal representation in spatial learning. *J Neurosci* 10:331–339.

Engen T. (1982). *The perception of odors*. Academic Press, New York.

Farbman AI. (1992). *Cell biology of olfaction*. Cambridge University Press, Cambridge.

Galef BG. (1990). An adaptionist perspective on social learning, social feeding, and social foraging in Norway rats. In: *Contemporary issues in comparative psychology*. Dewsbury DA, ed. Sinauer, Sunderland, Ma, 55–79.

Granger R, Staubli U, Ambros-Ingerson J, Lynch G. (1991). Specific behavioral predictions from simulations of the olfactory system. In: *Olfaction: A model system for computational neuroscience*. JL Davis, H Eichenbaum, eds. MIT Press, Cambridge, 251–264.

Gray JA. (1971). Medial septal lesions, hippocampal theta rhythm, and the control of vibrissal movement in the freely moving rat. *EEG Clin Neurophysiol* 30:189–197.

Haberly LB. (1985). Neural circuitry in the olfactory cortex: Anatomy and functional implications. *Chem Senses* 10:219–238.

Ketchum KL, Haberly LB. (1991). Fast oscillations and disperative propagation in olfactory cortex and other cortical areas: A functional hypothesis. In: *Olfaction: A model system for computational neuroscience*. JL Davis, H Eichenbaum, eds. MIT Press, Cambridge, 69–100.

Keverne EB. (1987). Pheremones. In: *Encyclopedia of neuroscience*. Vol II. G Adelman, ed. Birkhauser, Boston, 944–946.

Kuperstein M, Eichenbaum H, VanDeMark T. (1986). Neural group properties in the rat hippocampus during the theta rhythm. *Exp Brain Res* 61:438–442.

Larson J, Lynch G. (1986). Induction of synaptic potentiation in hippocampus by patterned stimulation involves two events. *Science* 232:985–988.

Larson J, Wong D, Lynch G. (1986). Patterned stimulation at the theta frequency is optimal for the induction of hippocampal long-term potentiation. *Brain Res* 368:347–350.

Leon M, Wilson DA, Guthrie KM. (1991). Plasticity in the developing olfactory system. In: *Olfaction: A model system for computational neuroscience*. JL Davis, H Eichenbaum, eds. MIT Press, Cambridge, 121–140.

Leonard CM. (1972). Connections of the mediodorsal nuclei. *Brain Behav Evol* 6:524–541.

Lynch G. (1986). *Synapses, circuits, and the beginnings of memory*. MIT Press, Cambridge.

Macrides F, Eichenbaum H, Forbes WB. (1982). Temporal relationship between sniffing and limbic theta rhythm during odor discrimination reversal learning. *J Neurosci* 2:1705–1717.

Murray EA, Gaffan D, Mishkin M. (1993). Neural substrates of visual stimulus-stimulus association in rhesus monkeys. *J Neurosci* 13:4549–4561.

Nauta WJH. (1972). Neural associations of the frontal cortex. *Acta Neurobiol Exp* 32:125–140.

Otto T, Eichenbaum H, Wiener SI, Wible CG. (1991a). Learning-related patterns of CA1 spike trains parallel stimulation parameters optimal for inducing hippocampal long term potentiation. *Hippocampus* 1:181–192.

Otto T, Schottler F, Staubli U, Eichenbaum H, Lynch G. (1991b). The hippocampus and olfactory discrimination learning: Effects of entorhinal cortex lesions on learning-set acquisition and on odor memory in a successive-cue, go/no-go task. *Behav Neurosci* 105:111–119.

Otto T, and Eichenbaum H. (1992a). Complementary roles of orbital prefrontal cortex and the perirhinal-entorhinal cortices in an odor-guided delayed non-matching to sample task. *Behav Neurosci* 106:763–776.

Otto T, Eichenbaum H. (1992b). Neuronal activity in the hippocampus during delayed non-match to sample performance in rats: Evidence for hippocampal processing in recognition memory. *Hippocampus* 2:323–334.

Pavlides C, Greenstein YJ, Grudman M, Winson J. (1988). Long-term potentiation in the dentate gyrus is induced preferentially on the positive phase of theta rhythm. *Brain Res* 439:383–387.

Perrett DI, Mistlin AJ, Chitty AJ. (1987). Visual neurons responsive to faces. *Trends Neurosci* 10:358–364.

Price JL, Carmichael ST, Carnes KM, Clugnet M-C, Kuroda M, Ray JP. (1991). Olfactory input to the prefrontal cortex. In: *Olfaction: A model system for computational neuroscience*. JL Davis, H Eichenbaum, eds. MIT Press, Cambridge, 101–120.

Ranck JB Jr. (1973). Studies on single neurons in the dorsal hippocampal formation and septum in unrestrained rats. *Exp Neurol* 41:461–555.

Rose GM, Dunwiddie TV. (1986). Induction of hippocampal long-term potentiation using physiologically patterned stimulation. *Neurosci Lett* 69:244–248.

Rudell A, Fox S, Ranck JB Jr. (1980). Hippocampal excitability phase-locked to the theta rhythm in walking rats. *Exp Neurol* 68:87–96.

Schacter DL. (1985). Multiple forms of memory in humans and animals. In: *Memory systems of the brain*. NM Weinberger, JL McGaugh, G Lynch, eds. Guilford Press, New York, 351–380.

Shepherd GM. (1972). Synaptic organization of the mammalian olfactory bulb. *Physiol Rev* 52:864–917.

Shepherd GM. (1991). Computational structure of the olfactory system. In: *Olfaction: A model system for computational neuroscience*. JL Davis, H Eichenbaum, eds. MIT Press, Cambridge, 3–42.

Staubli U, Ivy G, Lynch G. (1984). Hippocampal denervation causes rapid forgetting of olfactory information in rats. *Proc Natl Acad Sci USA* 81:5885–5887.

Stewart M, Fox SE. (1990). Do septal neurons pace the hippocampal theta rhythm? *Trends Neurosci* 13:163–168.

Sutherland RJ, Rudy JW. (1989). Configural association theory: The role of the hippocampal formation in learning, memory, and amnesia. *Psychobiology* 17:129–144.

Vanderwolf CH, Kramis R, Gillespie LA, Bland BH. (1975). Hippocampal rhythmic slow activity and neocortical low-voltage fast activity: Relations to behavior. In: *The hippocampus*. Vol. 2. *Neurophysiology and behavior*. RL Isaacson, KH Pribram, eds. Plenum Press, New York, 101–128.

Vertes RP. (1981). An analysis of brain stem systems involved in hippocampal synchronization and desynchronization. *J Neurophysiol* 46:1140–1159.

Wiener SI, Paul CA, Eichenbaum H. (1989). Spatial and behavioral correlates of hippocampal neuronal activity. *J Neurosci* 9:2737–2763.

Winson J. (1978). Loss of hippocampal theta rhythm results in spatial memory deficit in the freely moving rat. *Science* 201:160–163.

10 Perceptual Interpretation and the Neurobiology of Perception

A. S. Bregman

Since the occasion of this volume is a philosophical one, I will situate my research on auditory perception in a more general framework. Many people ask what neuroscience can tell us about how the mind works. I would like to reverse this question and ask what the mind can tell us about the brain. In particular, I would like to examine the human capacity of perception, particularly auditory perception, and ask what sorts of neural mechanisms could perform the desired tasks.

What is perception? Many people have offered their views on this topic. Mine is a functional one: perception is knowing the world through the energy pattern received by the senses. This does not distinguish it from cognition, but I will leave that distinction for another time. All I want to say here is that the task of understanding the world puts some special requirements on the process of perception. These requirements arise from the nature of the world itself.

COMPOSITIONAL PROPERTY OF THE REAL WORLD

We live in a peculiar sort of universe in which the detailed objects and happenings that fill it are actually manifestations of general principles interacting with one another. For example, the spectrum of light reaching my visual system from the table in front of me is the result of many factors, including the distribution of energy in the light source, the fact that surfaces can reflect light, the smoothness of the surface, the absorptive properties of the surface, the fact that nearby objects cast shadows, the fact that the color of shadows depends on the color of the light reflected from nearby objects, the nature of human eyes, and so on. Another way to say this is that individual phenomena are generated by a composition of more general principles or invariances in the world (Bregman, 1977).

Notice my wording: this is a property of the world, and not merely a property of how we know the world. If the world did not have this property of compositionality, science and all other forms of understanding would be impossible. It is generally recognized that science attempts to explain phenomena as manifestations of the interaction of general principles such as laws, universal constants, structures, and so on. This compositional strategy would mean nothing, and have no success, unless the universe were itself compositional. Because both the phenomena of the world and our explanations of them are compositional, the structure of scientific explanations matches the structure of the universe.

WHAT IS EXPLANATION?

We can say, then, that scientific explanation is the reconstruction of the to-be-explained phenomenon as a composition of simpler principles, parts, or influences and their interaction with one another. I would like to argue that all types of explanations and understandings are like this, not just scientific explanations. In everyday understanding, when we try to explain a person's behavior, we do so in terms of a composition built out of factors such as the various situational constraints, and the goals, beliefs, memories, powers, and so on that we attribute to that person. We say, in reply to the question, "Why did he take the bus?" that he (A PARTICULAR PERSON) wanted (A TYPE OF GOAL) to get to (A TYPE OF ACTION) San Francisco (A PARTICULAR PLACE) and he doesn't have (SOCIAL STATUS OF OWNERSHIP) a car (A PARTICULAR THING). Whereas this composition is unique to this exact event, the components that make it up (in capitals) are not unique but occur in our explanations in endlessly varying combinations. We account for the particular phenomenon as a composition of stable structures, events, principles, or other sorts of invariants.

THE UTILITY OF A COMPOSITIONAL EXPLANATION

The value of performing the task of explanation this way is that we carry around in our minds the properties of each generality (e.g., ownership in the behavioral example, or gravity in an example drawn from physics) and assume that these generalities carry their properties with them into all compositions. If particular events are simply generated by the composition of general principles, then by learning about how each principle works, we gain the power to predict and control specific events in which these factors participate.

HUMAN PERCEPTION AS EXPLANATION

I maintain that the perception carried out by each of our senses is a form of understanding or explanation that uses the strategy for understanding that I have outlined. That is, it understands particular phenomena by interpreting them as compositions of general factors (Bregman, 1977).

The raw datum that any sense has to deal with is the distribution of energy on its organ of reception: in vision, this is the distribution of optic stimulation across two retinas and how it changes over time, and in audition, the distribution of the activation of the hair cells in two cochleas and how it changes over time. Perception resembles an explanation in that it interprets these sense data as resulting from simpler underlying factors, acting together. We should always remember that the activation patterns on the sense organs are not random, but arise from a composition of external influences. It is important that we experience these external influences, not the sense data, and that we separate the distinct influences if possible. Suppose we consider the activity in two small areas, one on each retina, corresponding to a small region of the table in front of us. The lack of commonality in the regions seen by the two eyes is due to the shininess of the surface, a property that determines how light coming from different directions is reflected and virtual images are formed, and explains discrepancies in the colors registered on the two retinas. In this case what we want to see is the shininess of the surface, not the fact that the eyes are registering a different correspondence between surface texture and local regions of color.

What we really want to see, then, are the simple factors in the world, not the activities on our retinas. Most often, we are successful, and thus we can predict important facts about the situation. First of all we see a *surface*, a powerful fact that helps us understand the sense data. It allows prediction: it tells us that if an edge moves over time, so will the details of texture included in the surface to which the edge belongs. We also see its color-absorbing properties, which we call its color, and its albedo, which we call its shininess. This allows us to predict that if the object moves, the color will move along with it and will remain attached to the surface. So our visual system is "explaining" the array of sense data as the consequence of regular properties of objects and light, and "sees" these properties, not the light itself. All we see is the explanation, not the sense data that gave rise to it.

When I refer to sense data, I am not making the classic distinction that opposes sensations (primitive experiences) to perception (experience of the world). My opposition is between sense data, which is not an experience at all, but just neural activity, on the one hand, and perception, which is both experience and explanation, on the other.

DIFFICULTIES IN FINDING THE SIMPLE ELEMENTS THAT COMPOSE THE SCENE

Although it is advantageous for our percepts to serve as explanations of sensory input, the task of forming the explanations and seeing the simple factors in the world is not as easy as it might appear. The shapes that are made by the distribution of activation on our sense receptors may be only very indirect manifestations of the underlying forms. We can see this in vision in the case of shapes. Figure 10.1 shows a miniature world of two solid objects shaped like the letters A and B. We also see their projections on an enlarged schematic retina. Notice that the shapes on the retina are not the same as the true shapes of the objects. Instead, parts have been deleted by a

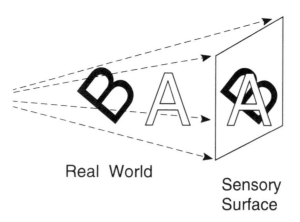

Figure 10.1 A miniature world and its projection onto a schematic retina (shown in upright orientation).

compositional process, called occlusion, which happens when other objects stand between an object and an observer.

A number of irregular contours are present in the projection; for example, those created in the disconnected regions of the B. The shapes of these contours are partly due to the shape of the B and partly to the shape of the A that occludes it. Perception explains the received light pattern as a composition of simpler factors, shapes, arrangement in space, occlusion, and rotation. Notice that all these factors participate together in explaining the input. The underlying structure of simple factors (the deep structure, as Chomsky would call it) is formed of components that cannot be assigned independently. For example, the B and the rotation go together to explain the visible B. If it is not a B, it does not have to be considered to be rotated. If there were a culture in which the form that we call a rotated B were itself a letter of normal orientation, then the notion of rotation would not have to be composed with the B to form a description that accounted for the sense data.

This sort of joint participation of simpler concepts in accounting for scenes is ubiquitous. It is often referred to as "analysis by synthesis," although it might be better to call it "understanding through composition." Its power lies in the fact that the deviation of the surface forms of the sense data from the canonical versions of those forms is not interpreted as random error but as the result of the action of other underlying factors. Therefore the deviation tells us something specific about the scene: if the visible fragments of the B are understood as having been fragmented because the B was occluded, this tells us something in addition to the fact that the form is acceptable as a B. It also tells us that the A is opaque.

COMPOSITIONS HAVE PREDICTIVE POWER

The compositional structure explains the redundancies in the distribution of activation of the receptor and permits prediction to take place about what

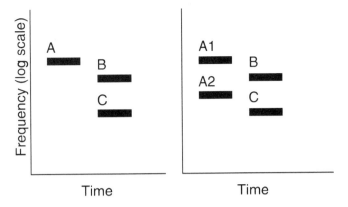

Figure 10.2 Left: a pure tone followed by a two simultaneous pure tones. Right: the same as the left panel except that a second pure tone accompanies the first one. Each panel shows one iteration in a repetitive cycle.

changes could be expected to occur. For example, it explains why separated regions have similar or related properties (because they are parts of the same object). It also permits the prediction that if one grasped one of these non-adjacent parts and pulled it, the other part would move in the same direction.

AUDITORY PERCEPTION AS COMPOSITION

We can now move to the field of audition and examine how the cues to the structure of the auditory scene tell the auditory system how to build the description of the scene, and how many of the changes that take place in our perception of these scenes can be understood as changes in a composition (Bregman, 1977, 1981).

The use of transformational concepts is very important to the strategy of dealing with scenes in terms of invariant entities. If deviations in the shape of some entity from one instant to the next can be attributed to transformations, then an invariant underlying form of the entity itself can be preserved. This is the basis for the perceptual constancies.

We have seen that visual perception uses transformations to account for scenes. Rotation and occlusion are two examples. However, there are also examples of the use of transformations (and the ensuing preservation of invariant entities) in auditory descriptions of scenes, for example, the transformation of pitch.

The first panel of figure 10.2 shows a tone with two frequency components, B and C, preceded by a single pure tone, A. This whole pattern is repeated over and over cyclically (Bregman and Pinker, 1978). If A is near B in frequency, as shown, the listener can often hear A and B as a sequence of pure tones, accompanied by a third sound, C. It is as if an interpretation has taken place in which the underlying concepts are a *pure tone* (A), repetition (where B is a repetition of A), *accompaniment* (C accompanies AB), and, finally, *pitch change* (A changes into B). This transformation of pitch is heard as a separate melodic pattern.

On the other hand, if A and B are far apart in frequency, a different interpretation emerges. A pure tone (A) is heard as alternating with a complex tone BC. The underlying concept of accompaniment is lost. Instead of C accompanying B, B and C are assigned to be parts of a more complex tone BC. The relation, *accompaniment*, has given way to the relation, *parts of*. The pitch transformation of A, causing it to become B, is also lost, even though there is still a frequency pattern in the sense data that might have been heard in that way. Instead we hear a melodic motion of A to BC taken as a whole. So a different arrangement of fundamental descriptive concepts has occurred under these circumstances. I believe that these concepts do not merely exist as separate words in the sentences we use when we verbally describe the experience, but are separate underlying factors in the experience itself.

Now we come to the second panel of the figure. It is exactly the same as the first panel, except that we have added another pure tone (A2), present at the same time as A (now called A1). The frequency ratio between A1 and A2 is arranged to be the same as the one between B and C. This time we hear a single complex sound, A1A2, moving down in frequency to become BC. The latter is heard as a repetition of A1A2, but at a lower frequency. The composition in this case is relatively simple. There is no *accompaniment*. At each moment there is only one (complex) sound. There is pitch *transformation* again, as A1A2 becomes BC. We have *repetition* again, but this time we do not hear A1 repeating with a pitch change, but the entire sound A1-A2 changing. Hearing the sound as undergoing a pitch transformation reduces the number of entities in the description; BC is not a different sound, but merely the repetition of A1A2, transformed in pitch.

Another example is illustrated in figure 10.3. If we play a pitch glide, repeatedly rising and falling in frequency, with breaks at the middle of the

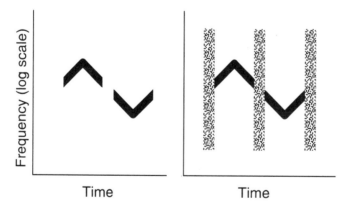

Figure 10.3 Left: a pure tone, rising and falling in frequency, with gaps in the rising and falling portions. Right: the same as the left panel except that noise bursts fill the gaps. Each panel shows one iteration in a repetitive cycle.

rising and falling portions, the listener will hear these breaks. The left-hand side of the figure shows a single cycle of this pattern. However, if we fill the breaks with noise bursts of the right intensity, as shown on the right, the listener will hear the glide travel through underneath the noise, although it does not actually do so. No breaks are heard (Dannenbring, 1976).

The resulting percept, when the continuity is heard through the noise, contains a number of transformations. For example, we hear a transformation of the same pure tone up and down in pitch. Once more, hearing the event as a transformation reduces the number of entities in the description, the parts before and after the noise being heard as a single changing sound. The notion of a single sound being transformed explains why different regions of time have similar simple spectra, and why the changes are smooth.

Occlusion is another transformational concept participating in the description of the sound pattern. In this example, the tone is heard as being occluded by the noise burst. Again, using the concepts of *transformation* and *occlusion* reduces the number of discrete entities. In fact there are only two entities, a pure tone and a noise burst. Making the perceptual composition is like forming the sentence, "a repeating noise burst interrupts an up-and-down gliding tone." (Incidentally, sentences also carry meaning by constructing a new meaning out of the interaction of the general meanings carried by their parts.)

Here is another example in auditory perception of using compositions to account for input. The phenomenon is called homophonic continuity (Warren, 1982; figure 10.4). The stimulus begins with a steady sound that, at a certain moment, begins to rise in intensity. It stays at the higher intensity for a short time, then drops back to the original value and continues on. The perceptual interpretation may differ, depending on whether the rise in intensity to the second level is abrupt or gradual. We hear a slow rise in intensity as a loudness transformation; that is, as a single sound rising in loudness. If the rise is abrupt, we hear this stimulus as having two component sounds: one

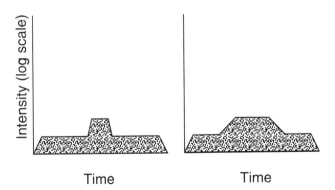

Figure 10.4 Stimulus for homophonic continuity. A long, steady noise burst is shown with an amplitude increment in the middle. On the left, the increment is abrupt and on the right, slow.

sound continuing at the same loudness, and a second sound joining the first one at the point of intensity increase, accompanying the first one for the duration of the increase, and disappearing at the point of intensity decrease. The perception of one changing sound will give way to that of two steady-loudness sounds when the changes are abrupt and the period of higher intensity is brief.

The change in perception can again be seen as a change in the compositional structure of the scene. With more abrupt transitions, the concept of accompaniment replaces the concept of loudness change in the composition, and two sounds replace one. This change affects the perception of the loudness of the stimulus. After the increase, in the first case we hear a single loud sound, whereas in the second we hear two softer ones. Intensity has been accounted for by a different composition of factors: in the one case by adding the transformation of *getting louder*, and in the second case by adding the notion of a second sound. This is not a cognitive phenomenon where we have arrived at an interpretation through reasoning. We actually hear the interpretation.

Let me go back to an earlier visual example before introducing the next auditory one. When we encounter the distribution of light on a table top, our perception explains the energy pattern reaching our eye as a composition of surface color, gloss, shape, shadows. Each of these factors is a separable part of our experience. We do not see the surface as changing in color where it is in a shadow. We just see it as being in a shadow. The shadow is seen as a separable causal influence in the scene. So are the gloss, shape, and texture of the surface.

COMPOSITION IN SPEECH AND SENTENCE PERCEPTION

The next example is in the domain of speech perception. Let us examine how our perception of an English sentence accounts for the intensity of a particular syllable in the sentence. Let us suppose that the sentence is composed by the speaker under the influence of a number of causal factors. The intensity of the syllable may be influenced by the pattern of stress in the word being spoken, which may, in turn come from two sources. The first is that, in English, each word has an assigned stress pattern (lexical stress), for example, PROduce, the noun, versus proDUCE the verb. The second influence may be that a contrast in ideas is being signified by the stress (contrastive stress), as in, "I want to proDUCE the result, not just let it happen." Third, loudness may be increased by the nervousness of the speaker. Fourth, it can be increased by background noise, since speakers attempt to maintain a fixed signal-to-noise ratio. Fifth, the intensity can be affected by the distance of the listener from the speaker, who wants to be heard. The boosts in intensity that result from all these influences are added together. To truly understand the event we have to parse the surface frequency and amplitude into these factors. The amplitude of a single syllable (together with neighboring amplitudes, as well as other acoustic variables) supplies evidence for all these causal factors at the same time. When we experience the event, only these causal factors appear, not the total intensity of the sound.

The account of perception that I have offered thus far is directly analogous to the account that Chomsky gave of the understanding of sentences (Bregman, 1981). His account was compositional in the same way. He pointed out that sentences were compositions of generative syntactic concepts, such as *noun phrase* or *question*, and that the job of a language understander was to recognize the deep structural forms that, in combination, shaped the sentence. Because the composition was complex, it was possible for two different deep structures to give the same surface structure. For example, in the sentence, "they are racing horses," the word "racing" may be a verb, the sentence meaning that some people are racing their horses. Alternatively, "racing" may modify "horses," the sentence telling what kind of horses they are. This ambiguity is a direct result of the fact that the surface form is a complex composition of simpler syntactic forms so that different selections and combinations can produce two or more results that look the same on the surface.

SURFACE AMBIGUITY IN VISUAL AND AUDITORY PERCEPTION

Visual and auditory perception also have to deal with surface ambiguity. Figure 10.5 may be seen as either a triangle occluded by a rectangle or as two irregular shapes attached to the borders of a rectangle. Our problem is to derive the simplest underlying form (the Gestaltists referred to this tendency to go for simple forms as the principle of *prägnanz*).

Here is an example of surface ambiguity in audition. Let us go back to the first panel of figure 10.2, in which a pure tone A alternates with a pair of pure tones AB. If we think of our perception of this event as a causal story about it, alternatives are possible. The first is that a pure tone A is alternating with a complex tone BC. Another is that a pure tone A undergoes a drop in pitch (to become B), while at the same time a second tone C appears and

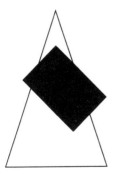

Figure 10.5 A display that can be seen either as a triangle occluded by a rectangle or as two irregular shapes attached to the borders of a rectangle.

accompanies it. So the sense data are on the surface, ambiguous. The problem is to derive the simplest underlying explanation by using innate rules of simplicity.

Differences in the Rules of Simplicity Between Vision and Audition

The rules of simplicity are different for vision and audition because light and sound have different properties, leading us to use them in different ways. Our eyes are mainly concerned with the reflection of energy, whereas our ears are concerned primarily with the sources of the energy.

The sun is the main emitter of light outdoors. However, in vision our main goal is not to use the emitted energy to find out about the sun; rather, we use it to find out about the objects that reflect the energy. The emission of light energy gives us little detail about the world; reflection gives most of the information. In audition, there is no constant noise source (analogous to the sun) whose reflections reveal the surface properties of objects. Even if there were, the human auditory system has no lens to focus the acoustic image so as to distinguish the fine details of surface reflective properties. Audition primarily uses the acoustic emissions that are generated when events occur and cause energy to be transferred. Reflections are used mainly to determine the properties of the enclosure in which the listener is situated, such as its gross size and acoustic "liveness."

Another difference has to do with opaqueness and transparency. In vision most bodies are opaque, a minority transparent. Therefore the main compositional process that the visual system has to deal with is the occlusion of further surfaces by nearer ones. Only occasionally does it have to deal with the kind of mixing together of information that we get with transparency. In audition, on the other hand, transparency rules the day. Since audition uses the energy emitted when events occur, and may pick them up at some distance, the effects of different sound sources add up in the air. Another way of saying this is that most sounds are transparent; that is, their contributions are not lost, but merely combined with the contributions of other events in the mixture of sound that reaches our ears. So the main compositional process dealt with by audition is that of mixing (summation of amplitudes).

Occasionally, the auditory system must deal with occlusion too. However, the occurrence of occlusion in sound is not usually due to the way the sound reaches our ears, but to the properties of the organ of hearing. Occlusion occurs only in the case of very loud sounds. Because the hearing sense is not linear, whenever a sound A becomes more intense, a softer sound, B, added to it has less and less effect on our sense apparatus. Therefore if A is very intense the effects of B become inaudible. In everyday language, A drowns out B. Thus, even though a perfectly linear system would not lose the effects of B, in our actual ears transparency is lost and occlusion occurs. In such cases the auditory system uses similarity and continuity to find out whether a soft sound, A, interrupted by a loud sound, B, actually continued underneath B. If a softer sound A1 occurs just before a brief louder sound B and another softer sound A2 occurs right after B, the plausibility of considering A1 and A2 as part of a single occluded sound A is assessed. If the right conditions are met, the two are heard as parts of a single sound, A, that continues underneath B.

Another difference between vision and audition is in the role of inertia. Inertia influences vision but not audition. We can see this in the cases of visual apparent motion and auditory melodic motion, which are otherwise comparable phenomena. In vision we can detect effects of inertia. Suppose we have a vertical column of lamps. If each one is briefly lit in succession from top to bottom, we see apparent movement from top to bottom. Suppose, then, that we start two simultaneous patterns of apparent motion, one from the top and the other from the bottom. What happens when they meet in the middle? There are two possible percepts: the motions can cross, or can bounce, the eye following each motion back from the middle point to the starting point. The dominant percept is crossing. This suggests that our visual sense expects motions to continue (i.e., for objects to have inertia).

The auditory analog is two patterns formed out of pure tones, one ascending and one descending, that cross in the middle. Again we can hear either a crossing of the two patterns, or a bouncing in which each melodic pattern turns around at the crossing point and returns to its beginning frequency. In audition, the bouncing percept is dominant (Tougas and Bregman, 1985). There seems to be no bias toward hearing a melodic trajectory continue in the same direction. The difference between the senses can be attributed to the physics of the situations. Actual motion, of which apparent motion is a cartoon, involves the movement of bodies that do have inertia; hence, the visual expectation. The changing of pitch, on the other hand, occurs as a result of changes in the length or tightness of vibrating bodies (e.g., our vocal cords), and there is no reason for a change to continue in the same direction. If anything, the change will run into some limit (as with the pitch of a voice) and return to a previous value. Hence our auditory system shows no bias favoring continuation.

Earlier, I proposed that the ambiguities in sense data (the linguist's surface ambiguity) were resolved by rules of simplicity of interpretation. We see from this discussion that these rules may differ across sense modalities.

THE BASIC PROBLEM IN AUDITION: SOUND MIXTURE

The rules of simplicity in audition derive from the problems faced by that sense. The main problem it has to deal with is the mixing of the energy from the many sounds present at the same time (Bregman, 1990). In a first step, the inner ear forms a frequency-based representation in which different frequencies are registered in different neural pathways. That is, the neural representation resembles the speech scientist's spectrogram, in which frequency is represented on the vertical axis, time on the horizontal axis, and intensity by the darkness of each frequency-time region. If sounds were presented only one at a time, this spectral representation might serve directly as a basis for recognition, different familiar sounds having different shapes in the frequency-by-time representation. However, in a mixture, how is the auditory system to know whether a particular frequency at a particular time has come from only one sound source or is the sum of the energy from two or more? The spectrogram of a mixture is equal to the sum of the spectrograms of all the constituent sounds in the mixture. The auditory system must parse the spectrum over time to recover separate descriptions of individual sounds. This can be viewed as a problem of grouping and allocation. Which bits of the neural spectrogram should be grouped as coming from the same environmental event? How much of the energy that has been registered in each region of frequency and time should be allocated to each environmental sound?

This seems to be a horrendous problem, but it is solved by taking into account certain simple relations that occur among the components whenever acoustic energy has arisen from a single source. These are regularities in the incoming array of sound that tell us, on a probabilistic basis, which parts of the sound have come from the same sound-producing event.

If the world is regular in certain ways, the simplest interpretation is one that respects these regularities. For example, an important class of sounds generates components that are multiples of a single frequency. The vibrations of the human vocal cords work this way. We can exploit this regularity to discover the appropriate grouping of components in the auditory mixture. So if we hear a set of components that are multiples of a single fundamental, and interpret it as the parts of a single sound, this interpretation respects the regularities of the world and is therefore a "simple" interpretation.

SEQUENTIAL SIMILARITY

A number of other properties of the incoming array of sound derive from the fact that it has come from a number of distinct sources. These properties can tell us, on a probabilistic basis, which parts of the sound have come from the same sound-producing event. Therefore, the auditory system can use them to decide how to group the components. One such property is sequential similarity. If we play a rapid series of tones, say 10 per second, of alternating high and low frequencies, as long as the high and low frequencies do not differ too much, say only by a couple of semitones, we allocate all of them to a single sound source and hear them as a coherent stream of sound. However, if the frequency difference gets quite large, say 10 to 15 semitones, we hear two separate streams of sounds, a high one and a low one (van Noorden, 1977). The auditory system, because of the rapid and large change in properties from one tone to the next, prefers to hear two streams, each with uniform properties. We can see from this example that the minimum change of properties over time is treated as a form of simplicity by the auditory system, allowing it to choose among alternative interpretations.

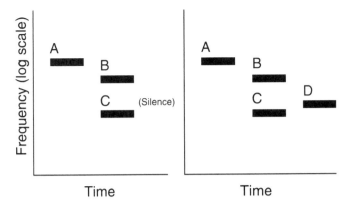

Figure 10.6 Competition between the sequential capturing of component B into a sequence A-B, and the integration of B into a unit formed of simultaneous sounds B and C. Each panel shows one iteration in a repetitive cycle.

COMPETITION OF INTERPRETATIONS AND THE CUMULATION OF EVIDENCE

Because of the large number of relations among the components of signals, one relation may favor one grouping of sense data whereas another favors a different grouping. The system deals with this disagreement by allowing the alternative groupings to compete with one another, the winner being the one for which the grouping is most strongly favored by all the regularities (cues) in the sense data.

An example of such a competition can be seen in figure 10.6. On the left is a cyclical pattern similar to the one in figure 10.2 (left panel), with the A tone set at a frequency in which it is a bit too high to capture B out of the BC mixture, and a silence inserted after the BC complex.

The strategy for getting A to be effective in capturing B can be seen as analogous to a problem in social psychology. Suppose Bob (B) and Carol (C) are going out together, but Alice (A) is interested in capturing Bob for herself. Her own charm is not strong enough to break up the Bob-Carol pair. What is her best strategy? Obviously, to introduce an attractive new man, Don (D), to Carol. Carol's attraction to Don will weaken the Bob-Carol bond, allowing Alice to snag Bob. In a similar way, if we introduce a fourth tone, D, near the frequency of C, the ensuing C-D sequential grouping will compete with, and weaken, the B-C fusion. This will allow A to capture B into an A-B sequential stream (Bregman and Tougas, 1989). We see then that the groupings are competitive. This competition of interpretations implies the existence in the nervous system of a field of competing claims that are resolved.

PROBLEMS FOR PHYSIOLOGICAL EXPLANATION

Now let us see what all this means for our ability to explain perception in physiological terms. I have mentioned an important functional property that the brain must embody if it is to perform perception. It must be able to carry out a compositional process.

This compositional process must embody two separate sorts of knowledge. The first is a representation of typical underlying causal factors, including the shapes of familiar forms, such as a voice, a tone, or a letter B, or the tendency for objects to throw shadows, the tendency of sounds to maintain their properties over time, and so on. The second type of knowledge concerns the ways in which the form that each underlying factor takes, in an actual situation, can change as other factors are composed with it. For example, the continuity of a sound may be violated if a loud enough interruption occurs, or the shape of a visible object can be altered if another form is placed between it and the viewer.

The neural system must be able to operate on a representation of a form (either visual or auditory), imposing on it the changes implied by the other causal factors in the situation. For example, if a sheet of paper is tilted away from the viewer, this implies that the retinal shapes of all the letters written on it will change in a regular way. The tilt accounts for the transformations of all the shapes. To understand that it does, the brain must have a way of imposing foreshortening on letter shapes and verifying that this would yield the retinal data. This requires a constructive capability of the sensory systems. I take it as true that we could interpret some sense data as a transformed version of a shape, even though we had never seen this particular shape affected by that particular transformation before (an example might be a cat occluding a pterodactyl). The existence of a general capacity to decide whether the details of some sense data are adequately explained by a composition requires a constructive ability.

What is being constructed? Obviously, the answer is a form, whether auditory, visual, or whatever. A form is not just a concatenation of features. We often hear the question, "How are features brought together in the brain?" But they are not merely brought together. An A and a tilt are not the same as a tilted A. The A and the tilt are composed, the tilt affecting the shape of the A. This composition is a very rapid process in which something novel is created out of primitive concepts, rules of composition, and rules of simplicity in a manner precise enough to match the sensory input. A nervous system that represented external events and objects through a system of fixed connections that were only slowly modified by experience could not achieve this result. The activity in the nervous system that forms representations must be *flexible, composable, and instantly modifiable*. Connections, as they are currently conceived, do not have these properties.

Networks of connections have been shown to be good classifiers, but dealing with compositions is not a problem of classification, but of creating an explanation, bearing in mind that an explanation is a composition of underlying factors. So far I have not heard of any connectionist network that could compose basic principles in a generative way and thereby achieve a match to sense data. Therefore, the formulation of a neural system that has these properties remains an important challenge for the physiological explanation of the human mind.

REFERENCES

Bregman AS. (1977). Perception and behavior as compositions of ideals. *Cognit Psychol* 9:250–292.

Bregman AS. (1981). Chomsky without language. *Cognition* 10:33–38.

Bregman AS. (1990). *Auditory scene analysis: The perceptual organization of sound*. MIT Press, Cambridge.

Bregman AS, Pinker S. (1978). Auditory streaming and the building of timbre. *Can J Psychol* 32:19–31.

Bregman AS, Tougas Y. (1989). Propagation of constraints in auditory organization. *Percept Psychophys* 46(4):395–396.

Dannenbring GL. (1976). Perceived auditory continuity with alternately rising and falling frequency transitions. *Can J Psychol* 30:99–114.

Tougas Y, Bregman AS. (1985). The crossing of auditory streams. *J Exp Psychol: Hum Percept Perform* 11:788–798.

Van Noorden LPAS. (1977). Minimum differences of level and frequency for perceptual fission of tone sequences ABAB. *J Acoust Soc Am* 61:1041–1045.

Warren RM. (1982). *Auditory Perception: A New Synthesis*. Pergamon Press, New York.

11 Formation of Perceptual Objects from the Timing of Neural Responses: Target-Range Images in Bat Sonar

J. A. Simmons

The biological sonar, or echolocation, of bats is an unusual and interesting perceptual system that has been studied with great success, largely from the perspective of neuroethology (Griffin, 1958; Pollak and Casseday, 1989; Popper and Fay, 1995; Suga, 1990). Although it might seem too exotic and too specialized to be a source of information about general principles of brain function, echolocation in fact has unexpected importance for the neurosciences because a crucial mechanism thought to be the basis for forming perceptual images is readily observed in bats. Specifically, the bat's biosonar system affords an opportunity to examine the role of the timing of neural responses as a fundamental dimension supporting the creation of images depicting the locations and the identifying features of objects in space. This circumstance intersects with a philosophical concern that is now being expressed in experimental neuroscience about how the different neural responses making up the brain's representation of objects in scenes are linked together actually to reconstruct these objects as images rather than merely to represent their constituent features separately.

BACKGROUND

The focus of this chapter is experimental demonstration of the emergence of discrete objects or entities in perception from the detection of temporal coherence of neural responses across sets of neurons. Coherence in the timing of responses across different neurons is presumed to play a crucial role in identifying which representations of particular features will to be linked together into the same entities in perception (see von der Malsburg, this volume). That is, diverse stimulus features are bound together into discrete perceptual objects because the responses that encode them are time locked to each other. It follows that, if the synchronization of responses leading to perception of a single object is broken up by displacing some responses to a different time relative to other responses, the original perceived object will itself break up to form two different objects that can be distinguished from each other along specific perceptual dimensions, defined by which neural responses have been displaced in time. This chapter describes the experimental break-up of the bat's image of a sonar target by temporal dissociation of neural responses contributing to that image.

Temporal binding of features to form whole objects has to be backed up by neuronal mechanisms for detecting coherence in responses across different neurons. This requires some means for sampling the time of occurrence of responses taking place in different neuronal pools and bringing together these samples into a new response that stands for coherence across the inputs. Echolocation by bats provides a valuable scientific example because these same neuronal mechanisms required for detecting temporal coherence in a general sense actually lead to formation of the most prominent dimension of the images the bat perceives. Echolocating bats perceive the depth of their surroundings—target distance or range—from the arrival time of sonar echoes (Simmons, 1989). To determine the magnitude of echo delay, the timing of responses evoked by each echo is explicitly compared with the timing of responses evoked by the preceding broadcast using a neuronal coincidence-detection scheme (Dear et al, 1993; Dear, Simmons, and Fritz, 1993; Simmons et al, 1995b; Suga, 1990; Sullivan, 1982). As a result of this comparison, the bat perceives an image with distance as its primary psychological dimension. The formation of these images can be observed by making psychophysical measurements on the perceived distance to targets in trained bats while adjusting the stimuli to manipulate the timing of responses. In effect, the grouping of responses on the basis of temporal coherence to form discrete entities in perception can be watched while it happens.

RECONSTRUCTING OBJECTS FROM THEIR REPRESENTATIONS

The Feature-Inventory Model of Perception

Until recently, our understanding of the role of neural responses in creating perceived images focused largely on the degree to which neurons exhibit response selectivity, or are tuned to a particular range of values along one or more stimulus parameters. Neurons are observed to respond vigorously only if the stimulus falls inside the cell's receptive field, defined from response rate or response probability (strength of response) as an excitatory segment of the range of possible values for some specific stimulus parameter. Because neurons differ in the degree to which their responses are selective to single stimulus features or combinations of features, different stimuli will evoke different levels (strengths) of responding across populations of cells. The diversity of receptive field properties across different neurons leads to a corresponding diversity in the sets of responses evoked by different stimuli. However, a difference in response strength across populations of neurons accounts only for the encoding of stimulus features; it leaves open the question of how the resulting dispersed ensemble of feature representations is reintegrated into perception of the intact stimulus. To form cohesive images, responses distributed across populations of cells somehow have to be "read out" together to determine the preponderance of their message about the stimulus. The convergence of information required to bring disparate feature representations into cohesive images thus is an essential aspect of perception that must be supported by mechanisms whose specific purpose is to achieve convergence as a process distinct from the feature representations themselves (see Damasio, this volume; von der Malsburg, this volume).

Perception of a stimulus is usually described in terms of an inventory of features developed across parallel populations of neurons having a wide variety of response selectivities (e.g., to color, orientation, motion, contrast). In this feature-inventory scheme, the content of perception depends on the amount of activity the stimulus evokes in different feature-selective neuronal populations. The process of identifying which inventory (i.e., stimulus) has occurred consists of determining the strengths of responses in different feature-selective neural channels and then registering the profile of response strengths across these channels. In effect, the resulting response-strength profile is the image created by the feature-inventory model; the content of the perceived image is derived from the particular combination of selective neural responses that occur for any given stimulus.

The Binding Problem in the Inventory Model

The chief difficulty with the feature-inventory model is that stimuli ordinarily occur in scenes that contain many objects together. A perceptual entity corresponds to an object whose feature representations manifestly are bound together into a unified reconstruction of the object itself, embedded in surroundings composed of other, often quite similar, objects. The representations of different features may overlap for different objects, yet it is the objects that are depicted in perception, not just their features. That is, although objects may share certain features in common, the representations of these features generally are apportioned to their corresponding entities in perception, not lumped together into illusory objects that are created by the overlap of particularly potent features. A number of discrete objects, each with its own features, commonly have to be incorporated into the same image and perceived individually as discrete components of the scene as a whole. All these objects are present together, so their features are extracted together, but how are individual feature profiles kept intact on an object-by-object basis to retain the integrity of parts of the scene in the image?

Feature Binding Through Temporal Coherence of Responses

The feature-inventory model uses an inherently spatial representational scheme based on the strength of responses. Neurons that are located in different places in brain structures respond differentially to stimuli, resulting in stimulus-dependent spatial patterns of activity spread across brain tissue. This spatial organization might be simple and maplike (e.g., a topographic display of some stimulus feature) or it might be complex and distributed, but it still is fundamentally a representation of response strengths by place. Historically, the perceptual role of the other principal response dimension—the timing of neural responses—has largely been relegated to specifying when the stimulus occurred rather than to specifying individual stimulus features. Now, however, recognition that the binding problem is a challenge to the feature-inventory model has brought increasing attention to the role of the timing of neural responses for the actual creation of perceived images.

In a general sense, because particular features must occur together if they are contained in the same stimulus object, the responses to these features will occur more or less at the same time. For example, responses evoked by the onset of a stimulus are transient or phasic events that necessarily have coherence with respect to each other because they are triggered by the same stimulus. The simultaneity of phasic neural responses encoding different features of the same stimulus probably is important for specifying that these features go together to form a perceptual entity (feature binding; see Singer, this volume). This is an extension of the question of "when the stimulus occurs" to include "when its identifiable features occur together." If the neural responses that encode specific features of some object all occur together within a specified time interval (the duration of a single binding window in the temporal binding hypothesis), the information they contain will be attributed to the same object in perception. However, if these responses become separated in time by some amount larger than the binding window, the information they contain will diverge in perception, still contributing to perception of the same features, but now in separate objects.

Because neural discharges in different cells presumably are the actual signals whose temporal coherence has to be monitored, the maximum possible width of the binding window probably is related to the width of the discharges themselves, which is roughly several hundred microseconds. Simultaneous arrival of multiple inputs at specialized coincidence-detecting neurons, each input with a width of several hundred microseconds, would define a critical interval of time, also several hundred microseconds wide, for deciding that simultaneity of those inputs did in fact occur. This consideration establishes an outer limit for the size of the binding window. However, although the time window for judging the simultaneity of responses in different neurons seems likely to have a maximum size corresponding to the width of the responses themselves, it could well have a much smaller effective size if only the onset or rise time of the neural response is being registered for each input. Without knowing just how short a piece of the rising edge of each neuronal action potential carries the bulk of the message that the response occurred, it is much more difficult to set a lower limit for the size of the time window required to determine that simultaneity occurred. This is an important consideration, because slight mismatches in response timing across inputs to coincidence-detecting neurons might contribute to distinguishing subtle differences in stimulus features or their grouping.

Responses to different features of the same stimulus clearly will be synchronized by the onset of the stimulus. However, even at the level of the receptors these responses might not actually occur simultaneously because different receptors could receive their parts of the stimulus at slightly different times (e.g., hair cells at different locations along the cochlear partition), or the locations of the receptors on the sensory surface (e.g., photoreceptors at different positions on the retina) could result in different lengths of afferent fiber paths along which responses must travel. Furthermore, after being initiated, phasic responses to stimulus onset would propagate upward along the central sensory pathway to trigger discharges in neurons at successively higher processing centers at progressively later times. Depending on the disparity among the levels at which different features are extracted, comparison of the timing of responses to different features might have to be made across corresponding disparities in time of many tens of milliseconds. Consequently, coincidence-detecting neurons can be expected to receive their inputs from different neuronal pools at different latencies to counteract differences in the timing of the responses actually evoked in these pools by the same stimulus. Such countervailing intrinsic latency differences incorporated in coincidence-detecting circuits would also have to be in the range of tens of milliseconds.

Testing the Temporal Feature-Binding Hypothesis

If temporal coherence indeed leads to binding of features into perceived objects, experiments to manipulate the timing of neural responses representing different features ought to affect the grouping of attributes within perceived objects. Changing the timing of responses to one set of features relative to another should produce predictable changes in the number of perceived objects and the features attributed to them, but only if the responses being manipulated actually can be identified as representing specific features of specific objects. This requirement reveals the first practical impediment to verifying that the timing of responses determines the detailed composition of perceived images—finding a particular sensory system on which to do experiments. The temporal binding hypothesis emerged chiefly from consideration of the distributed nature of the selectivity of visual neural responses to different stimulus features in contrast to the apparent unity of perceptual objects in scenes (Livingstone and Hubel, 1988). Consequently, wide acceptance of the temporal binding hypothesis is likely to depend on the degree to which it specifically can be demonstrated to occur in the visual system. However, conditions that reveal the temporal basis for binding may profitably be explored in other sensory systems where simplification of the stimulus features and image dimensions might make the initial demonstration easier to achieve.

The ideal sensory system in which to test the temporal binding hypothesis would represent a specific, identifiable perceptual dimension from the timing of neural responses itself. Changes in the timing of responses evoked by different objects should cause these objects to appear at different locations along this dimension. Furthermore, different objects that are present together would be distinguished from each other along this dimension from the timing of their responses. This example system should provide a view of image formation using response timing as computational data. The emergence of discrete objects along this perceptual dimension from registration of the timing of their responses across different neurons as occurring together would illustrate the formation of discrete entities in perceived images. Note that the neural responses themselves might well be dispersed to different latencies at different levels of processing or in different parts of neuronal circuits; detecting their coherence would require time-compensated convergence of inputs to coincidence-detecting neurons. The merging or the segregation of objects whose responses move closer together or farther apart in time at the coincidence detectors would trace the temporal dynamics of the process that binds responses together within a minimal window interval that defines simultaneity for perceptual purposes. In effect, this ideal sensory system would serve as a test bed for observing the calculus that integrates neural events into perceptual events.

Assuming that the proper sensory system can be found, there is a second practical impediment to verifying that the timing of neural responses is the key to grouping these responses and forming perceptual objects. Neural responses to a given stimulus do not simply occur all at the same time, to be followed somewhat later by responses to a different stimulus, so that responses to individual stimuli remain isolated from each other as discrete bursts of discharges. Instead, the responses even to sequentially presented stimuli are spread out in time so that they overlap appreciably. Because sensory systems consist of a series of sequentially and hierarchically organized processing stages, responses to any one stimulus in different neurons become distributed in time over a span of many tens of milliseconds depending on the location of the neurons in different processing sites, and also on their connections in neuronal circuits within each site. These sites, nuclei in the ascending pathway and areas in the cerebral cortex, presumably constitute successive levels of processing. They also represent delays imposed on latencies of responses traveling through the system, such that response latencies occur in sequence upward through the pathway and also from cell to cell within circuits at each level.

Taking the system as a whole, responses just to stimulus onset can be dispersed over 50 to 100 msec. Consequently, responses already set in train by the onset of a stimulus or by steady-state stimulation continue to occur until the entire span of latencies is exhausted, even after the stimulus is over. Moreover, even when two stimuli do occur at slightly different times, their responses frequently run concurrently in parallel neuronal subsystems, so that strict simultaneity of responses as a criterion for coherence not only might fail to group responses that really do belong together, but also might mistakenly group responses that do not belong together. Judgments of functional simultaneity of responses for binding purposes thus have to allow for offsets in absolute response time of as much as several tens of milliseconds to take into account the detailed organization of central sensory pathways and accumulating latency dispersion from one level of processing to the next. In effect, the actual function of latency dispersion within the sensory system has to be understood so that the contribution of responses at different latencies to the eventual image is known.

Transient or Oscillatory Responses as a Basis for Temporal Coherence

At its core, the most intractable aspect of the binding problem is apportioning information about the same features to different objects that are present together as part of one scene. The neuronal subpopulations whose responses make up the feature inventory may not be capable of subdivision into units corresponding to different objects on the basis of response strengths because the feature representations for the objects overlap too much. The crucial concept of the temporal model for binding is that the necessary subdivision could take place across response time rather than just across feature space (see Singer, this volume). If neural responses were clocked in a sequential fashion and this clocking kept track of, those responses to different features that occur at exactly the same time might be identifiable and serve as a basis for keeping the information they represent together as a cluster of features. These clusters would be defined by precise coherence of neural responses over a suitable interval of time, and the consequence of their identification as being coherent might be creation of cohesive units in perception. In principle, detecting temporal coherence would not be difficult; it would require only that coincidences of responses in different cells be registered as distinctive events. Neural mechanisms specifically designed for carrying out computations on the timing of responses have been observed in a number of different perceptual systems (Carr, 1993; Dear et al, 1993a; Dear, Simmons, and Fritz, 1993; Langner, 1992; Suga, 1990; Sullivan, 1982).

The clocking of responses could involve nothing more complex than the synchrony of phasic responses grouped together by the onset of a stimulus, which is a transient event. On-responses to the same stimulus would all be initiated more or less at the same moment, and they would propagate upward along the central sensory pathway to trigger discharges in neurons at successively longer, progressively more dispersed latencies that reflect the connections between cells at the same or different levels. Coincidences between responses occurring in neurons located at any combination of levels could be detected by bringing these responses together at the right times, that is, after compensating for their dispersed latencies at different sites. In the case of phasic responses to stimulus onset, the binding window would be the size of the time interval within which all responses are classified as belonging to the same object. (Here, the binding window refers to the span of time over which inputs arrive at the coincidence detectors, after the various dispersed latencies are compensated by the circuits comprising inputs to the coincidence detectors.) The subdivision of perception into different objects would be based on the number of discriminably different time intervals or binding windows into which the whole span of time encompassing all the dispersed latencies can be subdivided. If the timing of responses in two groups of neurons representing the same feature were to diverge by more than the width of the binding window, the information contained in these responses would diverge and be attributed to separate objects in perception.

Alternatively, the clocking of responses could involve more complicated temporal patterns of repetitive responses lasting for an appreciable period after stimulus onset, during a period of sustained stimulation. It is convenient to think of these longer-lasting representations as consisting of bursts of repetitive or oscillatory responses triggered by the occurrence of a stimulus, with the timing or phase of the oscillations being the key to registering coherence and segregating features of different objects that are present in the same scene. A number of parallel oscillators could be active at the same time within the same activated neuronal populations, just at different phases, to represent different objects that are present together. In this case, the binding window would be the size of the segment of phase space within which responses in different neurons are treated as being simultaneous. (Once again, the binding window refers to time or phase at the coincidence detectors, after latencies for responses being brought together are compensated for their likely dispersion.)

The subdivision of perception into different objects would be based on the number of oscillations with discriminably different phases that can be set up and allowed to run in parallel. In this case, if the phase of oscillations in two groups of neurons representing the same feature were to diverge by more than the width of the binding window, the information contained in these responses would diverge and be attributed to separate objects in perception. It is important to note that the responses being bound together do not have to be oscillatory. This is just one way to create parallel groups of responses which are clocked so they can be compared efficiently by their phase, but the responses do have to be regulated in their time of occurrence, and these times then do have to be compared by coincidence-detecting neuronal circuits or their equivalent.

Measuring Temporal Properties for Binding of Responses into Perceived Entities

The crucial insight of the temporal binding hypothesis is that the time of occurrence of brain activity in different local sites—the synchronized latencies of transient responses or the phase of oscillatory bursts of more sustained neural responses—might be the basis for subdivision of feature-selective responses on an object-oriented basis. This is a major conceptual step that is increasingly supported by hard evidence for the visual system. At the present time, while the very complicated problem of evaluating temporal binding in vision moves forward in different laboratories, it is worth stepping back from the problem to examine alternative avenues for verifying at least part of the hypothesis. What is required at this point is an unambiguous demonstration of the required temporal coincidence-comparison mechanisms in action for perception itself, for the formation of two perceptual entities out of one entity as a result of temporal divergence of sets of neural responses, complete with measurements of the width of the binding window and of the acuity with which the timing of a group of synchronized responses can be judged to have occurred. Can an ideal perceptual system be found for this purpose?

It would be particularly useful to have measurements of the duration of the binding window for perception, but a successful experiment requires equating a specific set of neural discharges caused by a stimulus object with a corresponding object in perception. In particular, it depends on knowing just which of two psychophysically distinguishable objects is represented by the time of occurrence of a given set of neural responses. Furthermore, it is essential that the perceptual system be intrinsically capable of determining the time of occurrence of sets of responses with greater accuracy than the width of the binding window itself. Otherwise, the measured binding window might reflect only the noisiness or jitter in perception of the time of occurrence of individual responses, instead of limitations inherent in the binding process. At the present time, these considerations severely restrict the choice of perceptual systems in which to conduct the demonstration.

The visual pathways become extremely complicated in the cerebral cortex, with parallel pathways of different lengths to different cortical areas representing both different visual features and different levels of processing. The temporal dispersion of responses across the cortex just to the onset of a visual stimulus is of the order of 50 to 100 msec, and sustained responses widen this span considerably. At any given moment after presentation of a stimulus, responses that are selective to a variety of different stimulus features will be taking place, while responses to the same features will be distributed in time over tens of milliseconds. How can the experimenter determine which of these responses have to be synchronized with each other to affect the formation of a perceived object that itself can be identified in the image?

The relevant responses might occur coherently but at somewhat different times according to the response latencies for propagation of information to different cortical locations, so strict simultaneity might not be the crucial factor for controlling perception. Coincidence-detecting neurons that receive inputs over pathways with different response latencies would be able to determine whether neurons representing different features were discharging together at specific times when their occurrences differ by the difference in the latencies of their inputs. Such delay-coincidence mechanisms play an important role in the auditory system (Carr, 1993; Dear et al, 1993; Dear, Simmons, and Fritz, 1993; Kuwabara and Suga, 1993; Suga, 1990; Sullivan, 1982). Thus, at the present time, an auditory example would seem useful for testing critical aspects of the temporal binding hypothesis if this test has to be carried out at the interface between behavioral and physiological methods. The auditory pathways of the brain are fully as complicated as those for vision (subcortical auditory pathways are especially complicated compared with those for vision), and they provide just as much troublesome dispersion of response latencies across different levels, of the order of 50–100 msec for auditory onset responses. The function of the progressively lagging latencies in auditory responses is understood, however, at least for several specific examples.

Response Timing and Neural Encoding of Stimulus Features

There is yet a further complication: the information to be bound together is assumed to consist of feature dimensions represented by neural receptive fields, which themselves are defined in terms of response strength, not response timing. Response timing is assumed to serve instead as the basis for binding. Whereas the timing of neural responses may well enter into binding, it might also enter into the coding of specific stimulus features along their feature dimensions. For example, does the amount of brightness in a stimulus change with small shifts in the timing of neural responses as well as with shifts in the population of neurons that are active? This would be a competing effect on perception—both the fusion of parallel feature representations and the actual perceived magnitude of one of the features would be determined by the timing of responses in different groups of neurons. In general, the possibility that some dimension of the perception itself might emerge from the timing of responses as well as from which neurons respond has received little attention. The chief difficulty appears to be finding examples in which the timing of responses in the central nervous system can unambiguously be associated with one of the perceived dimensions of an image.

To evaluate the role of response timing for creating discrete entities in perception thus requires getting control over both possibilities, that timing affects binding and also perception of feature magnitude, by finding a perceptual system in which both of these actions can be observed for the same images and experimentally dissociated. The sonar of bats offers a rare glimpse of how the timing of events in the brain affects the content of perceived images. In echolocation, the timing of neural responses determines the segmentation of a specific perceptual dimension, distance, into discrete objects to which different features are attributed, and it also determines the magnitude of the distance for each object. By great good fortune, some other aspect of responses carries information about the shape of objects and can be distinguished by its relation to distance for each separate object.

TARGET RANGING IN THE SONAR OF BATS

Echolocation Sounds of the Big Brown Bat

The big brown bat, *Eptesicus fuscus* ("dusky house-flier," mammalian order Chiroptera, family Vespertilionidae; Kurta and Baker, 1990), broadcasts frequency-modulated (FM) sonar sounds and can detect insect-size objects at distances up to about 5 m from their echoes (Kick, 1982). *Eptesicus* feeds on flying insects that it detects, tracks, identifies, and intercepts with the guidance of sonar. Figure 11.1 illustrates spectrograms of echolocation sounds broadcast by *Eptesicus*. These sounds contain frequencies from about 20 to 100 kHz in several harmonic FM sweeps, most prominently the first harmonic sweeping from 55 kHz down to 23 kHz, and the second harmonic sweeping from 100 kHz down to 45 kHz (Simmons, 1989). The durations of the sounds in figure 11.1 are from about 8 msec (a) to as short as 0.5 msec (f and g). The bat adjusts the length of each broadcast sound according to its distance from the target to keep the duration only slightly shorter than the delay of the echo (see figure 11.2A). The bat's ability to perceive insects and avoid obstacles to flight depends on its receiving echoes of these sounds. It broadcasts its sounds at rates of roughly 5 to 150 per second at different stages of its approach to a target, and forms an image for each emission and its associated series of echoes.

Target Range and Echo Delay

Echolocating bats determine the distance to objects (target range) from echo delay (Simmons, 1989; Suga, 1990). Experiments demonstrate that *Eptesicus* is

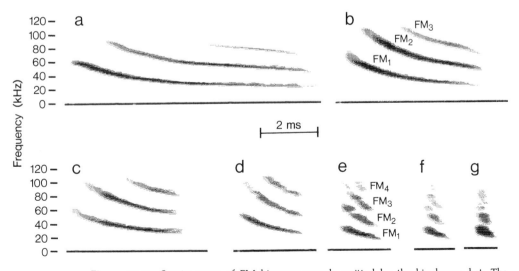

Figure 11.1 Spectrograms of FM biosonar sounds emitted by the big brown bat. The duration and the sweep structure change as the bat approaches the target.

exquisitely sensitive to small changes in the delay of successive echoes, and that the information responsible for this sensitivity evidently is conveyed up the auditory pathway by the timing of neural responses (Menne et al, 1989; Moss and Schnitzler, 1989; Moss and Simmons, 1993; Simmons et al, 1990). Moreover, the bat remembers information about the distance to different parts of a target from images having the psychological dimension of range (Simmons 1989; Simmons, Moss, and Ferragamo, 1990).

Figure 11.2A illustrates schematically the spatial and acoustic conditions for target ranging in echolocation. The bat emits a sonar sound that travels out to the target and then reflects back to the bat's ears. Each echo is essentially a delayed replica of the broadcast sound. The bat hears the emission directly as it is sent out, and, then, after the two-way travel time of the sound, it hears the echo. For echoes in air the value for this delay (t), is 5.8 msec per meter of target range. If *Eptesicus* can perceive targets as far away as 5 m, it must be able to process echoes at delays up to about 30 msec. Note that the duration of the broadcast sound is nearly as long as the echo's total delay. When approaching an insect, *Eptesicus* reduces the duration of its signals to keep the emission from overlapping with the echo. The sound's duration thus is just short of the two-way travel time of the echo, so the sound extends in space out to the target and most of the way back to the ears before ending. This extended duration results in responses to the earlier, higher-frequency sounds in each FM sweep occurring well before responses to later, lower-frequency sounds even start to occur. Because the bat's auditory responses are triggered frequency by frequency, the onset of responses representing each sound is dispersed over a span of time equal to the duration of the sound as a whole, which can be anywhere from 0.5 msec at the shortest target ranges to as much as 15 to 20 msec at the longest ranges.

Coincidence Detection as the Basis for Determining Echo Delay

The auditory system of *Eptesicus* responds first to the emission and then to the echo with a volley of neural discharges registering the time of occurrence of successive frequencies in the FM sweeps for each sound (Simmons et al, 1995b). The timing of responses evoked by the echo is compared with the timing of responses evoked by the preceding emission to determine the value of delay, t, and thus of target range. This comparison is carried out by delaying and dispersing responses within the auditory system to each frequency in the emitted sound to form a kind of short-term, dynamic memory for the FM sweeps. In the inferior colliculus, latencies start at about 5 msec and can extend up to about 25 to 30 msec or more (Haplea, Covey, and Casseday, 1994), the operating range of the bat's sonar. Responses to the emission thus are still in progress when responses to the echo start to occur. Latency dispersion is compounded by dispersion of responses to successive frequencies over the duration of each sound (see above). The timing of individual responses to each emission or echo thus falls within a span of

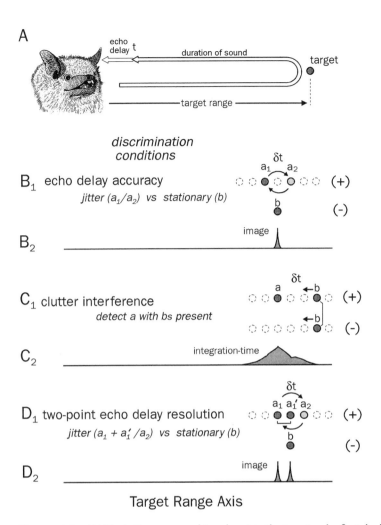

Target Range Axis

Figure 11.2 (A) The bat's sonar sound travels out to the target and reflects back to the bat's ears, where it is received after a delay (*t*) proportional to target range. The duration of each broadcast is usually only slightly shorter than the two-way travel time of echoes, so the bat virtually fills the path from its mouth out to the target and back to the ears with the sound. (B₁) Procedure for measuring the bat's echo-delay accuracy. The positive stimulus (+) is a series of jittering echoes (a_1 alternating with a_2) with a delay change (δt) that declines to zero in small steps; the negative stimulus is a series of echoes (*b*) at a fixed delay. (B₂) The bat's performance in percentage errors has a single, sharp peak located at the perceived arrival time of the jittering echoes when the jitter becomes too small to be detected (threshold $\delta t = 10$–15 ns; figure 11.3). (C₁) Procedure for measuring the bat's clutter-interference window. Positive stimulus (+) is a test echo (*a*) at a fixed delay, with additional cluttering echoes (*b*) at varying delays (δt); negative stimulus (−) is just the cluttering echoes (*b*). (C₂) The bat's performance in percentage errors has a broad peak (about ±350 μsec wide; figure 11.4) centered at the location of test echo (*a*) and tracing the region where cluttering echoes (*b*) interfere with detection of test echo (*a*). (D₁) Procedure for measuring the bat's sensitivity to two-point targets or double echoes, for 0, 10, 20, or 30 μsec time separations of double echoes (a_1, a_1'). As in B₁, positive stimulus (+) is a series of jittering echoes (a_1 alternating with a_2), and negative stimulus (−) is a series of fixed echoes (*b*) but the single echo (a_1) is replaced with the double echo ($a_1 + a_1'$). The jittering delay (δt) is now used to determine whether the bat perceives just one delay for the double echo or two delays. (D₂) The bat's performance in percent errors shows two peaks—one corresponding to a_1 and the other to a_1' at different separations (figure 11.5).

several tens of milliseconds, satisfying the requirement that the bat's responses mimic the latency dispersion found in other sensory systems.

Variously dispersed responses to the emission, which occur at characteristic latencies in each neuron, serve as inputs to coincidence-detecting neurons, and responses to the echo occurring somewhat later serve as the other inputs. When the air-path delay of the echo, t, matches the difference between the latencies of the emission and echo inputs to specific coincidence-detecting neurons, those cells respond to signify that a coincidence has occurred, indicating that an echo has been received at the corresponding delay.

Accuracy of Echo-Delay Perception

The perception of echo delay, t, as a dimension of sonar images (the range dimension) has been evaluated in several different types of behavioral experiments. In figure $11.2B_{1-2}$ the most basic type of experiment is illustrated; it measures the smallest change in echo delay that the bat can perceive from one echo to the next (echo delay accuracy). As shown schematically in figure $11.2B_1$, each bat is trained to discriminate between a stimulus consisting of echoes of successive sonar sounds that vary in delay between two values by the amount δt (a_1 and a_2) and another stimulus consisting of echoes that arrive at a stationary delay, b. The variable-delay echoes actually jitter in delay—the delay is changed from one emitted sound to the next, cycling back and forth from a_1 to a_2 (arrows in figure $11.2B_1$) so that the target appears to flutter from one range to another. In this case, the value of delay b is about 3 msec, which corresponds to a target range of about 0.5 m, and the values of a_1 and a_2 are respectively placed a few microseconds earlier and later than b. The bat is rewarded for choosing the jittering echoes ($+$) instead of the stationary echoes ($-$) in either a two-choice or a yes-no task (Menne et al, 1989; Moss and Schnitzler, 1989; Moss and Simmons, 1989; Simmons, 1979, 1993; Simmons et al, 1990). This procedure delivers the crucial stimulus characteristic—the shift in echo delay δt—from one emission to the next while the bat broadcasts a series of signals, so that the corresponding series of echoes will alternate in arrival time from one echo to the next by the amount δt. The size of δt is changed from one block of trials to another in small steps (from 50 μsec down to zero μsec) to determine the smallest echo-delay shift the bat can perceive in this echo-by-echo presentation.

As the separation of echoes a_1 and a_2 (δt) becomes progressively smaller, the bat's performance traces a remembered image (figure $11.2B_2$) from the percentage of errors it makes in this task (Simmons, 1979, 1993; Simmons et al, 1990). In effect, plotting the error rate for different values of δt yields an outline of the image of echo a_1 along the delay axis, with echo a_2 serving as a probe echo to compare with echo a_1. Several different experiments of this type have produced similar results; they reveal that the bat's limit for perceiving changes in echo delay around a value of roughly 3 msec for b is

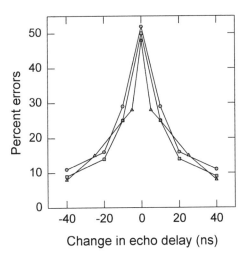

FINE ECHO DELAY ACUITY

Figure 11.3 Performance of three *Eptesicus* in jittered-echo task for measuring echo-delay accuracy (figure 2B$_1$). The width of the bat's image for the delay of a series of echoes is about 10 to 15 ns under optimum quiet conditions.

smaller than 0.5 μsec. One series of experiments pursued small enough delay steps to determine the bat's limiting acuity for echo delay (Simmons et al, 1990).

Figure 11.3 shows the performance of three *Eptesicus* in this jittered-echo task for delay changes up to ± 40 ns (yes, nanoseconds!). The limits of performance (threshold for 25% errors, or 75% correct responses) is 10 to 15 ns for detecting changes in delay, δt, around a value of $t = 3$ msec under quiet conditions. Moreover, in the presence of random noise deliberately introduced to establish a controlled echo signal-to-noise ratio of 36 dB, the bat can perceive changes as small as 40 ns. These jittered-echo experiments also reveal that *Eptesicus* can perceive changes in the phase of echoes relative to emissions, which, for FM sounds, amount to shifts of several microseconds in the relative timing of different parts of the FM sweeps. Thus, the bat's image of a series of echoes arriving at a single delay is very sharp, even though the sounds themselves are several milliseconds long (figure 11.1c–e; Simmons, 1993), and the neural responses to both the emissions and the echoes are spread over a span of 25 to 30 msec. The bat evidently can concentrate all the information it has about the timing of responses to a series of emissions and echoes, compressing the latency differences and coincidence detections into a single echo delay estimate that is as sharp as 10 to 15 ns. This extraordinary precision satisfies the requirement that the intrinsic timing acuity of the sensory system be significantly sharper than the width of the neural discharges themselves, which typically is several hundred microseconds.

Clutter Interference: Detection of one Echo in the Presence of other Echoes

The jittering-echo experiment illustrated in figure 11.2B$_{1-2}$ was carried out to measure the fine accuracy of echo-delay perception; the resulting acuity of 10 to 40 ns is the bat's hyperacuity for echo delay (analogous to visual hyperacuity; Altes, 1989). The experiment shown in figure 11.2C$_{1-2}$ (on clutter interference) is different. It measures the width of the time window around the arrival time of one test echo (in this case, a) for additional echoes, b, to interfere with detection of the test echo (Simmons et al, 1989). (Extraneous echoes that mask the presence of desired echoes are called clutter interference in radar or sonar systems.) The bat is trained in a two-choice task to detect echo a at a delay of $t = 3$ msec, and echo b is presented at delays that differ from echo a by the amount δt. The interfering echoes, b, are delivered with echo a at delays that vary from about 1 msec later to 1 msec earlier in small steps (δt thus varies by ± 1 msec around 3 msec). In this task, all the echoes are presented together each time the bat broadcasts a sonar sound, so the bat has no opportunity to hear echo a separate from echo b, as it has for separately delivered echoes a_1 and a_2 in the jitter task (figure 11.2B$_1$).

As the arrival time of echo b passes through the region occupied by echo a, the bat's performance at detecting echo a traces a zone of clutter interference that extends in time over a broad span around the arrival time of the echo to be detected (figure 11.2C$_2$). Figure 11.4 shows the average percentage errors for several bats in the clutter-interference experiment diagrammed in figure 11.2C$_1$. The width of this zone is about ± 350 μsec (at half-height

CLUTTER INTERFERENCE WINDOW

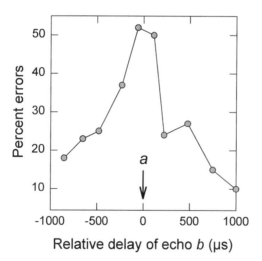

Figure 11.4 Average performance of five *Eptesicus* in clutter-interference experiment (figure 2C$_1$). The zone of clutter interference is about ± 350 μsec wide at its half-height.

J. A. Simmons

of curve). It defines a region of time within which neural representations of echoes *a* and *b* must coexist in the same format so that the arrival of one echo obscures the presence of the other. In effect, waveforms of two echoes that arrive within about 350 μsec of each other are combined into a single compound echo, so that the presence of the second echo is masked by the first. In terms of the bat's sonar receiver, the width of this clutter-interference window is the integration time for echo reception (Simmons et al, 1989), but it also is about the duration of individual neural discharges within the bat's auditory system, which are several hundred microseconds wide. It seems reasonable to suppose that two stimuli normally evoking separate volleys of neural discharges, but whose times of occurrence are closer together than the width of these neural discharges, must merge in perception because the separate volleys of discharges merge to form a single volley. Is the clutter-interference zone in figure 11.4 the binding window within which neural responses that occur simultaneously are grouped together to form one entity in perception?

Discrimination of Double Echoes with Closely Spaced Delays

The third type of behavioral experiment on echo-delay perception shown in figure 11.2D$_{1-2}$ measures the bat's ability to perceive two closely spaced echoes as having discrete, separate arrival times (two-point echo-delay resolution). This two-point threshold is important because the insects that bats seek as prey are made up acoustically of two or three primary reflecting points or surfaces (e.g., head, abdomen, wings) that each reflect a replica of the broadcast sound back to the bat (Kober and Schnitzler, 1990; Moss and Zagaeski, 1994; Simmons and Chen, 1989; Simmons, 1989). Echoes from real targets encountered frequently every night by flying bats consist of two or three closely spaced echo components separated by small delay intervals of only a few tens of microseconds at most. (Most insects have dimensions of only 1 to 2 cm, so their reflecting surfaces are close together along the range axis.) The simplest prototypical natural echo would thus be a double echo with a small delay separation of its two component reflections; target identification would be based on perception of the delay separation of the reflections.

Two experiments demonstrate that *Eptesicus* can discriminate between single echoes at a delay of about 3 msec and double echoes with an overall delay of about 3 msec, but a delay separation as small as 2 to 10 μsec (Mogdans and Schnitzler, 1990; Simmons et al, 1989). Although these experiments show that bats can distinguish among targets that reflect double echoes, the results address only whether the bat can "tell the difference" between a double echo and a single echo. They do not address whether the bat actually perceives the double echo as containing two reflected replicas of the broadcast sound, and, thus, whether the target actually contains two separate parts (e.g., a head and a wing). This is an important question because it indeed is possible for the bat to perceive that double echoes are different from single echoes without perceiving that they actually are double.

The Interference Spectrum of Overlapping Double Echoes

The two overlapping reflections making up the double echoes are separated by very short intervals of only a few tens of microseconds, well within the ± 350-μsec width of the clutter-interference zone or the integration time for echo reception (figures 11.2C_{1-2} and 11.4). Furthermore, the minimum separation the bat can detect is even smaller, in the region of 2 to 10 μsec depending on which experiment is considered. The duration of the bat's emissions is far larger than these delay separations; it is similar to the overall delay of the echoes (3 msec) rather than the difference as small as a few microseconds between the delays. Consequently, a double echo consists of two different reflected replicas of the broadcast sound arriving so close together that they overlap almost completely and are combined by the bat's inner ear into a single sound. These double echoes actually merge together on reception by the ear to form a single echo with a complex interference spectrum created by the mutual reinforcement or cancellation of the combined double-echo waveforms across different frequencies (Altes, 1984; Simmons, 1989).

The interference spectrum for the double echo as a whole contains a series of peaks and notches at specific frequencies related to the size of the delay separation of the two components of the echo. For example, the frequency spacing of the peaks and notches in the interference spectrum is equal to the reciprocal of this time separation. Because the inner ear's integration time is so long, the double echoes necessarily are treated as just one sound. As a result, the bat's discrimination of small changes in the delay separation of double echoes must be based on the interference spectrum of the overlapping waveforms and not on any direct measurement of their two constituent delays as separate, discrete events in time. That is, the double echoes must be received as having one arrival time plus one complex spectrum, not two arrival times.

This is the currently accepted description of how bats identify targets from their shape—they perceive the distance to the target from the one delay formed by the two overlapping echoes, and they identify the shape from the spectral coloration of the double echo caused by interference (Neuweiler, 1990). The missing piece of information, however, is whether the bat perceives shape itself as a spatial structure of the target, with its two reflecting points, or whether it merely perceives the echo spectrum as an auditory quality of a more abstract nature (coloration or timbre). Whereas the 350-μsec integration time demonstrates that the bat receives one echo delay plus one interference spectrum for a double echo, it might still be able to perceive the delays of both components of the double echo if it could "read" the spectral peaks and notches to determine their message about time, not just their messsage about frequency.

Resolution of Closely Spaced Echoes

Figure 11.2D$_1$ illustrates an experiment designed to probe deeper into the nature of the bat's perception of a double echo. It combines the jittered-echo procedure of figure 11.2B$_1$ with presentation of a double echo to determine whether the bat perceives a single numerical value for the delay of the double echo (that otherwise has a distinctive spectral coloration to distinguish it from a single echo), or whether it perceives two different delay values, one for each of the two components of the echo. In the basic jitter experiment (figure 11.2B$_1$), echo a_1 is alternated with echo a_2 to determine the smallest separation (δt) of the jittering echoes that the bat can perceive. The resulting performance (figure 11.2B$_2$) traces an image of echo a_1 using echo a_2 as a probe or pointer for locating the perceived delay value the bat's auditory system assigns to echo a_1. If a second echo, a_1', is added to echo a_1 at a small time separation (see figure 11.2D$_1$), the resulting compound waveform ($a_1 + a_1'$) is a double echo with a unique spectrum formed by interference between the two overlapping components. Now, when the double echo ($a_1 + a_1'$) is alternated with the single echo (a_2) at different time separations in the jitter task (δt is still the difference between echo a_1 and echo a_2, as in figure 11.2B$_1$), does the bat perceive an image with just one peak for the double echo, or does it perceive an image with an additional peak caused by separate registration of the delays of echo a_1 and echo a_1'? If each component of the double echo is perceived as having its own arrival time, the bat should make a significant proportion of errors when echo a_2 (the pointer) is aligned at the same delay as either component a_1 or component a_1'.

Figure 11.5 illustrates the performance (again, percentage errors) of two *Eptesicus* in a jitter experiment with double echoes (see figure 11.2D$_1$) having a delay separation of 0, 10, 20, or 30 μsec between a_1 and a_1', and with delays of a_2 spanning the region containing the double echoes ($\delta t = -10 \mu$sec to $+50 \mu$sec in figure 11.5; Simmons, 1993). First, when there is only a single echo instead of a double echo (delay separation of a_1 and a_1' is zero μsec), conditions are the same as in the basic jitter procedure shown in figure 11.2B$_1$. The bat makes a single error peak when echo a_2 falls at the time of arrival of echo a_1 (no a_1' is present) in the top graph in figure 11.5. (This curve is just a wider view of the same curve shown in fine detail around its center in figure 11.3; it is the image of a single echo.) However, when there really are double echoes, the bats clearly make a peak of errors at two different locations of a_2 corresponding to the location of a_1 at zero μsec and a_1' at 10, 20, or 30 μsec (remaining three graphs in figure 11.5). Because the jitter procedure explicitly tests a remembered image from one emission to the next, the bat must perceive the individual delays of both components of the double echo. This occurs despite the fact that the overlapping component echoes are far closer together than the width of the clutter-interference zone (figure 11.4). Experiments with yet smaller delay separations between a_1 and a_1'

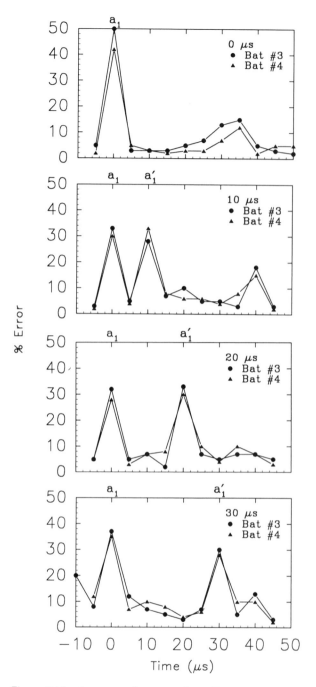

Figure 11.5 Average performance of two *Eptesicus* in two-point experiments (figure 2D₁). The bat can perceive the arrival time of each component in the double echo (a_1, a_1') for delay separations of 10, 20, or 30 μsec.

reveal that *Eptesicus* can resolve two echoes as having separate delays for differences as small as 2 μsec (Saillant et al, 1993).

The bat's ability to perceive closely spaced echo delays suggests a reason why it might need a high absolute acuity for echo delay in the range of 10 to 15 ns in quiet conditions (figure 11.3). To register two echoes that arrive close together in time as having separate delays (down to 2 μsec), the bat must be able to subdivide the perceived axis of delay into correspondingly fine delay steps. Without this fine-grain registration of delay, the numerical difference in delay between the two components of double echoes, and thus the small difference in distance to two reflecting surfaces in the target, would be obscured. The capacity to resolve closely spaced echoes as having different values for echo delay is crucial for locating each object in a complicated, realistic acoustic scene composed of multiple targets to be identified and tracked, and obstacles to be avoided. Bats do in fact manifest a need for surprisingly high temporal precision and resolution often during their nightly activities (Simmons et al, 1995a).

Transforming the Spectrum of Double Echoes into Two-Point Images

The bat's ability to perceive discrete delays as close together as 2 μsec is an example of hyperresolution because it is within the Rayleigh limit for the bat's signals. The frequencies broadcast by *Eptesicus* cover the band from about 20 to 100 kHz (figure 11.1); the shortest periods in these sounds are about 10 μsec, whereas the shortest delay separations the bat can perceive are about 2 μsec. *Eptesicus* can resolve two delays as separate events in time even when they are separated by less than the length of the shortest periods in the sounds. This ability demonstrates that it must have an intimate knowledge of the waveforms it broadcasts and the echoes it receives. Using this knowledge, the bat can exploit small differences between the transmitted and reflected signals to make extraordinarily fine inferences about the structure of targets. It uses this knowledge to deconvolve the double echoes to remove the limitations on echo processing originally caused by the relatively large ± 350-μsec width of the zone of clutter interference, or the integration time for echo reception (Saillant et al, 1993).

The goal of deconvolution is to recover information about the timing of closely spaced components of double echoes that has been lost in the time domain and shifted into the frequency domain by the overlap and mixing of these components. In simple terms, the bat's intimate knowledge consists of the frequencies and frequency spacing of the peaks and notches in the interference spectrum of double echoes, which the bat transforms back into an estimate of the time separation of overlapping echo components required to produce these peaks and notches through interference (Simmons, 1989). As a result, it perceives a component of the image for each component of the double echo, not just a single overall image for the combined components.

Eptesicus perceives both reflecting points in the target to exist at their respective ranges, which is quite different from perceiving merely that the target reflects echoes that are qualitatively distinct in their spectral features. The fact that the bat perceives the delay of the second echo of the pair for delay separations shorter than the 350-μsec integration time by deconvolution of the spectrum provides a tool for observing the boundary between events that are included inside the binding window and events that are excluded.

MANIFESTATION OF TEMPORAL BINDING IN ECHOLOCATION

Origin of Clutter Interference

Clutter interference occurs when a test echo (*a* in figure 11.2C$_1$) is obscured as a discrete signal by the arrival of other echoes (*b*) within a critical period of time around the test echo. In effect, all the responses that take place within this window are treated as responses to the same sound; that is, they are bound together as representing just one sound that has a particular spectrum, not two sounds. In the bat's auditory system, echoes are registered as separate sounds occurring at specific times by volleys of neural discharges that trace the frequencies of their FM sweeps (Pollak and Casseday, 1989; Simmons et al, 1995b; Suga, 1990). The minimum separation of two sounds required for each to evoke a separate volley of neural responses is about 300 to 500 μsec; this is called the recovery time for responses to the second sound (Covey and Casseday, 1991; Grinnell, 1963; Suga, 1964). The echo-detection task in figure 11.2C$_{1-2}$ appears to monitor this physiological recovery effect behaviorally. The discharges separately evoked by the test echo *a* and cluttering echoes *b* merge into a single volley if the sounds arrive closer together than 300 to 500 μsec, and the bat in fact cannot detect the test echo for separations shorter than 350 μsec. The curve in figure 11.4 traces the bat's behavioral recovery time, or integration time, in a two-echo task.

It is important to be sure that the $\pm$350-μsec width of the clutter-interference window (figure 11.4) does not merely reflect some limitation on the accuracy with which the bat can measure or enumerate the arrival times of echoes. The bat's ability to detect one set of echoes (*a* in figure 11.2C$_1$) is impaired if another set of echoes *b* arrives within about 350 μsec of the same arrival time (figure 11.4). Yet, the bat still has the ability to perceive very much smaller changes of a fraction of a microsecond in the delay of individual echoes (*a*$_1$ or *a*$_2$ in figure 11.2B$_1$; see figure 11.3) and it also can perceive separate delays for echoes that arrive as close together as a few microseconds (*a*$_1$ and *a*$_1'$ in figure 11.2D$_1$; see figure 11.5). The bat's fine acuity for echo delay and two-point resolution of different echo delays is far sharper than the size of the clutter-interference window, so there is no reason to believe that the relatively wide $\pm$350-μsec interference zone reflects some intrinsic inability of the bat to register arrival times precisely along its psychological scale of delay or range. The bat can cope with numerical values for the delays of more than one echo at a time on a very fine scale indeed. In effect the full time width of the responses that represent each echo is greater than the acuity with which it can locate or perceive shifts in the psychological center of these responses.

It also is important to see the significance of the ± 350-μsec length of the clutter-interference interval in relation to the length of the bat's sounds or the span of time over which neural responses take place to each emission and echo. This consideration leads to the conclusion that clutter interference must occur as a consequence of the action of neural coincidence detectors either succeeding or failing to detect the test echo as a separate sound from the cluttering echoes, demonstrating that clutter interference is a specific instance of temporal binding in the sense described above. The raw waveforms of the test and cluttering echoes themselves are several milliseconds long because the overall delay of the echoes (t) is about 3 msec and the bat adjusts its emissions to approximate this length (figure 11.2A). These echo waveforms of course overlap at delay separations of several milliseconds or less, whereas clutter interference only appears at much shorter separations; echoes have to be closer together than 1 msec for even a weak interference effect to appear (figure 11.4).

The span of time encompassing neural responses to the emitted sound or to the echoes is even longer than the duration of the FM sweeps. Individual frequencies in the FM sweeps of emissions and echoes are dispersed over the duration of the sounds, which is several milliseconds, and the responses to these frequencies are further dispersed over a span of 30 msec or more by the system of progressively lengthening and expanding latencies in the bat's auditory system (Haplea, Covey, and Casseday, 1994). Consequently, the two series of responses evoked by the emission and by the echoes run concurrently for a considerable length of time, at least for 25 msec after the onset of responses to the echoes (Simmons et al, 1995b).

Clutter interference does not occur just because the echo waveforms overlap, and it does not occur just because the lengthy series of neural responses evoked by these sounds overlap. Instead, it occurs because the effective width of the burst of responses evoked by each emission-echo pair of sounds is only about ± 350 μsec after the slopes of the FM sweeps and the dispersal of response latencies all are taken into account. The bat's images reflect only the difference in time between the emission and the echoes, or the distance to targets, not the relatively spread-out pattern of discharges evoked by each sound. The only responses that can extract this difference to remove the slope of the sweeps and also the dispersal of absolute latencies in *Eptesicus* are the responses of the coincidence detectors that compare individual discharges to the emission and the echo at various different latencies (Dear et al, 1993; Dear, Simmons, and Fritz, 1993). In echolocating bats, the auditory system's coincidence detectors create a display of target range because each coincidence detector is tuned to a specific echo delay whose value is the difference in time between the latencies of its inputs—a response to the emission at one latency (from 5 to about 30 msec; Simmons et al, 1995b) and a response to the echo at a different, shorter latency. The bat perceives a target at a specific range because echoes at the corresponding delay activate coincidence detectors tuned to that delay value (Riquimaroux, Gaioni, and Suga, 1991).

Can Temporal Binding Be Demonstrated in Echolocation?

If two echoes arrive farther apart than the integration time or binding window of ± 350 μsec, they each evoke a volley of discharges. Each volley then activates coincidence detectors tuned to the corresponding echo delay value. Clutter interference most likely occurs because the separate volleys of discharges making up the neural representations of two echoes collide and become intermingled into a single volley from which the coincidence detectors extract a single value for the delay of echoes rather than the two delays present in the original sounds. Therefore, the width of the clutter-interference window corresponds to the limit for detection of one versus two independent sets of responses in time. Can this collision of responses in time be demonstrated directly in the bat's images? The circumstance that the time scale for clutter interference, or integration time, is coarse but the time scales for echo delay acuity and two-point resolution are very fine sets the stage for an important contribution by the bat and its unusual perceptual system to our understanding of temporal binding.

Because the bat's perceptual acuity is better than its clutter-interference zone, we can ask the bat itself to examine the structure of the images of double echoes it perceives, using its own intrinsic temporal precision to tell us how the information contained in these images is apportioned along the scale of delay or range. It turns out that we can demonstrate behaviorally that the width of the clutter-interference zone corresponds to the width of the window that defines the time of occurrence of a single volley of neural discharges. To the bat, this is the binding window for a target as a discrete event along the axis of distance.

Amplitude-Latency Trading of Echo Delay

Because the bat perceives the distance to objects from the time that elapses between the volley of neural responses to the emission and the volley of responses to the echo, its perception of the delay of echoes will be vulnerable to any change in the timing of the discharges themselves. Of course, if the delay of the echo changes, the timing of discharges to the echo changes, too, and the bat correctly perceives the result as a change in the distance to the target (Simmons, 1973). However, the timing of neural responses to sounds can be altered without changing the actual time at which the sound is presented. Specifically, if the amplitude of the stimulus is reduced, the latency of the neural responses will be lengthened (Pollak, 1988; Pollak et al, 1977; Pollak and Casseday, 1989). This effect is called amplitude-latency trading, and it has been demonstrated to occur in the target-ranging process used by *Eptesicus* (Simmons, 1993; Simmons et al, 1990; Simmons, Moss, and Ferragamo, 1990).

Physiological measurements show amplitude-latency trading to be about 15 to 20 μsec for each decibel of amplitude change (written as -15 to -20 μsec/dB because a decrease in amplitude lengthens latency). This physiological effect leads to the prediction that changing the amplitude of echoes should cause the bat to perceive echoes at a different delay, and in fact the bat's image of echo a_1 in figure 11.3B$_1$ shifts by about -17 μsec/dB (Simmons, Moss, and Ferragamo, 1990). The whole curve shown in figure 11.5 for zero-μsec delay separation (top graph) shifts to the right by 17 μsec either when echo a_1 is decreased by 1 dB or when echo a_2 is increased by 1 dB (Simmons et al, 1990). This amplitude-latency trading effect is observed with single echoes (a_1). What happens to the image of a double echo ($a_1 + a'_1$; see figure 11.5 for 10-, 20-, or 30-μsec delay separations) when either of the two components is changed in amplitude?

Experimental Dissociation of Double-Echo Images

The Predictions   Two separate echoes will evoke separate volleys of discharges as long as they arrive farther apart than some minimal interval, which has been measured physiologically to be in the range of 300 to 500 μsec. The question is, does the width of the clutter-interference zone measured behaviorally in figure 11.4 correspond to this interval? If the two echoes are far enough apart to evoke neural discharges whose latencies register their arrival time for target ranging, they both should undergo amplitude-latency trading. However, changing the amplitude of just one of the two echoes should change the perceived delay of only that echo because the latencies for the discharges evoked by the two echoes are independent. The specific prediction is that, in the image of a double echo, changing the amplitude of echo a_1 should move the first peak in the bat's error curve to a new location by -15 to -20 μsec/dB, and changing the amplitude of echo a'_1 should move the second peak. However, if the two echoes are close enough in delay that the discharges to the second echo are obscured or fail to occur, then changing the amplitude of echo a'_1 should not produce a shift in the second error peak because that peak in the bat's performance curve is not derived from the timing of an independent volley of discharges evoked by echo a'_1. Instead, because the second error peak is derived from the spectral peak-and-notch deconvolution of the overlapping components in the double echo (Saillant et al, 1993), it should stay in the same location when the amplitude of echo a'_1 changes. A perceived delay shift should not occur for echo a'_1 because the frequencies at which spectral peaks and notches are located by interference should not change as the amplitude of one of the echoes is changed. In this case, the second error peak for echo a'_1 depends on the discharges evoked by the first echo, a_1, for its absolute time value because these are the responses that carry information about the spectral peaks and notches for the double echo as a whole. (No responses occur directly to the second echo at all; it just modulates the pattern of responses evoked by the first echo.) Only a change in the amplitude of echo a_1 should shift the error peak for echo a_1' to a new delay, and then both error peaks should move together (Simmons, Moss, and Ferragamo, 1990).

Whether the error peak for the second echo a_1' shifts according to amplitude-latency trading thus becomes a test for whether the second echo is represented by its own volley of discharges or is instead extracted from the spectral peaks and notches in the double echo as a whole. The specific prediction is that the second error peak for a double echo should undergo amplitude-latency trading by itself only if the delay separation of the two echoes is larger than the integration time of 350 μsec. At shorter delay separations, the second error peak should instead undergo amplitude-latency trading in tandem with the first error peak.

The Results   The prediction described was tested in double-echo experiments with different time separations of the two echo components. The procedures are the same as diagrammed in figure 11.2D$_1$, but with larger delay separations of the two echoes ($a_1 + a_1'$) and a correspondingly wider span of values for the delay of the pointer echo, a_2. Now the two components are separated by 20, 300, or 500 μsec to provide a span of separations ranging from shorter than the clutter-interference time (20 μsec) to roughly equal to the clutter interference time (300 μsec) and finally to longer than the clutter-interference time (500 μsec). (In figure 11.5 the double-echo separations of 10, 20, or 30 μsec were all shorter than the clutter-interference time to demonstrate that the bat could perceive both echo delays even for very short delay intervals.) Figure 11.6 shows typical results from a series of double-echo jitter experiments with *Eptesicus*. (The time axis of figure 11.6 shows the delay of echo a_2 in figure 11.2D$_1$ relative to the delay of the second component, a_1'. That is, zero on the horizontal axis is the arrival time of echo a_1'. Echo a_1 still arrives at a delay of about 3 msec and is earlier than echo a_1' by 20, 300, or 500 μsec.)

In figure 11.6A, the performance curve for a 20-μsec echo-delay separation contains two large error peaks, one at -20 μsec for a_1 and the other at zero μsec for a_1'. Similarly, the performance curves for the 300-μsec delay separation (figure 11.6C) and the 500-μsec delay separation (figure 11.6F) show error peaks at the delays of both a_1 (at -300 μsec in C and -500 μsec in F) and a_1' (at zero μsec in C and F). As already indicated in figure 11.4, the bat can perceive the delay of the second component of the double echo at small delay separations, and now figures 11.6C and F show that it can also perceive the second component at longer delay separations. So, at delay separations of 20, 300, or 500 μsec, the bat's image of a double echo depicts the two components at their corresponding arrival times. The most important question, however, is how these error peaks are affected by changes in the amplitude of echo a_1'.

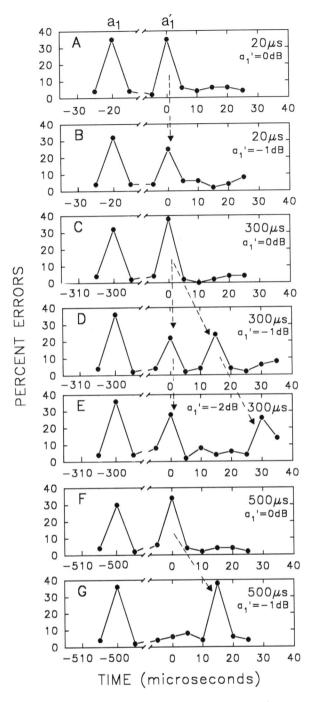

Figure 11.6 Performance of one *Eptesicus* in a series of two-point experiments with different echo-delay separations for a_1 to a_1' of 20 μsec (A), 300 μsec (C), or 500 μsec (F). The experiment tested the occurence of amplitude-latency trading in the image of the second component (a_1') at each separation (20 μsec in B, 300 μsec in D and E, 500 μsec in G). At 20 μsec no trading shift occurred (A, B), at 500 μsec a full shift occurred (F, G), whereas at 300 μsec half the image shifted and half did not (C, D, and E), to split the image into two parts.

To start with the 500-μsec delay separation, figure 11.6G shows that a 1-dB reduction in the amplitude of the second echo a_1' results in a shift in the second error peak by about 15 μsec to the right (sloping arrow from F to G). The bat thus perceives the arrival time of echo a_1' as being about 15 μsec later if the amplitude of this echo is made weaker by 1 dB. The occurrence of amplitude-latency trading for the second error peak at a 500-μsec delay separation in figure 11.6G indicates that echo a_1' evokes its own volley of neural discharges independent of the discharges evoked by echo a_1, and that the bat judges the arrival time of the second component of the double echo from the latencies of these discharges. (Not shown is the amplitude-latency shift for a_1 itself, which occurs independently.) Thus, a double-echo delay separation of 500 μsec indeed results in two independent sets of neural responses whose times of occurrence can be perceived as separate objects in the bat's images.

In contrast, at a delay separation of only 20 μsec in figure 11.6B, the second error peak does not shift to a different time when echo a_1' is reduced by 1 dB (vertical arrow from A to B). The bat thus does not form this second delay estimate from the timing of neural discharges evoked by echo a_1' itself. Instead, the information used to form the second delay estimate is carried by neural discharges evoked by the double echo as a whole and timed to occur with respect to echo a_1, not echo a_1'. (Changing the amplitude of echo a_1 shifts the locations of both error peaks by 15 μsec; for economy, this is not shown in figure 11.6.)

The crucial result is found at an intermediate delay separation of 300 μsec, which is about equal to the width of the clutter-interference zone (figure 11.4). At the 300-μsec delay separation, a curious thing happens to the bat's image of the double echo. The second error peak corresponding to the delay of echo a_1' splits into two error peaks when the amplitude of echo a_1' is reduced by 1 dB (figure 11.6D) or by 2 dB (figure 11.6E). One of these peaks remains at the same location as echo a_1' (vertical arrows in C, D, and E). This partial peak behaves similarly to the peak for echo a_1' at the short 20-μsec delay separation (figures 11.6A and B). In contrast, the other error peak that splits off from the second error peak in figure 11.6C moves by 15 μsec to a longer delay for a 1-dB echo amplitude change and moves by 30 μsec for a 2-dB change (sloping arrows in C, D, and E). This shifting peak behaves similarly to the error peak for echo a_1' at the long 500-μsec delay separation (figures 11.6F and G).

Thus, at a delay separation close to the integration time for echo reception, two distinct types of representations for the second echo component a_1' are created and coexist side by side. One of these representations consists of an independent volley of neural discharges to the second echo, and the part of the image produced from this representation undergoes amplitude-latency trading (sloping arrows in C, D, and E). The other representation consists of the spectral peaks and notches caused by overlap of the two echo components, and the part of the image produced from this representation does not undergo amplitude-latency trading (vertical arrows in C, D, and E). Instead, it is linked by amplitude-latency trading to the time of occurrence of responses to the first component, echo a_1.

Clutter Interference Is Temporal Binding, but Images Can still Contain Fine Details about Scenes

The bat's use of the timing of neural discharges evoked by emissions and echoes to determine target range makes its psychological scale of distance a test bed for evaluating temporal mechanisms of binding because the bat defines the existence of targets along the scale at least partly by the independent occurrence of these volleys of discharges. This condition satisfies the requirement stated in the introduction that objects in perception have to be equated both with objects in stimuli and with the timing of neural responses to examine whether binding occurs from synchrony of responses. The question about temporal binding in echolocation thus focuses on the collision of volleys of discharges to form a single volley during clutter interference. Figure 11.6 demonstrates this phenomenon at the level of perception, using the bat's own temporal precision itself rather than microelectrodes to make the desired observations.

By placing the time separation of the two echoes (a_1 and a_1') directly astride the integration time window at 300 μsec, the opposing mechanisms of binding and unbinding can be observed in action. The error peak for echo a_1' that shifts to different times due to amplitude-latency trading is based on the timing of neural discharges. The emergence of this shifting peak (sloping arrows) from within the second error peak in figures 11.6C through E represents temporal segregation or unbinding of responses to form a discrete echo-delay estimate—in effect, a separate object in the bat's perceptions. The error peak that fails to shift (vertical arrows) represents information that remains bound to the earlier set of discharges to echo a_1. This part of the image is produced by processing of spectral information carried by responses to the double echo as a whole, and reveals that other mechanisms besides the timing of responses can create an object in perception, too.

These other mechanisms strictly are deconvolution processes because they operate within the integration time window; in echolocation they correspond to transformation of the interference spectrum of overlapping echoes back into the time domain (Saillant et al, 1993). Deconvolution processes are capable of subdividing the binding window into small segments so that several objects can be depicted in images of scenes without being limited by the binding window itself. In fact, the bat's extraordinarily accurate echo delay (figure 11.3) and two-point resolution (figure 11.5) reveal that quite a large number of independent perceptual entities can be maintained in the images by a combination of accurate registration of time and sophisticated processing of feature information (in this case, spectral peaks and notches), as is proposed for binding in vision. These results in bats should dispel any worries that the width of the temporal binding window is a serious impediment to perception of details in scenes because it might prevent discriminations of parts of objects by lumping together all of the features whose responses are contained in the window.

ACKNOWLEDGMENTS

Research carried out in the past 10 years has been supported by ONR, NSF, NIMH, NIH, McDonnell-Pew, DRF, and SDF. Some of the colleagues who have worked on this project in the past five years are R. A. Altes, F. H. Bouffard, S. P. Dear, M. J. Ferragamo, J. B. Fritz, T. Haresign, D. N. Lee, T. A. McMullen, C. F. Moss, P. A. Saillant, and J. M. Wotton.

REFERENCES

Altes RA. (1984). Texture analysis with spectrograms. *IEEE Trans Sonics Ultrasonics* SU-31: 407–417.

Altes RA. (1989). Ubiquity of hyperacuity. *J Acoust Soc Am* 85:943–952.

Carr CE. (1993). Processing of temporal information in the brain. *Annu Rev Neurosci* 16:233–243.

Covey E, Casseday JH. (1991). The monaural nuclei of the lateral lemniscus in an echolocating bat: Parallel pathways for analyzing temporal features of sound. *J Neurosci* 11:3456–3470.

Dear SP, Fritz J, Haresign T, Ferragamo M, Simmons JA. (1993). Tonotopic and functional organization in the auditory cortex of the big brown bat, *Eptesicus fuscus*. *J Neurophysiol* 70:1988–2009.

Dear SP, Simmons JA, Fritz J. (1993). A possible neuronal basis for representation of acoustic scenes in auditory cortex of the big brown bat. *Nature* 364:620–623.

Griffin DR. (1958). *Listening in the Dark*. Yale University Press, New Haven, CT (reprinted in 1986 by Cornell University Press, Ithaca NY).

Grinnell AD. (1963). The neurophysiology of audition in bats: Temporal parameters. *J Physiol* 167:67–96.

Haplea S, Covey E, Casseday JH. (1994). Frequency tuning and response latencies at three levels in the brainstem of the echolocating bat, *Eptesicus fuscus*. *J Comp Physiol A* 174:671–683.

Kick SA. (1982). Target detection by the echolocating bat, *Eptesicus fuscus*. *J Comp Physiol* 145:431–435.

Kober R, Schnitzler HU. (1990). Information in sonar echoes of fluttering insects available for echolocating bats. *J Acoust Soc Am* 87:874–881.

Kurta A, Baker RH. (1990). *Eptesicus fuscus*. *Mamm Species* 356:1–10.

Kuwabara N, Suga N. (1993). Delay lines and amplitude selectivity are created in subthalamic auditory nuclei: The brachium of the inferior colliculus of the mustached bat. *J Neurophysiol* 69:1713–1724.

Langner G. (1992). Periodicity coding in the auditory system. *Hearing Res* 60:115–142.

Livingstone M, Hubel D. (1988). Segregation of form, color, movement, and depth: Anatomy, physiology, and perception. *Science* 240:741–749.

Menne D, Kaipf I, Wagner I, Ostwald J, Schnitzler HU. (1989). Range estimation by echolocation in the bat *Eptesicus fuscus*: Trading of phase versus time cues. *J Acoust Soc Am* 85:2642–2650.

Mogdans J, Schnitzler HU. (1990). Range resolution and the possible use of spectral information in the echolocating bat, *Eptesicus fuscus*. *J Acoust Soc Am* 88:754–757.

Moss CF, Schnitzler HU. (1989). Accuracy of target ranging in echolocating bats: Acoustic information processing. *J Comp Physiol A* 165:383–393.

Moss CF, Simmons JA. (1993). Acoustic image representation of a point target in the bat, *Eptesicus fuscus*: Evidence for sensitivity to echo phase in bat sonar. *J Acoust Soc Am* 93:1553–1562.

Moss CF, Zagaeski M. (1994). Acoustic information available to bats using frequency-modulated sounds for the perception of insect prey. *J Acoust Soc Am* 95:2745–2756.

Neuweiler G. (1990). Auditory adaptations for prey capture in echolocating bats. *Physiol Rev* 70:615–641.

Pollak GD. (1988). Time is traded for intensity in the bat's auditory system. *Hearing Res* 36:107–124.

Pollak GD, Casseday JH. (1989). *The neural basis of echolocation in bats*. Springer-Verlag, New York.

Pollak GD, Marsh DS, Bodenhamer R, Souther A. (1977). Characteristics of phasic on neurons in inferior colliculus of unanesthetized bats with observations relating to mechanisms for echo ranging. *J Neurophysiol* 40:926–942.

Popper AN, Fay RR, eds. (1995). *Hearing by bats. Springer handbook of auditory research*. Springer-Verlag, New York.

Riquimaroux H, Gaioni SJ, Suga N. (1991). Cortical computational maps control auditory perception. *Science* 251:565–568.

Saillant PA, Simmons JA, Dear SP, McMullen TA. (1993). A computational model of echo processing and acoustic imaging in frequency-modulated echolocating bats: The spectrogram correlation and transformation receiver. *J Acoust Soc Am* 94:2691–2712.

Simmons JA. (1973). The resolution of target range by echolocating bats. *J Acoust Soc Am* 54:157–173.

Simmons JA. (1979). Perception of echo phase information in bat sonar. *Science* 207:1336–1338.

Simmons JA. (1989). A view of the world through the bat's ear: The formation of acoustic images in echolocation. *Cognition* 33:155–199.

Simmons JA. (1993). Evidence for perception of fine echo delay and phase by the FM bat, *Eptesicus fuscus*. *J Comp Physiol A* 172:533–547.

Simmons JA, Chen L. (1989). The acoustic basis for target discrimination by FM echolocating bats. *J Acoust Soc Am* 86:1333–1350.

Simmons JA, Freedman EG, Stevenson SB, Chen L, Wohlgenant TJ. (1989). Clutter interference and the integration time of echoes in the echolocating bat, *Eptesicus fuscus*. *J Acoust Soc Am* 86:1318–1332.

Simmons JA, Ferragamo M, Moss CF, Stevenson SB, Altes RA. (1990). Discrimination of jittered sonar echoes by the echolocating bat, *Eptesicus fuscus*: The shape of target images in echolocation. *J Comp Physiol A* 167:589–616.

Simmons JA, Ferragamo MJ, Saillant PA, Haresign T, Wotton JM, Dear SP, Lee DN. (1995a). Auditory dimensions of acoustic images in echolocation. In: *Hearing by bats. Springer handbook of auditory research*. AN Popper, RR Fay, eds. Springer-Verlag, New York, pp. 146–190.

Simmons JA, Moss CF, Ferragamo M. (1990). Convergence of temporal and spectral information into acoustic images of complex sonar targets perceived by the echolocating bat, *Eptesicus fuscus. J Comp Physiol A* 166:449–470.

Simmons JA, Saillant PA, Ferragamo MJ, Haresign T, Dear SP, Fritz J, McMullen TA. (1995b). Auditory computations for biosonar target imaging in bats. In: *Auditory computation. Springer handbook of auditory research*. HL Hawkins, TA McMullen, AN Popper, RR Fay, eds. Springer-Verlag, New York, pp. 401–468.

Suga N. (1964). Recovery cycles and responses to frequency modulated tone pulses in auditory neurons of echolocating bats. *J Physiol* 175:50–80.

Suga N. (1990). Cortical computational maps for auditory imaging. *Neural Networks* 3:3–21.

Sullivan WE. (1982). Neural representation of target distance in auditory cortex of the echolocating bat *Myotis lucifugus. J Neurophysiol* 48:1011–1032.

12 Audition: Cognitive Psychology of Music

S. McAdams

The earlier chapters in this volume discussed several levels of both the nervous system and psychological phenomena. A lot of these dealt with relatively simple perceptual structures whose extension in time is quite limited, with the exception of some of the demonstrations by Bregman, which often last several seconds. Of course, once one starts to talk about the perception of much larger-scale structures such as music, the time domain quickly telescopes beyond durations that can be dealt with in short periods of processing, and we have to call into play all kinds of relationships over very large time scales on the order of tens of minutes or even hours. It is thus of great interest to both psychology and neuroscience to try to understand how larger-scale temporal structures such as music are represented and processed by human listeners. These psychological mechanisms are necessary for the sense of global form that gives rise to expectancies that in turn may be the basis for affective and emotional responses to musical works (Meyer, 1956; Sloboda, 1992).

One of the main goals of auditory cognitive psychology is to understand how humans can "think in sound" outside the verbal domain (McAdams and Bigand, 1993). Within the field of contemporary auditory cognition research, music psychology has a very important status. This field in its current form situates itself strongly within the cognitive framework in the sense that it postulates internal (or mental) representations of abstract and specific properties of the musical sound environment, as well as processes that operate on these representations. For example, sensory information related to frequency is transformed into pitch, is then categorized into a note value in a musical scale, and ultimately is transformed into a musical function within a given context. Some research has begun to address how these computations can be implemented, focusing on the nature of the input and output representations as well as on the algorithms used for their transformation. A still smaller number of researchers are studying the way in which these representations and algorithms are instantiated biologically in the human brain (Marín, 1982; Zatorre, 1989; Peretz, 1993). This chapter presents research that lays the functional base for more neuropsychologically oriented work.

The processing of musical information may be conceived globally as involving a number of different stages (figure 12.1, McAdams, 1987; Bigand, 1993a; Botte, McAdams, and Drake, 1995). (I should emphasize that this diagram is not to be interpreted as a proposition for a stagelike serial processing conception of musical cognition. Although one would like, for purposes of systematic exploration, to decompose logically the response of the brain into its basic elements, these conceptual elements may not actually be instantiated by distinguishable processing stages.) After the spectral analysis and transduction of acoustic vibrations in the auditory nerve, the auditory system appears to employ a number of mechanisms (primitive auditory grouping processes) that organize the acoustic mixture arriving at the ears into mental "descriptions" (see Bregman, this volume). These descriptions represent events produced by sound sources and their behavior through time. Research has shown that the building of these descriptions is based on a limited number of acoustic cues that may reinforce one another or give conflicting evidence. This state of affairs suggests the existence of some kind of process (grouping decisions) that sorts out all of the available information and arrives at a representation (that is as unambiguous as possible) of the events and sound sources that are present in the environment. According to Bregman's (1990) theory of auditory scene analysis, the computation of perceptual attributes of events and event sequences depends on how the acoustic information was organized at an earlier stage. Attributes of individual musical events include pitch, loudness, and timbre, and those of musical event sequences include melodic contour, pitch intervals, and rhythmic pattern. Thus a composer's control of auditory organization by a judicious arrangement of notes can affect the perceptual result.

Once the information is organized into events and event streams, complete with their derived perceptual attributes, what is conventionally considered to be music perception begins. The auditory attributes activate abstract knowledge structures that represent in long-term memory the relations between events that have been encountered repeatedly through experience in a given cultural environment. That is, they encode various kinds of regularities experienced in the world. Bregman (1993) described the regularities present in the physical world and believes that their processing at the level of primitive auditory organization is probably to a large extent innate. There are, however, different kinds of relations that can be perceived among events, at the level of pitches, durations, timbres, and so on. These structures would therefore include knowledge of systems of pitch relations such as scales and harmonies, temporal relations such as rhythm and meter, and perhaps even timbre relations derived from the kinds of instruments usually encountered, as well as their combinations. The sound structures found in various occidental cultures are not the same as those found in Korea, Central Africa, and Indonesia, for example. Many of the relational systems have been shown to be hierarchical, and I will return to this point later.

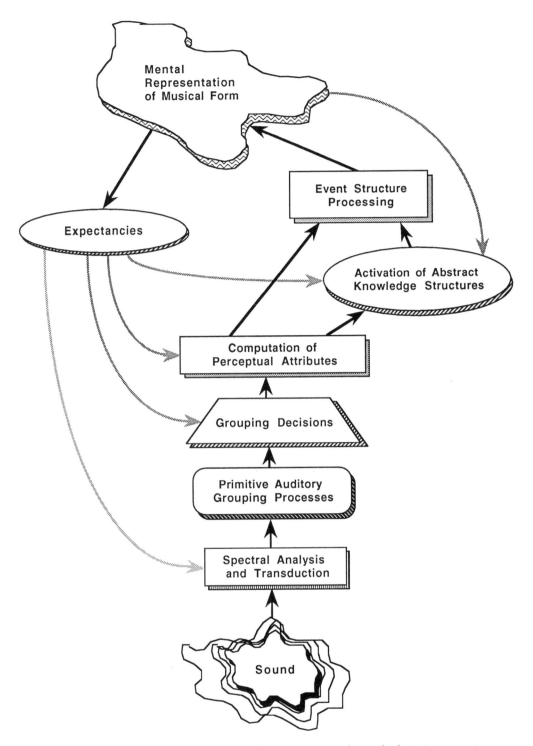

Figure 12.1 Schema illustrating the various aspects of musical information processing.

So the raw perceptual properties associated with musical events and groups of events activate the structures that have been acquired through acculturation, and the events thus acquire functional significance and evoke an interpretive framework: the key of F♯ major and a waltz meter, for example. A further stage of processing, event structure processing, assembles the events into a structured mental representation of the musical form as understood up to that point by the listener (McAdams, 1989). Particularly in Western tonal and metric music, hierarchical organization plays a strong role in the accumulation of a mental representation of musical form. At this point there is a strong convergence of rhythmic-metric and pitch structures in the elaboration of an event hierarchy in which certain events are perceived to be stronger, more important structurally, and more stable. The functional values that events and groups of events acquire within an event hierarchy generate perceptions of musical tension and relaxation or, in other words, musical movement. They also generate expectancies about where the music should be going in the near future based both on what has already happened and on abstract knowledge of habitual musical forms of the culture, even for pieces that one has never heard before. In a sense, we are oriented by what has been heard and by what we "know" about the musical style to expect a certain type of event to follow at certain pitches and at certain times (Dowling, Lung, and Herrbold, 1987).

The expectancies drive and influence the activation of knowledge structures that affect the way we interpret subsequent sensory information. For example, we start to hear a certain number of pitches, a system of relations is evoked and we infer a certain key; we then expect that future information that comes in is going to conform to that key. A kind of loop of activity is set up, slowly building a mental representation that is limited in its detail by how much knowledge one actually has of the music being heard. It is also limited by one's ability to represent things over the long term, which itself depends on the kind of acculturation and training one has had. It does not seem too extreme to imagine that a Western musician could build up a mental structure of much larger scale and greater detail when listening to a Mahler symphony that lasts one and half hours, than could a person who just walked out of the bush in Central Africa. The reverse would be true for the perception of complex Pygmy polyphonic forms. However, on the one hand we are capable of hearing and enjoying something new, suggesting inborn precursors to musical comprehension in all human beings that makes this possible. On the other hand, what we do hear and understand the first time we encounter a new musical culture is most likely not what a native of that culture experiences.

The expectancies generated by this accumulating representation can also affect grouping decisions at the basic level of auditory information processing. This is very important because in music composition, by playing around with some of these processes, one can set up perceptual contexts that affect the way the listener will tend to organize new sensory information. This process involves what Bregman (1990) called schema-driven processes of auditory organization. Finally, there is some evidence now that attentional processes can affect the way information is processed in the auditory periphery by way of the efferent projections innervating the outer hair cells in the cochlea (Puel, Bonfils, and Pujol, 1988; Giard et al, 1994), although their role in everyday perception is not yet clear. Whereas the nature and organization of these stages are probably similar across cultures in terms of the underlying perceptual and cognitive processing mechanisms involved, the higher-level processes beyond computation of perceptual attributes depend quite strongly on experience and accumulated knowledge that is necessarily culture specific.

Let us now take a closer look at each of these areas. I cannot possibly do justice to the vast amount of research that has been conducted in music psychology in the last 25 years or so within the space of this chapter. I can only present a very brief overview of a few selected topics to demonstrate how it is possible to do rigorous experimental research on such an ephemeral beast as musical experience. The majority of the material focuses on the more specifically musical areas of abstract knowledge structures and event structure processing.

ABSTRACT KNOWLEDGE STRUCTURES

Auditory comprehension and many aspects of auditory perception are based on generalizations that have been learned from specific experience. These generalizations include implicit knowledge that results from an acculturation within a given acoustic and sociocultural environment. They are abstract in the sense that they are not specific to a given musical pattern that one hears. For example, the key of C major is an abstraction. An infinite number of specific melodies can be realized within the system of pitch relations that is called a scale in music.

So on the one hand, abstract knowledge structures comprise systems of relations between musical categories that form the basis on which the musical syntax of a given culture is developed, such as pitch categories, scale structures, and tonal and harmonic hierarchies. These systems imply the existence of psychological processes of categorization, abstraction, and coding of relations among categories, as well as the functional hierarchization of these relations.

And on the other hand, learned generalizations from musical forms realized in time can comprise a lexicon of abstract patterns that are frequently encountered in a given culture, such as prototypical melodic forms, harmonic progressions, or formal schemes of musical structure like Western sonata form or Indian rāg form. A pattern lexicon would imply the abstraction and coding of structures that underly the surface of heard events. The main difference between abstract systems of relations between musical categories such as scales and tonal hierarchies and a lexicon of abstract patterns such as formal musical schemas is that the former are a sort of hierarchical alphabet "out of time" from which elements can be drawn to build musical materials, whereas the

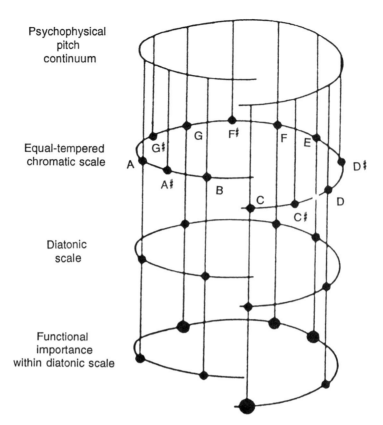

Psychophysical
pitch
continuum

Equal-tempered
chromatic scale

Diatonic
scale

Functional
importance
within diatonic scale

Figure 12.2 Different levels of representation of musical pitch in Western tonal music (from top to bottom): spiral representing the psychophysical pitch continuum with octave equivalence; categorization of pitch continuum into the 12-note equal-tempered chromatic scale; selection of a diatonic 7-note scale from the chromatic scale; functional interpretation of certain notes as being more stable or perceptually important than others (context of C major in this case). (From Dowling and Harwood, 1986, figure 4.14. © Academic Press. Adapted with permission.)

latter are sequential schemes that can be elaborated with these constituent elements.

What follows focuses primarily on systems of pitch relations in Western tonal music (Krumhansl, 1990; McAdams, 1989; Bigand, 1993a). All humans perceive a large continuum of pitch (figure 12.2, level 1). However, the pitch systems of all cultures consist of a limited set of pitch categories that are collected into ordered subsets called scales. In the Western equal-tempered pitch system, all diatonic scales of 7 notes (figure 12.2, level 3) are derived from an alphabet of the 12 chromatic notes within an octave (figure 12.2, level 2). The pitches of adjacent notes in the chromatic scale are separated by a semitone that corresponds to a frequency difference of approximately 6%. The octave is a special interval (2:1 frequency ratio) at which two pitches, although separated along the pitch dimension, seem to have something in common, or are perceived to be equivalent. In all cultures that name the pitches in scales, two pitches separated by an octave are given the same name (*do re mi fa sol la ti do* or C D E F G A B C in the Western system, and *Sa Re Ga Ma Pa Dha Ni Sa* in the Indian system). Young infants (Demany and Armand, 1984) and white rats (Blackwell and Schlossberg, 1943) make errors in pitch discrimination for pitches separated by an octave, suggesting that octave equivalence may be a universal feature of the mammalian auditory nervous system.

A given scale is defined by the pattern of intervals between the pitch categories. A major scale has the pattern 2—2—1—2—2—2—1 in numbers of semitones between scale steps (figure 12.3, upper panel). One type of minor scale, called natural minor, has the pattern 2—1—2—2—1—2—2 (figure 12.3, lower panel). Within a scale a functional hierarchy often exists among the pitches (figure 12.2, level 4), as well as among chords that can be formed of the pitches. In the Western tonal pitch system, some pitches and chords, such as those related to the first and fifth degrees of the scale (e.g., C and G are the tonic and dominant notes of the key of C major) are structurally more important than others (figure 12.3). This hierarchization gives rise to a sense of key. In fact, when chords are generated by playing several pitches at once, the chord that is considered to be most stable within a key, and in a certain sense to "represent" the key, comprises the first, third, and fifth degrees of the scale. In tonal music, one can establish a sense of key within a given major or minor scale and then move progressively to a new key (a process called modulation) by introducing notes from the new key and no longer playing those from the original key that are not present in the new key. Such phenomena suggest that a functional hierarchy also exists among the keys that affects a listener's perception of tonal movement in a piece of music, as well as his or her local interpretation of the function of given pitches and chords. Let us now look more closely at examples of research that have studied the mental structures underlying these music theoretical principles.

Pitch Scales

The pattern of intervals, or set of frequency ratios between notes in a scale, is relatively stable within a given culture. This led Jordan and Shepard (1987) to hypothesize that, in a manner similar to the way objects are represented as rigid structures in the brain allowing us to perform mental rotations of the object (Shepard and Metzler, 1971), the scale is mentally represented as a sort of rigid template of pitch intervals. As a consequence, all perception and memory for relations between pitches by normal listeners of a culture are assimilated to the structure of the appropriate template.

To test this hypothesis, Jordan and Shepard presented a modified major scale to listeners in which all the intervals were stretched such that the octave fell a semitone high, for example, on C# rather than C (figure 12.4). They then presented probe tones derived from the normal major scale starting on

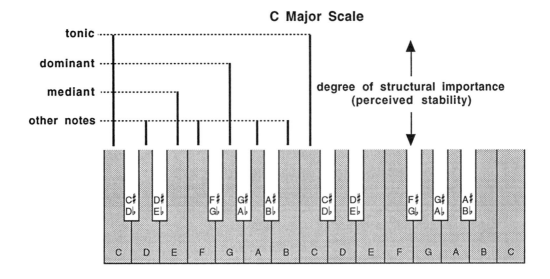

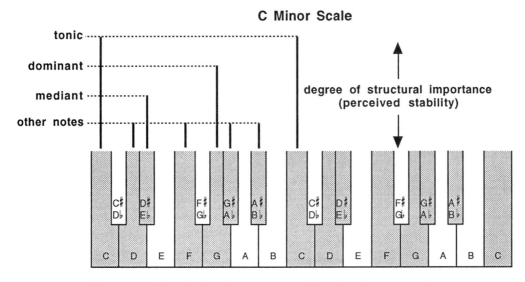

Figure 12.3 Piano keyboard representation of the scales of C major and C minor. Notes in each scale are shaded. The relative importance of the first (tonic, C), fifth (dominant, G), and third (mediant, E) degrees of the scale is illustrated by the length of the vertical bars. The other notes of the scale are more or less equally important, followed by the chromatic notes that are not in the scale (unshaded).

C, the major scale starting on C♯, or the actual stretched scale. They asked listeners to rate the degree to which the tone appeared to belong to the scale heard previously. Nonmusician listeners behaved as if they had continually adjusted a rigid template to accommodate the gradually shifting scale. At the end of the scale, such a template would be positioned on C♯. In fact, the notes derived from the C♯ major scale had higher ratings than those of either the C major or the stretched scales. Obviously, since scales differ from

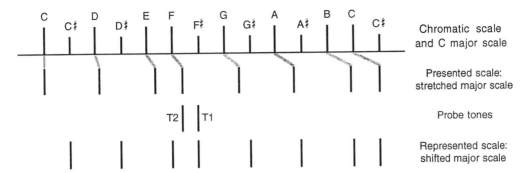

Figure 12.4 This diagram illustrates the chromatic scale from which the C major scale (longer vertical lines) is derived, the stretched major scale (starting on C and ending on C#) presented to listeners by Jordan and Shepard (1987), and the shifted major scale template thought to represent the framework against which listeners judged the fittingness of probe tones (positioned on C# major). Listeners' judgments indicate that the fittingness of probe tones was judged with respect to a shifted major scale template rather than in relation to a perfect pitch memory of the stretched scale. For example, tone T1 (fourth note of the shifted scale) would be judged as well fitted, whereas T2 (fourth note of the stretched scale) would be judged as poorly fitted even though T2 was actually present in the context stimulus and T1 wasn't.

culture to culture, such templates are learned through experience with the structure of the scales within one's own culture, and these results would therefore be expected to differ among cultures.

Pitch Hierarchies

Factors other than the simple logarithmic distance between pitches affect the degree to which they are perceived as being related within a musical system. The probe tone technique (Krumhansl, 1979) has been quite useful in establishing the psychological reality of the hierarchy of relations among pitches at the levels of notes, chords, and keys. In this paradigm, some kind of musical context is established by a scale, chord, melody, or chord progression, and then a probe stimulus is presented (figure 12.5). Listeners are asked to rate numerically either the degree to which a single probe tone or chord fits with the preceding context, or the degree to which two notes or chords seem related within the preceding context. This technique explores the listener's implicit comprehension of the function of the notes, chords, and keys in the context of Western tonal music without requiring them to explicate the nature of the relations.

Notes: The Tonal Hierarchy   If we present a context, such as a C major or C minor scale, followed by a single probe tone that is varied across the range of chromatic scale notes on a trial-to-trial basis, a rating profile of the degree to which each pitch fits within the context is obtained (Krumhansl and Kessler, 1982). This quantitative profile, when derived from ratings by musician

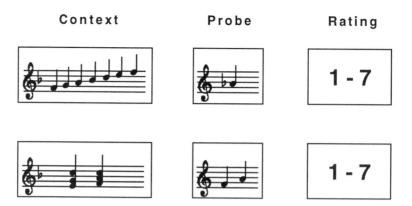

Figure 12.5 Schema of the probe-tone technique developed by Krumhansl (1979). A context-establishing stimulus is followed either by a probe tone that is rated for its fittingness with the context, or by a pair of events whose degree of relatedness is rated with respect to the context. Ratings are made on a numerical scale.

listeners, fits very closely to what has been described intuitively and qualitatively by music theorists (figure 12.6). Note the importance of the tonic note that gives its name to the scale, followed by the dominant or fifth degree and then the mediant or third degree. These three notes form the principal triad or chord of the diatonic scale. The other notes of the scale are of less importance, followed by the remaining chromatic notes that are not within the scale. These profiles differ for musicians and nonmusicians. For the latter, the hierarchical structure is less rich and can even be reduced to a simple proximity relation between the probe tone and the last note of the context.

Krumhansl (1990) showed that the hierarchy of tonal importance revealed by these profiles is strongly correlated with the frequency of occurrence of notes within a given tonality (the tonic appears more often than the fifth than the third, and so on). It also correlates with various measures of tonal consonance of notes with the tonic, as well as with statistical measures such as the mean duration given these notes in a piece of music, the tonic often having the longest duration. These correlations suggest that the acquisition and appreciation of a stable mental representation of the tonal hierarchy could be based initially on simple statistical and psychoacoustic properties of the musical surface. The importance of basic sensory qualities such as dissonance (related to the psychoacoustic attribute roughness) should not be underestimated (Plomp and Levelt, 1965; Kameoka and Kuriyagawa, 1969). They form what Mathews et al (1987) called the "acoustic nucleus" from which higher-level musical functions evolved. Although the higher-level functions are specific to a given culture, they may have common origins across cultures in a given result of sensory processing.

Chords: The Harmonic Hierarchy within a Key   Within a key, chords can be constructed on each note of the scale by superimposing intervals of a major or minor third (four and three semitones, respectively), such as C-E-G

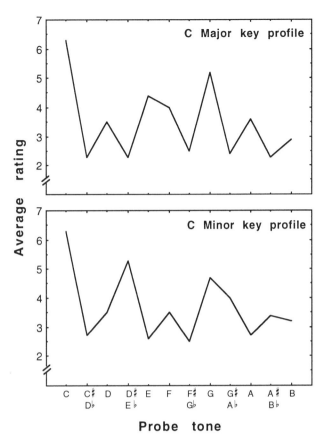

Figure 12.6 Major and minor profiles derived with the probe-tone technique from fitting-ness ratings by musician listeners. (From Krumhansl and Kessler, 1982, figure 2. © American Psychological Association. Adapted with permission.)

giving the C major triad, or A-C-E giving the A minor triad. A harmonic hierarchy similar to the tonal hierarchy was demonstrated for chords and cadences (Krumhansl, 1990). The harmonic hierarchy orders the function of chords within a key according to a hierarchy of structural importance. This gives rise to one of the particularly rich aspects of Western tonal music: harmonic progression. In the harmonic hierarchy, the tonic chord (built on the first degree of the scale) is the most important, followed by the dominant (built on the fifth degree) and the subdominant (built on the fourth degree). These are followed by the chords built on the other scale degrees. Less stable chords, that is, those that have a lesser structural importance, have a tendency to resolve to chords that are more stable. These movements are the basis of harmonic progression in tonal music and also create patterns of musical tension and relaxation. Moving to a less stable chord creates tension, and resolving toward a more stable chord relaxes that tension. Krumhansl (1990) showed that the harmonic hierarchy can be predicted by the position in the tonal hierarchies of the notes that compose the chords.

The establishment of a tonal context has a great deal of influence on the perception of relations between chords. If listeners are asked to rate the relatedness of two chords either independently of a context or within the context of two different keys, their relatedness varies as a function of the harmonic context (Bharucha and Krumhansl, 1983). In figure 12.7, the relatedness judgments have been analyzed by a multidimensional scaling technique that positions each chord in a Euclidean space, such that chords judged as being closely related are near one another and those judged as being less related are farther apart. Note that in the absence of a tonal context (i.e., within the context of random presentation of all the chord pairs), the chords C major and G major (I and V, respectively, on the left side of the middle panel), have a similar relation to that between the chords F# major and C# major (I and V, respectively, on the right side of the middle panel); in other words, they are the same distance apart in this two-dimensional representation of the relatedness judgments. However, note that in the C major context, the I and V chords of C major are perceived as more closely related than are the I and V chords of F# major, whereas in the F# major context the reverse is true, despite the fact that acoustically the pairs of events were identical. This result suggests that relatedness depends on the harmonic context within which the chords are interpreted. These relations are considered to determine the harmonic expectancies that can be measured in listeners and also reflect the frequency of occurrence of chord progressions in tonal music.

Krumhansl (1990) has also demonstrated quite elegantly that the hierarchies for notes and chords can be used to predict listeners' mental representations of relations among keys. These relations would represent the next higher level in the hierarchical knowledge structure concerning the syntax of pitch relations in tonal music.

Neuropsychological Data on Pitch Hierarchies   Research has been conducted on patients with neurological disorders to determine whether the processing of harmonic hierarchies is lateralized in the brain. Bharucha and Stoeckig (1986) developed a priming task in which a prime chord is played, followed by a target chord whose relation to the prime is either close or far away in the harmonic hierarchy. One of the notes in the target chord is mistuned, and the listener is to judge simply whether the chord is in tune or out of tune. In normal listeners, the interaction between chord relatedness and intonation judgments is strong. Greater accuracy on related trials is found for in-tune chords, and greater accuracy on unrelated trials is found for out-of-tune chords. These results are robust across musician and nonmusician populations. They imply that a harmonic context primes the processing of chords related within an established context, compared with chords that are distantly related within the context. Increased sensitivity to related targets is manifested, as is a bias toward judging related targets to be more stable or consonant.

A variant of this test was designed for two right-handed callosotomy (split-brain) patients such that harmonic perception in each hemisphere could

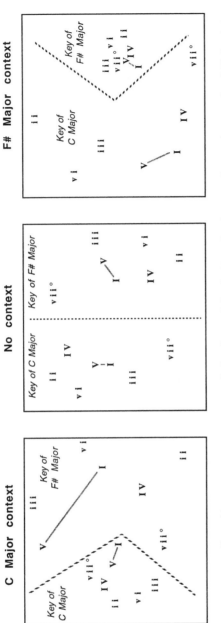

Figure 12.7 Effect of key context on perception of relatedness of chords. Note the changing distance between I and V chords in both keys as a function of context. These chords are closely related when they are the tonic and dominant chords of an established key but are distantly related when out of context. The Roman numerals indicate the degree of the scale on which the triad is based. Major chords are represented by upper-case numerals, minor chords by lower-case numerals, and diminished chords by °. (From Bharucha and Krumhansl, 1983, figure 1. © Elsevier Science Publications. Adapted with permission.)

be tested independently (Tramo, Bharucha, and Musiek, 1990). Only the right hemisphere manifested the normal interaction between intonation-detection accuracy and harmonic relatedness of prime and target chords. This result suggests that associative auditory functions that generate expectancies for harmonic progression in music are lateralized within the right hemisphere. Zatorre (1989) demonstrated elegantly that the processing of musical pitch also seems to be lateralized in the right hemisphere. Further work is required to determine how pitch computation and processes involved in the generation of harmonic expectancies interact computationally in the brain.

The Possibility of Developing Timbral Hierarchies

Timbre is the auditory attribute that distinguishes sounds presented under similar conditions and having the same pitch, loudness, and duration. For speech sounds, we might consider vowels and consonants to represent a certain space of timbral variation. It is clear for anyone who listens to poetry read aloud that timbre plays an æsthetic role that is analogous to that of pitch in music. Rhyme and alliteration, as well as modulations in the space of vowel and consonant qualities, provide a rich palette for sculpting sound around the meaning that is carried in words. One might wonder, therefore, whether the kinds of perceptual and cognitive possibilities and constraints that operate for pitch and duration (allowing them to be the most widely used auditory dimensions that carry musical form) can be generalized to other auditory attributes such as timbre.

Until the middle of the nineteenth century, the role that timbre played in music was either one of carrying a melodic voice and allowing it to be distinguished from other voices, or one of signaling section boundaries by changes in instrumentation. It thus primarily had a role as an attribute according to which sound events could be grouped or segregated on the basis of their similarity. With the advent of the symphony orchestra, timbre became an object of musical development in its own right, and composers began to build up composite timbres with sophisticated orchestration techniques (Boulez, 1987). In the latter half of the twentieth century, first electronic and then digital sound synthesis techniques suddenly gave the musician undreamed-of control over this auditory attribute. Composers were no longer obliged to work with the "found objects" of the orchestra, but could compose the sound from the inside. This opened the door to a structural use of timbre that in principle could come to rival that of pitch. However, there is no theory, or even a common practice, in such uses of timbre. Thus many composers, while discovering the occasional stunning result by creative intuition, admit that they have no systematic approach to integrating timbre into a musical discourse.

The development in cognitive psychology of multidimensional scaling techniques has allowed us to begin to penetrate the nature of this multifarious attribute. Following from pioneering work by Grey (1977), Krumhansl (1989)

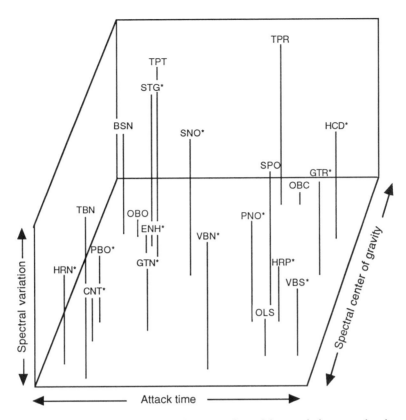

Figure 12.8 Three-dimensional timbre space derived from multidimensional scaling of dissimilarity judgments on 21 synthesized timbres by Krumhansl (1989). Axes are labeled with acoustical correlates to the perceptual dimensions analyzed by Krimphoff et al (1994). Sounds with significant distinctive features not accounted for by their distance from other timbres in the three-dimensional space are marked with an asterisk. HRN = French horn; TBN = trombone; CNT = clarinet; PBO = pianobow (bowed piano); BSN = bassoon; OBO = oboe; ENH = English horn; GTN = guitarnet (guitar-clarinet hybrid); STG = bowed string; TPT = trumpet; SNO = striano (bowed string-piano hybrid); VBN = vibrone (vibraphone-trombone hybrid); PNO = piano; OLS = oboleste (oboe-celeste hybrid); SPO = digitally sampled piano; HRP = harp; TPR = trumpar (trumpet-guitar hybrid); VBS = vibraphone; OBC = obochord (oboe-harpsichord hybrid); GTR = guitar; HCD = harpsichord.

found that in dissimilarity judgments between timbres, musician listeners tend to base their judgments on about three main perceptual dimensions plus a number of distinctive features that belong to individual timbres (figure 12.8). We recently succeeded in finding acoustic parameters that correlate very strongly with the position of the timbres along these dimensions (Krimphoff, McAdams, and Winsberg, 1994), which means we can now build sound-synthesis devices that have powerful perceptual controls on them. The continuous dimensions include the attack quality (horizontal axis), which distinguishes plucked and struck sounds from blown and bowed sounds and is correlated with the logarithm of the attack time; brightness (depth axis), which distinguishes sounds containing a greater preponderance of high frequencies from those whose spectra are limited to lower frequencies and is correlated with the spectral center of gravity (amplitude-weighted mean frequency); and the degree of variation in global spectral envelope among adjacent frequency components (vertical axis). We have yet to analyze acoustically the distinctive features that are suggested for certain timbres, but they certainly involve acoustic characteristics that are not generally shared among the timbres tested. These features are what distinguishes most clearly sound sources from one another and may well be involved in what allows their recognition (McAdams, 1993). The common dimensions may be candidates for the development of musical structure, although their respective degrees of salience vary among classes of listeners (McAdams, Winsberg, Donnadieu, DeSoete, and Krimphoff, 1995).

But more to the point about timbre as a structuring force in music, we asked the following related questions (McAdams and Cunibile, 1992): can listeners perceive relations among timbres in a way that allows recognition of that relation itself when played with different timbres? And can these relations be derived from the timbre space described above? In more musical terms these questions translate as: do listeners perceive timbre intervals in a way analogous to pitch intervals, and can these intervals be defined with respect to timbre space?

To investigate this, we performed experiments using what one might call a timbre-analogies task originally developed by Ehresman and Wessel (unpublished data, 1978). We define a timbre interval as a vector between two points in the space (figure 12.9). The vector represents the degree of change along each underlying perceptual dimension and corresponds closely to the notion of pitch interval that has been shown to be so crucial to the mental representation of melody and harmony. For example, it is well established in music psychology that a melody (a pattern of pitch intervals) can be transposed (translated to a different starting pitch) and still be easily recognized if the interval pattern remains the same. Analogously for timbre, to find a similar interval starting from a different timbre in the space, one has simply to translate the vector, keeping the same length and orientation. In geometrical terms, this operation is equivalent to finding two other points that form a parallelogram with the two original points.

Our results showed that both composers and nonmusician listeners can perform the task, although the musicians' judgments are generally more coherent with the timbral vector hypothesis. This study suggests that relations between timbres in this space can be perceived in their own right. Such developments may lead to a demonstration of the psychological plausibility of establishing timbre scales and melodies, and perhaps even of timbral hierarchies (Lerdahl, 1987). Although it is only a preliminary study, and actually poses more questions than it answers due to the considerable variability among listeners, it opens the possibility that psychological research can give some useful conceptual tools to the practising composer.

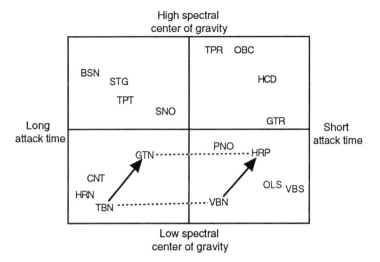

Figure 12.9 Timbral intervals may be conceived of as vectors in timbre space, shown as two-dimensional. The vectors represent the degree of change between two timbres along each salient perceptual dimension. The perception of an interval presupposes the brain's capacity to extract relational information from the sensory representation of the pair of timbres. An interval equivalent to TBN-GTN may be found starting from VBN by finding a point that best completes a parallelogram with the three other points; HRP in this case. (For abbreviations see figure 12.8.)

EVENT STRUCTURE PROCESSING

For numerous activities that last long enough to surpass largely our capacity to perceive everything in one fell swoop, understanding their temporal structure depends on an efficient abstract representation of the various parts and the relations between them. This representation often assumes a hierarchical form, probably for reasons of coding efficacy. In auditory research, the hierarchical representation of long event sequences is now being studied intensively in the realm of music cognition. A hierarchical mental structure implies several levels of coding. In the case of music, which involves event structures in time, this further implies several levels of temporal structure.

Two types of hierarchical structures can be distinguished in music. In a grouping hierarchy, sets of successive elements form groups that are recursively clustered with adjacent groups into higher level groups. All events of a group at a given level are carried upward to the next grouping level. In a reductional hierarchy, a structural level corresponds to a certain degree of abstraction of the relations, proceeding from local to global. Less important events at one level are reduced out at higher levels where only the hierarchically more important events appear. A representational unit that emerges at a higher level thus derives from a longer time span than those of lower levels.

Beyond a certain time span, it would no longer be a question of short-term perceptual processes that rely on working memory, but rather of longer-term cognitive processes that rely on permanent memory. A description of the operations by which these levels of representation are constructed, and by which their contents are determined, is the theoretical subject of musical syntax processing. Such a theory is related to cognitive music psychology as linguistics is related to psycholinguistics. The music cognition community had the good fortune to have been offered a formalization of a grammatical theory of tonal music by Lerdahl and Jackendoff (1983). I will use this theory as a framework for discussing experiments on the processing of large-scale musical structures, despite some of its neo-Chomskyan limitations.

A Generative Theory of Tonal Music

The main principle of Lerdahl and Jackendoff's (1983) theory is that an event sequence (presumably already organized into auditory events and streams according to processes akin to auditory scene analysis) is processed by a system of rules that constitute the musical grammar of a given style. This system gives rise to a structured mental description that represents the musical form as perceived and understood by a listener versed in the heard musical idiom. The theory that describes this system of rules comprises four main components (figure 12.10).

The first component parses the event stream into a grouping hierarchy. Groups of smaller time spans are embedded in groups of longer time spans recursively. In parallel, the second component analyzes the sequence into a hierarchical metric structure of alternating strong and weak beats that occur regularly in time. Strong beats at one level become beats at the next level. It is thus a reductional hierarchy in which weak beats are progressively reduced out. These two analyses converge to give a hierarchical segmentation of the event stream into time spans. The third component assigns a reductional hierarchy of structural importance to the pitches in each time span as a function of their position in the segmentational structure. An important pitch at one level is carried upward to the next level, leaving behind the pitches that are subordinate to it. In this way the representation of melodic patterns is reduced to the pitches that have a structural importance, hence the label time-span reduction for this component. It should be noted that the level to which such a reduction can reasonably take place is probably limited by constraints on working memory, although this subject has only recently begun to be studied in music psychology.

Stability and salience conditions that play a role in determining structural importance are based on abstract musical knowledge represented in the form of tonal and harmonic hierarchies as discussed previously, or on psychoacoustic properties that make a given event stand out with respect to its neighbors. Thus pitch and rhythm information converges in the elaboration of the event hierarchy at this stage.

Finally, the event hierarchy serves in the development of the last hierarchical representation, called prolongational reduction in the theory. This component expresses the melodic and harmonic tension and relaxation as well as

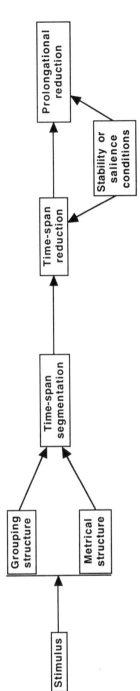

Figure 12.10 Major components of Lerdahl and Jackendoff's generative theory of tonal music.

the continuity and progression of the musical discourse. It is strongly based on the degree of relatedness of structurally important pitches and chords. Closely related chords produce a prolongation of the current state of tension or relaxation, whereas more distantly related chords can progress to greater tension or greater relaxation. Let us now examine in more detail the experimental results related to each of these theoretical components.

Perceptual Segmentation of Sound Sequences

The rules for grouping described by Lerdahl and Jackendoff essentially correspond to the Gestalt principles of temporal proximity and qualitative similarity (figure 12.11). Salient changes in duration, articulation, pitch register, and intensity or timbre, among others, can provoke a perceptual segmentation. Deliège (1987) tested these rules on constructed sequences as well as on

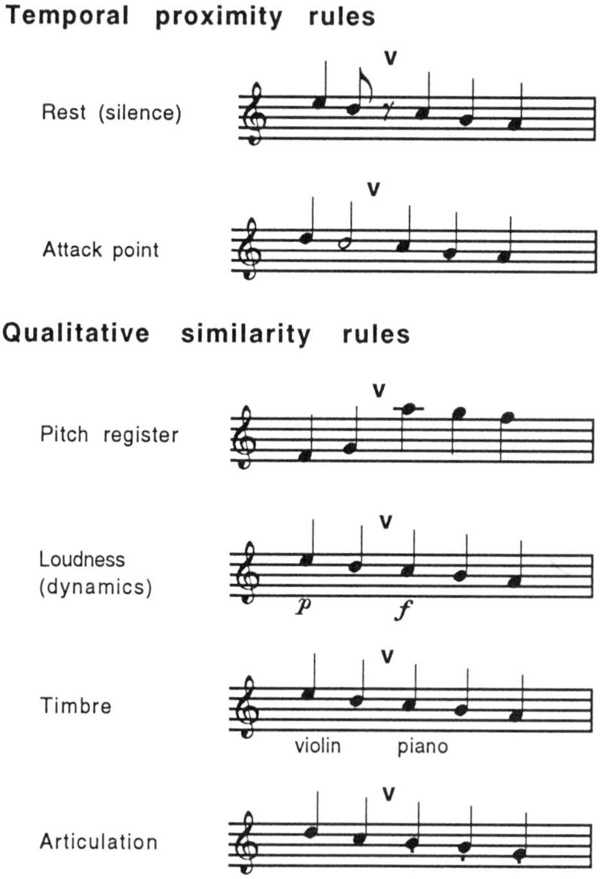

Figure 12.11 Examples of temporal and qualitative segmentation according to the grouping rules of Lerdahl and Jackendoff (1983). In the temporal proximity rules, a change in duration of a note (rest) or of the time interval between note onsets (attack point) can provoke a segmentation. In the qualitative similarity rules, an abrupt change in pitch register, loudness, timbre or articulation (legato [long notes] vs staccato [short notes]) can also result in segmentation.

musical fragments taken from the tonal repertoire. She asked listeners to indicate where they heard group boundaries in the sequence. In general the results conformed fairly well to the predictions of the theory, although the correspondence was stronger for musicians than nonmusicians.

Similar principles were shown to be responsible for larger-scale segmentations of musical sections (Clarke and Krumhansl, 1990; Deliège and El Ahmadi, 1990), where changes in pitch register, rhythmic density, instrumentation, and musical texture can signal section boundaries. These studies also showed that more levels of grouping can be demonstrated for musically trained listeners, and that higher-level groups are judged to have a stronger segmentation at their boundaries. The existence of groups as a mental representation was demonstrated experimentally; for example, it is more difficult for adult subjects to detect a temporal gap between groups than within groups. This was verified for infants and preschool children (Thorpe et al, 1988) in short sequences, and for 4.5- to 6-month-old babies listening to musical phrases from pieces by Mozart (Krumhansl and Jusczyk, 1990).

One of the important musical by-products of grouping is the occurrence of subjective accents. These occur on isolated events, on the second of two events in a group, and on the first and last of a string of events (Povel, 1984).

Extraction of a Metric Schema

The second component of Lerdahl and Jackendoff's theory concerns establishing a metric structure. There are processes that lead a listener to feel a regular pulse or beat that underlies a succession of sound events and to interpret those that are equally spaced in time as stronger than the others (e.g., every other event is perceived as accented). This impression of a regular alternation between strong and weak beats is called meter. It can be organized hierarchically (figure 12.12) if at the level of the regularly spaced strong beats one can still hear an alternation between strong and weak beats (e.g., every other event is strong, but every fourth event is even stronger). Meter is thus an abstraction that implies complex cognitive processes that extract

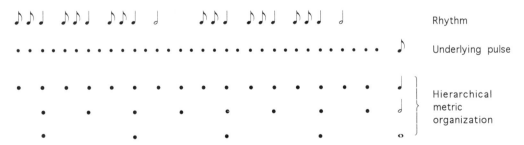

Figure 12.12 Metric organization of a rhythm pattern. An underlying pulse is determined from the smallest time interval of which the other intervals are integer multiples. For this rhythm, the lower metric levels are binary subdivisions of higher levels. The metric strength of an event is determined by the number of levels of the metric hierarchy that coincide with it.

(or detect) global temporal regularities at several levels. The cues on which meter extraction is based are far from being understood completely, but a few basic principles have been discovered.

For a given sequence of events, listeners first extract a regular pulse at a certain tempo such that the majority of the perceived events fall on a beat rather than between beats. Work by Fraisse (1963) and more recently by Drake and Botte (1993) showed that a preferred tempo for the beat level exists at about 1.7 beats/second (interonset time 600 msec) or a musical tempo marking of 100/minute, though for musicians the range can be larger, extending from 100 to 900 msec. Next, on the basis of accents produced by the grouping structure, the listener tries to infer a metric structure in which every N beats is accented, where N is usually 2, 3, or 4. For example, in a waltz, it is relatively easy to extract the underlying pulse on the basis of the event sequence and then determine that one out of every three is accented, thus giving a characteristic ternary meter. Povel (1984) showed that if the accents resulting from the grouping structure are regularly spaced, a meter is easily inferred from a sequence, and the rhythmic pattern is also more easily remembered and reproduced (figure 12.13). When several possible beat structures can be fit to a given sequence, the sense of meter is more ambiguous and the pattern itself is more difficult to remember and reproduce. These results suggest that patterns that fit unambiguously to a given metric scheme have an internal representation that is more precise.

Povel also proposed that this mechanism implies a kind of hierarchy of adjustable internal clocks that organize the rhythmic sequence into a beat hierarchy and that can adapt to changes in tempo. Tempo fluctuations are called rubato in music; but, despite these fluctuations, we do not have any trouble following the beat structure. That this is so is evidenced by the fact that people do not tend to stumble over the beat when dancing to even the most fluctuating Viennese waltzes. Similar dramatic fluctuations can be found in the music of many cultures. A particularly remarkable example is the gamelan music of Java. The extraction of pulse and metric hierarchy is a highly culture specific phenomenon, as Arom (1991) described for the complex polyrhythms played by the Aka Pygmies in central Africa.

Once a metric framework is well established, it can organize a temporal sequence even when few notes fall directly on the beats. This is called syncopation, and it gives a particularly exciting feel to a lot of African and Latin American music as well as to various styles of jazz. In these types of music, the long periods where many important notes fall off the beat create a great rhythmic tension that is suddenly released when a strong beat of the underlying meter is reaffirmed by a note falling directly on it.

Hierarchical Representation of Event Structures

In Lerdahl and Jackendoff's theory, a convergence of grouping and metric structures gives rise to a hierarchical segmentation of the event sequence into

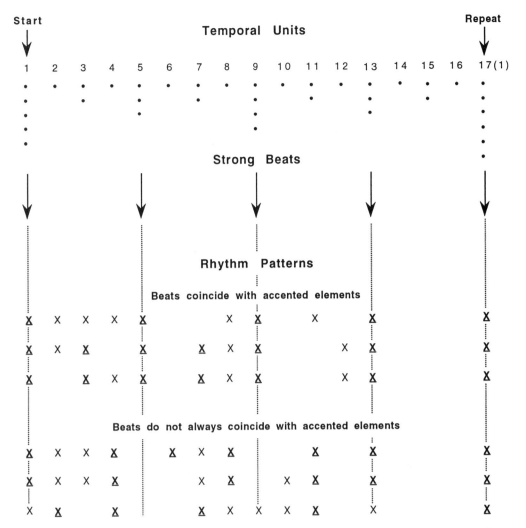

Figure 12.13 Examples of correspondence and conflict between subjective accents resulting from grouping and from the underlying meter. Events in a rhythmic pattern are marked with an X. Underlined Xs are heard as accented due to the grouping structure. (From Handel, 1989, figure 11.4. © MIT Press. Adapted with permission.)

time spans. Few experiments have studied the process by which this convergence is accomplished. However, the theory predicts that lower-level segments (having shorter time spans) will be defined predominantly by the metric structure, and higher-level segments will be determined by the grouping structure. Based on this segmented structure the theory hypothesizes a level of analysis at which the segmentational hierarchy is interpreted with respect to the tonal hierarchy represented in abstract memory, and arrives at a hierarchical representation of the structural importance of each note in the sequence as determined by the rules of the musical system of the culture. In this analysis, an important note at one level becomes an element at the next

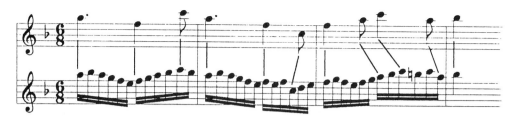

Figure 12.14 Theme and elaborated variation played by the violins in Beethoven's Sixth Symphony. The theme may be considered a structural "reduction" of the variation.

level up. This process translates the sense that some kind of perceptual similarity exists between musical fragments that may be different at the surface level, but identical at some higher hierarchical level where the ornamental notes have been reduced out in the representation. Such is the case in many theme and variations compositions (figure 12.14).

Serafine et al (1989) made an elegant demonstration of the psychological reality of a hierarchical mental representation of musical passages. They took melodies composed by Bach and simplified them to different degrees by a process similar to the time-span reduction in Lerdahl and Jackendoff's theory. For each reduction, "foil" reductions were also constructed that were similar to the "true" ones but included notes from the original melody that implied a different harmonic progression. Listeners had to identify the reductions that best corresponded to the original melody. That is, can one recognize the reduced version that corresponds to a given melody? Identification was better for the less-reduced structures, indicating certain limits in the hierarchical level at which such direct comparisons between melodies and reductions can be made. In a similar experiment (Bigand, 1990) listeners were able to judge the similarity between melodies that had different surface characteristics but that were derived from the same underlying structure, as would be the case in the recognition of the relation between different variations on a theme.

Schemas of Musical Tension and Release

The last component of Lerdahl and Jackendoff's theory is prolongational reduction that tries to account for the perception of movement between tension and relaxation in tonal music. According to the theory, on the basis of the time-span reduction presented above, a listener organizes the events into a coherent structure as they would be heard within a hierarchy of relative importance of the notes: less important notes are subordinated in a specific way to more important notes. Western tonal music is clearly organized on the basis of a hierarchical structuring of tension and relaxation. To move from an important or stable note to a less stable note creates tension. A movement in the other direction creates relaxation or a resolution of the tension. According to Lerdahl and Jackendoff, the degree to which an event evokes relaxation depends on its place within the tonal hierarchy, on the group to which it belongs, on its rhythmic value, and on its metric position; in other words, on its importance within the event hierarchy. This hypothesis of reduction then states that the hierarchical representation is instantiated by the strongest elements at a certain level and by their elaboration at lower levels with weaker elements. The event hierarchy is interpreted in terms of tension and relaxation in a way that ensures that each temporal region represents both a tensing and a relaxing within the progression from its beginning to its end at a given level of the hierarchy. So the greatest sense of tensing or relaxing would occur at the point at which several hierarchical levels attain a maximum of tension or of relaxation.

As with time-span reduction, little research has explicitly tested this hypothesis, but there are nonetheless a few encouraging results. Bigand (1993b) observed that melodies constructed such that their underlying structures evoke the same tension-relaxation hierarchy are perceived as being more similar than melodies that have similar surface features but different underlying structures. Musicians and nonmusicians are able to estimate the degree of tension and relaxation of a given note in a melody with remarkable precision and with very good agreement. Figure 12.15 shows the average estimates of musical tension given by listeners in response to two melodies that differed only in their rhythmic structure. These estimations corresponded very well qualitatively to the structures predicted by the theory.

In addition, a change in the rhythmic structure strongly affects the tension-relaxation hierarchy in terms of the independent contributions to the event hierarchy of the tonal hierarchy and the time-span segmentation. Notes that have a strong position in the tonal hierarchy tend to fall on strong beats in the melody in the upper panel and on weak beats in the lower panel. It is worth noting that for several runs of notes that have identical rhythmic structures in the two melodies, the fact that the position within the meter is different engenders large differences in perceived musical tension. This confirms the musician's intuition that the final percept depends on the convergence of both temporal and pitch information.

CONCLUSION

I hope to have shown in this extremely brief, whirlwind tour of research in the cognitive psychology of music that the complexity of structural processing revealed by this research rivals that of linguistic processing, even in what are conventionally called naive listeners. In both cases, humans possess elaborate long-term representations of abstract properties of the communicative structures that are acquired within a given cultural and linguistic environment. These structures are activated by auditory event sequences derived in early processing from acoustic stimulation. The resulting interpretations of the value or function of the different events are in turn subjected to a rich panoply of operations that affect the coding and elaboration of structures of signification. The perception and meaning of any given acoustic event is thus

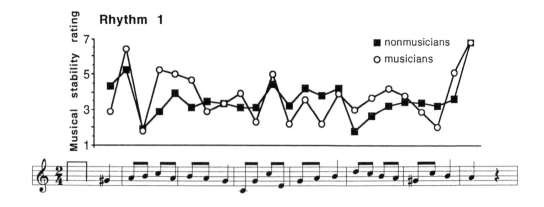

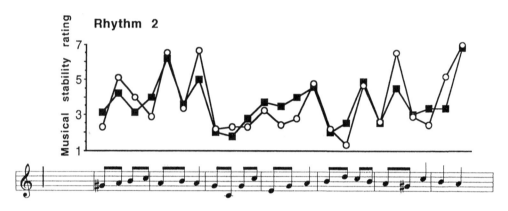

Figure 12.15 Musical stability profiles for musicians and nonmusicians. Higher ratings indicate greater stability or relaxation and lower ratings greater tension. The same melodic pattern was presented with two different rhythms that engendered significant changes in stability ratings. (From Bigand, 1993b, figure 7. © Harwood Academic Press. Adapted with permission.)

strongly affected by the whole context in which it appears. This, of course, raises numerous issues that remain to be addressed concerning the context-sensitive processing of complex acoustic structures by the human brain.

ACKNOWLEDEGMENTS

I thank I. Gold, L. Wiskott, E. Fernandez Espejo, and E. Bigand for helpful discussions on material in this chapter.

REFERENCES

Arom S. (1991). *African polyphony and polyrhythm: Musical structure and methodology.* Cambridge University Press, Cambridge.

Bharucha JJ. (1987). Music cognition and perceptual facilitation: A connectionist framework. *Music Perception* 5:1–30.

Bharucha JJ, Krumhansl CL. (1983). The representation of harmonic structure in music: Hierarchies of stability as a function of context. *Cognition* 13:63–102.

Bharucha JJ, Olney KL. (1989). Tonal cognition, artificial intelligence, and neural nets. *Contemp Music Rev* 4:341–356.

Bharucha JJ, Stoeckig K. (1986). Reaction time and musical expectancy: Priming of chords. *J Exp Psychol: Hum Percep Perform* 12:1–8.

Bigand E. (1990). Abstraction of two forms of underlying structure in a tonal melody. *Psychology of Music* 18:45–60.

Bigand E. (1993a). Contributions of music to research on human auditory cognition. In: *Thinking in sound: The cognitive psychology of human audition.* S McAdams, E Bigand, eds. Oxford University Press, Oxford, 231–277.

Bigand E. (1993b). The influence of implicit harmony, rhythm, and musical training on the abstraction of "tension-relaxation schemas" in tonal musical phrases. *Contemp Music Rev* 9:123–138.

Blackwell HR, Schlossberg H. (1943). Octave generalization, pitch discrimination, and loudness thresholds in the white rat. *J Exp Psychol* 33:407–419.

Botte MC, McAdams S, Drake C. (1995). La perception des sons et de la musique. In: *Perception et Agnosies: Séminaire Jean-Louis Signoret.* B Lechevalier, F Eustache, eds. De Boeck, Brussels, 55–99.

Boulez P. (1987). Timbre and composition—Timbre and language. *Contemp Music Rev* 2:161–172.

Bregman AS. (1990). *Auditory scene analysis: The perceptual organization of sound.* MIT Press, Cambridge.

Bregman AS. (1993). Auditory scene analysis: Hearing in complex environments. In: *Thinking in sound: The cognitive psychology of human audition.* S McAdams, E Bigand, eds. Oxford University Press, Oxford, 10–36.

Clarke EF, Krumhansl CL. (1990). Perceiving musical time. *Music Perception* 7:213–252.

Deliège I. (1987). Grouping conditions in listening to music: An approach to Lerdahl and Jackendoff's grouping preference rules. *Music Perception* 4:325–60.

Deliège I, El Ahmadi A. (1990). Mechanisms of cue extraction in musical groupings: A study of Sequenza VI for Viola Solo by Luciano Berio. *Psychology of Music* 18:18–44.

Demany L, Armand F. (1984). The perceptual reality of tone chroma in early infancy. *J Acoust Soc Am* 76:57–66.

Dowling WJ, Harwood D. (1986). *Music cognition.* Academic Press, Orlando, FL.

Dowling WJ, Lung KM, Herrbold S. (1987). Aiming attention in pitch and time in the perception of interleaved melodies. *Percep Psychophys* 41:642–656.

Drake C, Botte MC. (1993). Tempo sensitivity in auditory sequences: A tentative model of regularity extraction. *Percep Psychophys* 54:277–286.

Fraisse P. (1963). *Psychology of time.* Harper, New York (translated from *Psychologie du temps.* Presses Universitaires de France, Paris, 1957).

Giard MH, Collet L, Bouchet P, Pernier J. (1994). Signs of auditory selective attention in the human cochlea. *Brain Res* 633:353–356.

Grey JM. (1977). Multidimensional perceptual scaling of musical timbres. *J Acoust Soc Am* 61:1270–1277.

Handel S. (1989). *Listening: An introduction to the perception of auditory events*. MIT Press, Cambridge.

Jordan D, Shepard RN. (1987). Tonal schemas: Evidence obtained by probing distorted musical scales. *Percep Psychophys* 41:489–504.

Kameoka A, Kuriyagawa M. (1969). Consonance theory. Part II. Consonance of complex tones and its calculation method. *J Acoust Soc Am* 45:1460–1469.

Krimphoff J, McAdams S, Winsberg S. (1994). Caractérisation du timbre des sons complexes. II. Analyses acoustiques et quantification psychophysique. *J. Physique* 4(C5):625–628.

Krumhansl CL. (1979). The psychological representation of musical pitch in a tonal context. *Cognitive Psychology* 11:346–374.

Krumhansl CL. (1989). Why is musical timbre so hard to understand? In: *Structure and perception of electroacoustic sound and music*. S Nielzén, O Olsson, eds. Excerpta Medica, Amsterdam, 43–53.

Krumhansl CL. (1990). *Cognitive foundations of musical pitch*. Oxford University Press, Oxford.

Krumhansl CL, Jusczyk PW. (1990). Infants' perception of phrase structure in music. *Psychol Sci* 1:70–73.

Krumhansl CL, Kessler E. (1982). Tracing the dynamic changes in perceived tonal organization in a spatial representation of musical keys. *Psychol Rev* 89:334–368.

Lerdahl F. (1987). Timbral hierarchies. *Contemp Music Rev* 2(1):135–160.

Lerdahl F, Jackendoff R. (1983). *A generative theory of tonal music*. MIT Press, Cambridge.

Marín OSM. (1982). Neurological aspects of music perception and performance. In: *The psychology of music*. D Deutsch, ed. Academic Press, New York, 453–478.

Mathews MV, Pierce JR, Roberts LA. (1987). Harmony and new scales. In: *Harmony and tonality*. J Sundberg, ed. Royal Swedish Academy of Music, Stockholm, 59–84.

McAdams S. (1987). Music: A science of the mind? *Contemp Music Rev* 2(1):1–61.

McAdams S. (1989). Psychological constraints on form-bearing dimensions in music. *Contemp Music Rev* 4:181–198.

McAdams S. (1993). Recognition of sound sources and events. In: *Thinking in sound: The cognitive psychology of human audition*. S McAdams, E Bigand, eds. Oxford University Press, Oxford, 146–198.

McAdams S, Bigand E, eds. (1993). *Thinking in sound: The cognitive psychology of human audition*. Oxford University Press, Oxford.

McAdams S, Cunibile JC. (1992). Perception of timbral analogies. *Philos Trans R Soc Lond Biol Sci* 336:383–389

McAdams S, Winsberg S, Donnadieu S, DeSoete G, Krimphoff J. (1995). Perceptual scaling of synthesized musical timbres: Common dimensional specificities and latent subject classes. *Psychol Res* 58:177–192.

Meyer LB. (1956). *Emotion and meaning in music*. University of Chicago Press, Chicago.

Parncutt R. (1989). *Harmony: A psychoacoustical approach*. Springer-Verlag, Berlin.

Peretz I. (1993). Auditory agnosia: A functional analysis. In: *Thinking in sound: The cognitive psychology of human audition*. S McAdams, E Bigand, eds. Oxford University Press, Oxford, 199–230.

Plomp R, Levelt WJM. (1965). Tonal consonance and critical bandwidth. *J Acoust Soc Am* 38:548–560.

Povel DJ. (1984). A theoretical framework for rhythm perception. *Psychol Res* 45:315–337.

Puel JL, Bonfils P, Pujol R. (1988). Selective attention modifies the active micromechanical properties of the cochlea. *Brain Res* 447:380–383.

Serafine ML, Glassman N, Overbeeke C. (1989). The cognitive reality of hierarchic structure in music. *Music Perception* 6:397–430.

Shepard RN, Metzler J. (1971). Mental rotation of three-dimensional objects. *Science* 171: 701–703.

Sloboda JA. (1992). Empirical studies of emotional response to music. In: *Cognitive bases of musical communication*. MR Jones, S Holleran, eds. American Psychological Association, Washington, DC, 33–46.

Thorpe LA, Trehub SE, Morrongiello BA, Bull D. (1988). Perceptual grouping by infants and preschool children. *Dev Psychol* 24:484–491.

Tramo M, Bharucha J, Musiek F. (1990). Music perception and cognition following bilateral lesions of auditory cortex. *J Cognitive Neurosci* 2:195–212.

Zatorre RJ. (1989). Effects of temporal neocortical excisions on musical processing. *Contemp Music Rev* 4:265–278.

13 Toward a Neurobiology of the Mind

P. S. Churchland

For the ancient Greeks, philosophy embraced a vast range of questions about the natural world.[1] For example, what is the nature of change such that water can freeze or wood burn? What is the nature of the moon and the stars, and where the did the Earth come from? What is the fundamental thing that all stuff and objects are made of? How do living things reproduce? In addition, of course, they raised questions about themselves—about what it is to be human, to perceive and think, to reason and feel, to plan and decide.

Advances in natural philosophy—what we now call physics, chemistry, astronomy, and biology—have been spectacular, especially in the last 300 years. In these domains, science has in hand many answers that are rather well worked out. These answers are backed by a substantial body of experimental data, an interconnectedness of explanatory theory, and an unprecedented range of technological implementations of the theoretical principles. In short, the scientific program has succeeded in discovering at least the basic principles that explain an impressive range of natural phenomena. To be sure, physics, chemistry, geology, astronomy, and so forth are by no means complete, and lots of questions remain, some of which are deeply baffling.

By contrast, many questions concerning the nature of the mind have remained largely intractable since their first systematic discussion by the ancient Greeks. What is the nature of knowledge, and how is it possible to represent the world? What are consciousness and free will? What is the self, and how is it that some organisms are more intelligent or more adept than others? It is not surprising that an established empirical and theoretical foundation in this domain has eluded us for so long. For in order to understand what we are and how we work, we must understand the brain and how it works. Yet the brain is exceedingly difficult to study, and research on any significant scale is critically dependent on advanced technology.

Unlike celestial mechanics or evolutionary biology, where groundbreaking achievements could be made with relatively simple instruments, neuroscientific progress was severely restricted until the advent of cellular physiology, the light microscope, the electron microscope, and techniques that would selectively stain single cells. Because neural signaling and neural integration are fundamentally electrochemical events, progress required the means for detecting and manipulating microelectric events. This meant progress was essentially dependent on the theory and techniques of modern electronics. Although physicians since ancient times had made important clinical observations about their brain-damaged patients, these observations could not transcend the merely intriguing stage as long as we remained ignorant of the microorganization of nervous systems, the nature of neuronal function, and the computational capacities of neural networks.

Within this century, and especially within the last three decades, a number of scientific developments dramatically altered the status of mind-brain questions, moving them from the shelf labeled well-nigh-impenetrable-mystery to that labeled difficult-but-tractable. There is a gathering sense that some of the major pieces of the puzzle are falling into place, and that basic neurobiological explanations for certain psychological phenomena are now within reach.

The general developments are threefold.

• There has been a spectacular blossoming of data describing nervous systems. New neuroscientific techniques have made possible very detailed structural and functional descriptions of nervous systems at many levels of organization (figure 13.1). This has helped dislodge certain misconceptions about the brain, for example, that the only dreams we have are the dreams we remember. It has estimated the number of neurons in the human brain (about 10^{12}) and the number of synapses (about 10^{15}). It has discovered that awareness can be divided by separating the cerebral hemispheres, and that the receptive fields of individual sensory neurons are nothing like as fixed and stable through learning and injury as was supposed (Kaas, Merzenich, and Killackey, 1983, Ramachandran, 1993). The data have also catalyzed theorizing. For example, the detailed results concerning patterns of connectivity and cell types in the visual cortex inspired hypotheses concerning how circuits compute the direction and velocity of a moving stimulus (Hildreth and Koch, 1987), and how the curvature of a line can be detected by cells using signals from orientation-selective cells in cortical area V1.

• Increasingly subtle and sophisticated behavioral studies in experimental psychology and ethology have greatly deepened our understanding of what exactly are the psychological capacities, thereby clarifying the molar phenomena for which neurobiology seeks mechanisms.

• Computer modeling approaches that permit effective simulation of neural networks have led to computational discoveries concerning how networks of neuronlike units, with synapselike connections and a parallel organization, can accomplish certain complex tasks such as associative memory and pattern recognition. Since cognitive functions appear to be system-level properties, and in that sense are emergent properties, this research promises to be an important bridge between basic neuroscience and experimental psychology (Churchland and Sejnowski, 1992).

It is not that we now have clear and complete neurobiological answers to traditional philosophical questions. Rather, the philosophical significance de-

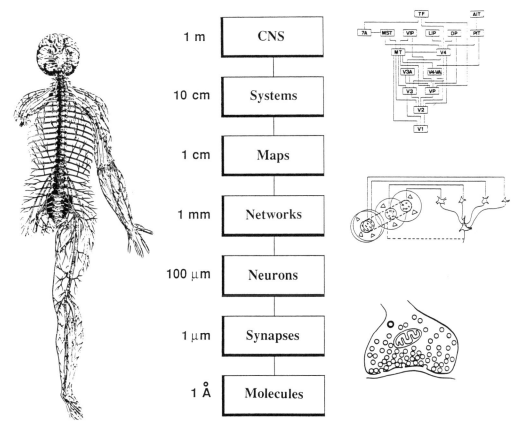

Figure 13.1 Schematic illustration of levels of organization in the nervous system. The spatial scales at which anatomical organization can be identified varies over many orders of magnitude. Icon to the left depicts the "neuron man," showing the brain, spinal cord, and peripheral nerves. Icons to the right represent structures at distinct levels: (top) a subset of visual areas in visual cortex; (middle) a network model proposing how ganglion cells could be connected to "simple" cells in visual cortex; and (bottom) a chemical synapse. (From Churchland and Sejnowski, 1992)

rives from the nature of the progress recently made and what it presages for future progress. These achievements rest on insightful use of a variety of techniques, broadly neuroscientific in scope, that are converging on problems about the mind. The convergent data have begun to suggest experimentally constrained hypotheses (see Llinás, Merzenich, and Singer, this volume), and newly developing techniques, such as positron emission tomography (PET), magentoencephalography (MEG), and magnetic resonance imaging (MRI), both anatomical and functional, are providing information about brain function at a level above the level of the single cell.

Neurobiological data bearing upon such time-honored philosophical issues as the nature of representation, consciousness, and perception are beginning to be available, and philosophers cannot speculate fruitfully on these issues in ignorance of the data. That the data are relevant in this context has the same rationale as the relevance of data in any context of inquiry. Thus, philosophers concerned with the nature of space and time cannot ignore Einstein's theory of special relativity and the physics of space and time, and philosophers concerned with the nature of life cannot ignore molecular biology. Although this parallel is now generally adopted within the subfield of philosophy of science, it is frequently rejected within the wider discipline, where philosophers are apt to assume that humans are special in ways that put human mental life beyond scientific understanding entirely (Taylor, 1985), or at least beyond the reach of neuroscience (Fodor, 1990; Searle, 1992).

Humans *are* special in certain respects, and the human brain appears to be the most complex brain on the planet. Remarkable capacities notwithstanding, we, like every other organism, evolved from simpler organisms. Consequently, our cognition, awareness, and motor control are not likely to be radically dissimilar to the cognition, awareness, and motor control of other mammals. From a biological perspective, those features that do distinguish us from our nearest living evolutionary relatives are more likely to be minor modifications on the basic design than a top-to-bottom innovation (Finlay and Darlington, 1995). Evolution, as Francois Jacob reminded us, does not proceed by redesigning from scratch, but by modifying what is already in place.

In addition, the biological perspective invites us to see higher functions within the wider framework of the basic requirements for survival, and survival is crucially dependent on sensorimotor control. Constraints on cognitive design derive from a world of hungry predators and unwilling prey, and the organization of cognitive functions is not independent of the motor functions they serve. Consciousness and cognition are not made in Plato's heaven, but in the competitive Darwinian world where small improvements in sensorimotor control give an organism a predatory and reproductive edge. Having the Darwinian lesson truly sink in is perhaps the most important element in loosening the bonds of the traditional philosophical approach that dismisses neurobiology as irrelevant to understanding our nature.

WHAT IS REDUCTIONISM?

Aiming for a scientific understanding of mental phenomena in terms of underlying brain mechanisms is reductionist in spirit.[2] The aim rests on the presumption that understanding the neurobiological mechanisms is not a frill but a necessity if we want to understand how we see, think, and make decisions. What I mean by a reductionist strategy in this context is basically what is meant elsewhere in science: we aim to explain macro-level phenomena in terms of micro-level phenomena. Whether science will finally succeed in reducing psychological phenomena to neurobiological phenomena is, needless to say, an empirical question.

The fundamental rationale behind this research strategy is straightforward: if you want to understand how a thing works, you have to understand not only its behavioral profile, but also its basic components and how they are organized to constitute a system. If you do not have the engineering designs available for reference, you resort to reverse engineering, the tactic of taking a part a device to see how it works (Churchland and Sejnowski, 1989). Because many philosophers who agree on the brain-based nature of the soul nonetheless rail against reductionism as ridiculous, it may be useful to explain in a bit more details what I do and, most emphatically, do not mean by a reductionist research strategy (see also Schaffner, 1993).

Clearing away the negatives first, I do not mean that a reductionist research strategy implies that a *purely bottom-up strategy* should be adopted. As far as I can tell, no one in neuroscience thinks that the way to understand the nervous system is first to understand everything about the basic molecules, then everything about every neuron and every synapse, and continue ponderously thus to ascend the various levels of organization until, at long last, one arrives at the uppermost level—psychological processes. Nor is there anything in the history of science that says a research strategy is reductionist only if it is purely bottom-up. That characterization is really just a straw man. The research behind the classic reductionist successes—explanations of thermodynamics in terms of statistical mechanics, of optics in terms of electromagnetic radiation, of hereditary transmission in terms of DNA—certainly did not conform to any purely bottom-up research directive.

As far as neuroscience and psychology are concerned, my view is simply that it would be wisest to conduct research on many levels simultaneously, from the molecular through to networks, systems, brain areas, and, of course, behavior. Here as elsewhere in science, hypotheses at various levels can coevolve as they correct and inform one another (PS Churchland, 1986). Neuroscientists would be silly to make a point of ignoring psychological data, for example, just as psychologists would be silly to make a point of ignoring all neurobiological data.

Second, by reductionist research strategy I do not mean that there is something disreputable, unscientific, or otherwise unsavory about high-level descriptions or capacities per se. It seems fairly obvious, to take a simple example, that certain rhythmic properties in nervous systems are network properties resulting from the individual membrane traits of various neuron types in the network, together with the way the set of neurons interact. Recognition that something is the face of Arafat, for another example, almost certainly emerges from the responsivity profiles of the neurons in the network plus the ways in which those neurons interact. "Emergence" in this context is entirely nonspooky and respectable, meaning, to a first approximation, property of the network. Determining precisely what the network property is for some particular feat will naturally take quite a lot of experimental effort. Moreover, given that neuronal behavior is highly nonlinear, the network properties are never a simple sum of the parts. They are some function—some *complicated* function—of the properties of the parts. High-level capacities clearly exist, and high-level descriptions are therefore necessary to specify them.

Eliminative materialism refers to the hypothesis that materialism is most probably true, and that many traditional aspects of explanation of human behavior are probably not adequate to the reality of the etiology of behavior (PM Churchland, 1981). The standard analogy here is that just as caloric fluid was useful but fundamentally mistaken in understanding thermal phenomena (conduction, convection, radiation), so some psychological categories currently invoked may be somewhat useful but fundamentally mistaken in fathoming behavioral etiology. Other existing characterizations of capacities may have a core of adequacy but undergo major redrawings, in something like the way Mendel's notion of factor came to be modified by genetics into the notion of gene, which itself was modified and deepened by developments in molecular biology. Some categories such as "attitude" are extremely vague and might be replaced altogether; others, such as "is sleeping" have already undergone a fractionation as electroencephalographic (EEG) and neurophysiological research revealed important brain differences in various stages of sleep. Categories such as "memory," "attention," and "reasoning" are similarly undergoing revision as experimental psychology and neuroscience proceed (PS Churchland, 1986). It remains to be seen whether there is a neurobiological reality to sustain notions such as "belief" and "desire" as articulated by modern philosophers such as Fodor (1990) and Searle (1992), although Paul Churchland and I have argued that revision here too is most probable. Certainly the revisionary prediction too is an empirical hypothesis and one for which empirical support already exists (PS Churchland and Sejnowski, 1992).

The possibility of nontrivial revision and even replacement of existing high-level descriptions by neurobiologically harmonious high-level categories is the crux of what makes eliminative materialism eliminative (PS Churchland, 1987; PM Churchland, 1993; Bickle, 1992). By neurobiologically harmonious categories I mean those that permit coherent, integrated explanations from the whole brain on down through neural systems, big networks, micronets, and neurons. Only the straw man is so foolish as to claim that there are no high-level capacities, no high-level phenomena (PM Churchland and PS Churchland, 1990). In its general aspect, my point here merely reflects this fact: in a profoundly important sense we do not understand exactly what, at its higher levels, the brain really does. Accordingly, it is practical to earmark even our fondest intuitions about mind-brain function as revisable hypotheses rather than as transcendental absolutes or introspectively given certainties. Acknowledgment of such revisability makes an enormous difference in how we conduct psychological and neurobiological experiments, and in how we interpret the results.

Finally, and at the risk of redundancy, may I emphasize that reductionism does not imply the vanity or unreality of macro-level phenomena that are successfully explained, and hence reduced, by micro-level phenomena. Consider several classic examples of reductionist success in science: explanations of thermodynamics in terms of statistical mechanics, explanation of optics in terms of electromagnetic radiation, and the explanation of heritability of phenotypic traits in terms of DNA, RNA, and protein synthesis. Have thermodynamics, optics, or behavioral genetics been cast aside? Or, to meet the worry even more directly, did temperature, light, or phenotypical traits cease to be granted reality? Not at all. For many good and serious scientific as well as practical reasons, thermodynamic descriptions (e.g., copper conducts heat better than tin), optical descriptions (e.g., indices of refraction), and phenotypical descriptions continue to play a crucial role in our thinking and in our understanding.

But aren't these categories really just otiose? One may ask. Not at all. Perceptually, our brains are tuned to the macro level—to the level of middle-sized objects and processes (Quine, 1961; Roche, 1981; Lakoff, 1987). Macro-level descriptions are here to stay. As for the reality of reduced phenomena, note that temperature, for example, is every bit as real a property as mean molecular kinetic energy. Indeed, that is what temperature in a gas *is*. So if the microphenomenon is real, the macroproperty with which it is identical has better be also.

IS THE REDUCTIONIST GOAL IMPOSSIBLE?

Over the last several decades a number of philosophers expressed reservations concerning the reductionist research goal of discovering the neurobiological mechanisms for psychological capacities, including the capacity to be conscious. Consequently, it may be useful to consider the basis for some of these reservations to determine whether they justify abandoning the goal, or whether they should even dampen our hopes about what might be discovered about the mind-brain. I will consider five main classes of objections. As a concession to brevity, my responses will be ruthlessly succinct, details being sacrificed for the sake of the main gist.

Impossible Because the Goal Is Absurd (Incoherent)

One set of reasons for dooming the reductionist research strategy is summed up thus: I simply cannot imagine that seeing blue or feeling pain, for example, could consist in some pattern of activity of neurons in the brain, or, more bluntly, I cannot imagine how you can get awareness out of meat. There is sometimes considerable filler between the its-unimaginable premise and the it's-impossible conclusion, but as far as I can tell, the filler is typically dust that cloaks the fallacious core of the argument (McGinn, 1990; Searle, 1992; Penrose, 1994; Wright, 1995).

Given how little in detail we currently understand about how the human brain "en-neurons" any of its diverse capacities, it is altogether predictable that we should have difficulty imagining the neural mechanisms. When the human scientific community was comparably ignorant of such matters as valence, electron shells, and so forth, natural philosophers could not imagine how to explain the malleability of metals, the magnetizability of iron, and the rust resistance of gold in terms of underlying components and their organization. Until the advent of molecular biology, many people thought it was unimaginable, and hence impossible, that being a living thing could consist in a particular organization of dead molecules. "I cannot imagine," said the vitalists, "how you could get *life* out of *dead* stuff."

From the vantage point of considerable ignorance, failure to imagine some possibility is only that: failure of imagination—one psychological capacity among others. It does not betoken any metaphysical limitations on what we can come to understand, and it cannot predict anything significant about the future of scientific research. After reflecting on the awesome complexity of the problem of thermoregulation in homeotherms such as ourselves, I find I cannot imagine how brains control body temperature under diverse conditions. I suspect, however, that this is a relatively uninteresting psychological fact about me, reflecting merely my current state of ignorance. It is not an interesting metaphysical fact about the universe or even an epistemological fact about the limits of scientific knowledge.

A variation of the cannot-imagine proposal is expressed as "we can never, never know ...," or "it is impossible ever to understand ...," or "it is forever beyond science to show that...." The idea here is that something's being impossible to conceive says something decisive about its empirical or logical impossibility. I am not insisting that such proposals are never relevant. Sometimes they may be. But they are surprisingly high-handed when science is in the very early stages of studying a phenomenon.

The sobering point here is that assorted "a priori certainties" have, in the course of history, turned out to be empirical duds, however obvious and heartfelt they were in their heyday. The impossibility that space is non-Euclidean, the impossibility that in real space parallel lines should converge, the impossibility of having good evidence that some events are undetermined, or that someone is now dreaming, or that the universe had a beginning, each slipped its logical noose as we came to a deeper understanding of how things are. If we have learned anything from the many counterintuitive discoveries in science it is that our intuitions can be wrong. Our intuitions about ourselves and how we work may also be quite wrong. There is no basis in evolutionary theory, mathematics, or anything else for assuming that pre-scientific conceptions are essentially scientifically adequate conceptions.

A third variation on this nay, nay, never theme draws conclusions about how the world must actually be, based on linguistic properties of certain central categories in current use to describe the world. Permit me to give a boiled-down instance: the category mental is remote in meaning—means something completely different—from the category physical. It is absurd therefore to talk of the brain seeing or feeling, just as it is absurd to talk of the mind having neurotransmitters or conducting current. Allegedly, this categorial absurdity undercuts the very possibility that science could discover that feeling pain is activity in neurons in the brain. The epithet "category error" is sometimes considered sufficient to reveal the naked nonsense of reductionism.

Much has already been said on this matter elsewhere (Feyerabend, 1981), and I shall bypass a lengthy discussion of philosophy of language with three brief points. First, it is rather far-fetched to suppose that intuitions in the philosophy of language can be a reliable guide to what science can and cannot discover about the nature of the universe. Second, meanings change as science makes discoveries about what some macrophenomenon is in terms of its composition and the dynamics of the underlying structure. Third, scientists are unlikely to halt their research when informed that their hypotheses and theories sound funny relative to current usage. More likely they will say this: the theories might sound funny to you, but let me teach the background science that makes us think the theory is true; then it will sound less funny. It may be noted that it sounded funny to Copernicus' contemporaries to say the Earth is a planet and moves; it sounded funny to say that heat is molecular motion or that physical space is non-Euclidean, or that there is no absolute downness, and so forth.

That a scientifically plausible theory sounds funny is a criterion only of its not having become common coin, not of its being wrong. Scientific discoveries that a certain macrophenomenon is a complex result of the microstructure and its dynamics are typically surprising and typically sound funny—at first. Obviously none of this is positive evidence that we can achieve a reduction of psychological phenomena to neurobiological phenomena. It says only that sounding funny does not signify anything, one way or the other.

A fourth variation on this theme is favored by physicists who see the mystery of consciousness, and sometimes free will as well, as requiring a fundamental change in science at its deepest level, namely, physics itself (Penrose, 1989, 1994; Chalmers 1995, Bennett, Hoffman, and Prakash, 1989). Essentially, the idea is this: we can now tell that the mysteriousness of consciousness is so profound as to imply that neuroscience cannot provide the explanations, however much more is known about the brain. What is really needed is a new, revolutionized physics. Just how that physics should go to enjoy the explanatory power of existing physics *and also* explain consciousness is a matter sketched in only the boldest of strokes, if at all.

Roger Penrose conjectures that the key advance in physics will have something to do with a theory of quantum gravity, although how that might shed light on consciousness is not revealed. David Chalmers conjectures that information may be a basic property of the universe, thereby requiring a rewriting of physics, but like Penrose, his new physics is tantalizingly pie-in-the-sky, as is the secret of how his version of a new physics, were it to exist, might actually explain consciousness, how it might achieve what he says neuroscience cannot ever achieve.

Is a revolution in physics the Great Hope for explaining consciousness? Perhaps, but I would not invest heavily in that venture just yet. First, we need some positive reason to think that is where the gold is, not merely a flat-footed perplexity in the face of a mystery. Second, mysteries do not come with their degree of profoundness pinned to their shirts. We cannot tell just by stewing in the mystery of consciousness, that however much we learn about the brain, the mystery of consciousness will remain utterly unsolved (Grush and Churchland, 1995). Sometimes in science, problems that seem easy, such as the precession of the perihelion of Mercury, turn out to be very hard and require fundamental changes in theory, whereas others that seem very difficult, such as the composition of the stars or what a protein is, turn out to be more tractable than was feared, once new techniques make new observations possible. From the vantage point of ignorance, how profound a mystery seems to be is an unreliable index of how profoundly revolutionary its solution may really be. Is it possible that consciousness might be irreducible in the way that electrical properties turn out to be? Possibly, yes. But bet-money-on-it *probable*? No. In *Matter and Consciousness* (1988), Paul Churchland responded thus to the proposed analogy between consciousness and electromagnetism:

Unlike electromagnetic properties which are displayed at all levels of reality from the subatomic level on up, mental properties are displayed only in large physical systems that have evolved a complex internal organization. The case for the evolutionary emergence of mental properties through the organization of matter is extremely strong. They do not appear to be basic or elemental at all. (p. 13)

The main, if rather humdrum and unglamorous, reason for thinking consciousness is a neurobiological phenomenon is that so far as is known, you need a well-functioning nervous system to have it. Moreover, as far as humans are concerned, we can also state, albeit crudely and only at the systems level, the conditions that are jointly sufficient for consciousness. Quite simply, volcanoes, atoms, and ferns are just out of luck as far as consciousness is concerned. Granted, none of this entails that Penrose, Chalmers, and like-minded physics investors are indeed wrong. My main point is solidly pragmatic: relative to the data available so far, the go-for-a-new-physics strategy is as empirically unappealing for the problem of consciousness as it was for the problem of life. I wish the new physicists all the best of luck, and as soon as a new physics is on the table—which may take some time—wisdom counsels we fairly assess whether it will help solve various problems in biology.

Impossible Because of Multiple Realizability

The core of this objection is that if a macrophenomenon can be the outcome of more than one mechanism (organization and dynamics of components), then it cannot be identified with any one mechanism, and hence reducing it to the (singular) underlying microphenomenon is impossible. This objection seems to me totally uninteresting to science. Again, permit me to ignore important details and merely summarize the main thrust of the replies.

1. Explanations, and therefore reductions, are domain relative. In biology? it may be fruitful first to limn the general principles explaining some phenomenon seen in diverse species, and then figure out how to account for interspecies differences, and then, if desirable, how to account for differences across individuals within a given species. Thus the general principles of how hearts or stomachs work are figured out, perhaps based on studies of a single species, and particularities can be resolved thereafter. Frog hearts, macaque hearts, and human hearts work in essentially the same general way, but there are also significant differences, apart from size, that call for comparative analyses. Consider other examples: (a) from the general solution to the copying problem that emerged from the discovery of the fundamental structure of DNA, it was possible to undertake explorations of how differences in DNA could explain certain differences in the phenotype; (b) from the general solution to the problem of how neurons send and receive signals, it was possible to launch detailed exploration into the differences in responsivity profiles of distinct classes of neuron (Flanagan, 1996).

2. Once the mechanism for some biological process has been discovered, it may be possible to invent devices to mimic those processes. Nevertheless, invention of the technology for artificial hearts or artificial kidneys does not obliterate the explanatory progress on actual hearts and actual kidneys; it does not gainsay the reductive accomplishment. Again, the possibility that hereditary material of a kind different from DNA might be found in things elsewhere in the universe does not affect the basic scaffolding of a reduction on this planet. Science would have been much the poorer if Crick and Watson had abandoned their project because of the abstract possibility of Martian hereditary material or artificial hereditary material. In fact, we do know the crux of the copying mechanism on Earth, namely, DNA, and we do know quite a lot about how it does its job. Similarly, the engineering of artificial neurons and artificial neural nets (ANNs) facilitates and is facilitated by neurobiological approaches to how real neurons work; the engineering undertakings do not mean the search for the basic principles of nervous system function is misguided.

3. There are always questions remaining to be answered in science, and hence coming to grasp the general go of a mechanism, such as the discovery of base-pairing in DNA, ought not be mistaken for the utopian ideal of a complete reduction, a complete explanation. Discoveries about the general go of something typically raise hosts of questions about the detailed go of it, and then about the details of the details. To signal the incompleteness of explanations, perhaps we should eschew the word reduction in favor of "reductive contact." Hence we should say the aim of neuroscience is to make rich reductive contact with psychology as the two broad disciplines coevolve. I experimented with this recommendation myself, and although some philosophers warm to it, scientists find it quaintly pedantic. In any case, let me apply more cumbersome locution and say here that reductive contact between molecular

biology and macrobiology has become steadily richer since 1953, although many questions remain. Reductive contact between psychology and neuroscience has also become richer, especially in the last decade, although it is fair to say that by and large the basic principles of how the brain works are poorly understood.

4. What precisely are supposed to be the programmatic sequelae to the multiple realizability argument? Is it that neuroscience is irrelevant to understanding the nature of the human mind? Obviously not. That neuroscience is not necessary to understand the human mind? One cannot deny that it is remarkably useful. Consider the discoveries concerning sleep, wakeness, and dreaming; the discoveries concerning split brains, humans with focal brain lesions, the neurophysiology and neuroanatomy of the visual system, and so on. Is it perhaps that we should not get our hopes up too high? What precisely is too high here? Is it the hope that we will discover the general principles of how the brain works? Why is that too high a hope?

Impossible if the Brain Causes Consciousness

Nay-saying the reductionist goal while keeping dualism at arm's length is a maneuver requiring great delicacy. John Searle's strategy is to say that although the brain causes conscious states, any identification of conscious states with brain activities is unsound. Traditionally, it has been opined that the best the reductionist can hope for are correlations between subjective states and brain states. This is followed by the claim that although correlations can be evidence for causality, they are not evidence for identity. Searle tried to bolster the traditional objection by saying that whereas α-β identifications elsewhere in science reveal the reality behind the appearance, in the case of awareness, the reality and the appearance are inseparable—there is no reality to awareness except what is present in awareness. There is, therefore, no reduction to be had.

Synoptically, here is why Searle's maneuver is unconvincing: he fails to appreciate why scientists ever opt for identifications rather than always going with mere correlations. What analysis shows is that depending on the data, cross-level identifications to the effect that α is β may be less troublesome and more comprehensible scientifically than supposing thing α causes (separate) thing β. This is best seen by example (PM Churchland, 1994, 1995).

Science as we know it says electrical current in a wire is not caused by moving electrons; it is moving electrons. Genes are not caused by chunks of base pairs in DNA; they are chunks of base pairs (albeit sometimes distributed chunks). Temperature is not caused by mean molecular kinetic energy; it is mean molecular kinetic energy. Reflect for a moment on the inventiveness required to generate explanations that maintain the nonidentity and causal dependency of electric current and moving electrons, genes and chunks of DNA, and heat and molecular motion. Unacquainted with the relevant convergent data and explanatory successes, one may suppose this is not so difficult.

Enter Betty Crocker.

In her microwave oven cookbook, Betty Crocker offers to explain how a microwave oven works. She says that when you turn the oven on, the microwaves excite the water molecules in the food, causing them to move faster and faster. Does she, as any high school science teacher knows she should, end the explanation here, perhaps noting, "increased temperature just is increased kinetic energy of the constituent molecules"? She does not. She goes on to explain that because the molecules move faster, they bump into each other more often, which increases the friction between molecules, and, as we all know, friction causes heat. *Betty Crocker still thinks heat is something other than molecular KE; something caused by but actually independent of molecular motion.*[3] Why do scientists not think so too?

Roughly, because explanations for heat phenomena—production by combustion, by the sun, and in chemical reactions; of conductivity, including conductivity in a vacuum, the variance in conductivity in distinct materials, and so on—are vastly simpler and more coherent on the assumption that heat is molecular energy of the constituent molecules. By contrast, trying to make the data fit with assumption that heat is some other thing caused by speeding up molecular motion is like trying to nail jelly to the wall.

If one is bound and determined to cleave to a caloric thermodynamics, one might, with heroic theory-constructing effort, pull it off. Converts, however, are improbable. The cost in coherence with the rest of scientific theory, not to mention with other observations, is extremely high. What would motivate paying that cost? Perhaps an iron-willed, written-in-blood resolve to maintain unsullied the intuition that heat *is what it is and not another thing*. In retrospect, and knowing what we now know, the idea that anyone would go to exorbitant lengths to defend heat intuition seems rather a waste of time.

In the case at hand, I am predicting that explanatory power, coherence, and economy will favor the hypothesis that awareness just is some pattern of activity in neurons. I may turn out to be wrong. If I am, it will not be because an introspectively based intuition is immutable, but because the science leads us in a different direction. If I am right, and certain patterns of brain activity are the reality behind the experience, this fact does not in and of itself change my experience and suddenly allow me (my brain) to view my brain as an MRI scanner or a neurosurgeon might view it. I will continue to have experiences in the regular old way, although to understand the neuronal reality of them, my brain needs to *have* lots of experiences and undergo lots of learning.

Finally, barring a jump to the dualist's horse, the idea that there has to be a bedrock of subjective appearance on which reality-appearance discoveries must ultimately rest is faintly strange. It seems a bit like insisting that "down" cannot be relative to where one is in space; down is down, by gosh and by golly. Or like insisting that time cannot be relative, that either two events happen at the same time or they do not, and that's that.

Humans are products of evolution; nervous systems have evolved in the context of competition for survival, in the struggle to succeed in the four Fs: feeding, fleeing, fighting, and reproducing. The brain's model of the external world enjoys improvement through appreciating various of reality-appearance distinctions; in short, through common critical reason. In the nature of things, it is quite likely that the brain's model of its internal world also allows for appearance-reality discoveries, at least because such distinctions would be a necessity for outwitting clever prey and predators, not to mention clever conspecifics. Even though the brain did not evolve to know the nature of the sun as it is known by a physicist, or to know itself as it is known by a neurophysiologist, in the right circumstances, it can come to know them anyhow (PM Churchland, 1993).

Impossible Because Consciousness Is a Virtual Machine

This is the view of Dennett (1992). Like Searle, Dennett is no dualist. Unlike Searle, who thinks that quite a lot, if not all, about consciousness can be discovered by neuroscience, Dennett has long been convinced that study of the brain itself—its physiology and anatomy—is largely a waste of time as far as understanding the nature of consciousness and cognition is concerned. Simplified, the crux of his idea is this: humans become conscious as they acquire language and learn to talk to themselves. What happens in this transformation is that a parallel machine (the neural networks of the brain) simulates a serial machine (operations are performed one at a time, in a sequence, according to rules, which may be recursive.)

By acquiring a language and then learning to speak silently to oneself, one allegedly creates a consciousness virtual machine in the brain. Dennett explains what this by means of a pivotal analogy: it is like creating a virtual machine for simulating piloting a plane on your desktop computer by installing software such as *Flight Simulator*. Consciousness bears the same relation to the brain as running the flight simulation bears to the events inside the computer.

Dennett's methodological moral is unambiguous: just as we cannot hope to learn anything much about the flight simulator (it scope and limits, how it works) by studying the computer's innards while it is running *Flight Simulator*, so we cannot hope to learn much about consciousness by studying the brain's innards while it is conscious. If we want to know about *Flight Simulator* and its many properties, the best we can do is study its performance; in a sense, there really is not anything else to *Flight Simulator* than its performance. We find it fruitful in talking about *Flight Simulator* to say things like "its altimeter registers altitude," but this does not mean that there is something in my computer that really is high in the sky or something that measures how high it really is. Such talk is simply an economical, convenient way of making sense of the computer's screen performance when it is running *Flight Simulator* software.

Ditto (more or less) for consciousness, in Dennett's view. The brain is the hardware on which the consciousness "software" runs, hence looking at the brain itself is not going to teach us much about the software itself. Even as it is mistaken to suppose the computer has a little runway hidden tucked inside that is rolled out when I press a button, so it is mistaken to think the brain really does anything like fill in the blind spot or fill in during seeing subjective motion as in a movie (PS Churchland and Ramachandran, 1993). Dennett believes he has shown us that there really is not so much in the way of inner experience to be explained after all. As with *Flight Simulator*, if we want to know about consciousness and its properties, it is performance under a variety of conditions that must be studied. Based on the performance we can of course infer the various computational properties of the software. *And that is all there will be to explaining consciousness.* Consequently, the tools of experimental psychology will suffice. The details of neuroscience might tell us something about how the software runs on the brain; that will not tell us anything about the nature of consciousness, but only about how the brain runs software. This, in capsule, is my understanding of the conviction that inspired Dennett to his book's title, *Consciousness Explained*.

How plausible is the Dennett story? My criticism here draws on work of Paul Churchland (1995) and focuses mainly on this question: is it remotely reasonable that, when we are conscious, the parallel machine (the brain) is simulating a serial machine? As an archival preliminary, however, note that Dennett's package has been subjected to intense and careful analysis. First, his claim that acquisition of human language is a necessary condition of human consciousness has been repeatedly challenged and thoroughly criticized (Flanagan, 1992; Block, 1993). Endlessly it has been noted that this seems to imply that preverbal infants are not conscious; that other animals such as chimpanzees and oranges are not conscious; that subjects with global aphasia or left hemispherectomies are not conscious. Briefly, Dennett's response is that, indeed, nonverbal subjects are not aware in the way a fully verbal human is aware; for example, they cannot think about whether interest rates will go down next month. Unfortunately, his response is tangential to the criticism. The issue is whether preverbal children and animals can be conscious of colors, sounds, smells, spatial extent, motion, being dizzy, feeling pain, and so on, in rather like the way I am conscious of them.

Second, Dennett's according preeminent status to linguistic activity and his correlative debunking of sensory experiences (e.g., filling in), feelings, and nonlinguistic cognition generally have been subjected to a constant barrage of complaints (Flanagan, 1992; Block, 1993; Searle, 1992). Regrettably, I can give here only a highly truncated version of the long and sometimes convoluted debates between Dennett and various critics. The heart of the complaints is that Dennett wrongly assumes that performance is all that needs explaining, that explaining *reports* of conscious experience is tantamount to explaining conscious experience itself. Dennett's core response here has been to wave off the complainers as having failed properly to understand him, scolding them for being still in the grip of bad old conceptual habits implying homunculi, ghosts in the machine, furtive Cartesianism, and kindred mistakes. Suffice to say that Dennett's if-you-disagree-you-have-misunderstood stance, although conceivably true of some critics, does not appear true of all.

Is a virtual serial machine necessary to get a one-after-another temporal ordering? Not at all. For example, it has been well known for at least eight years that neural nets with recurrent loops can yield temporal sequencing and do so very economically and elegantly (Singh, 1992; Mozer, 1992; Sutton, Mamelak, and Hobson, 1992). For a recent example, beautiful work in using real-valued genetic algorithms to evolve continuous-time recurrent neural networks capable of sequential behavior and learning has been done by (Beer 1995a,b; Beer and Gallagher, 1992) and other sequencing work has been done by Mozer (1992). Clearly, sequencing tasks per se do not imply the existence of a simulated serial machine (PS Churchland and Sejnowski, 1992).

Is a virtual serial machine necessary to get rule-following behavior as seen in linguistic performance? Not at all. Again, as Elman (1991) showed, recurrent neural nets can manage this very well (Mozer and Bachrach, 1991; Pollack, 1991; Giles et al, 1992; Jain, 1992; Pinkas, 1992; Sumida and Dyer, 1992). Is a virtual serial machine necessary to restrict a certain class of operations to one at a time? Not at all. First, a special class of operations could be the output of one network, albeit a widely distributed network. Second, they could be the output of a winner-take-all interaction between nets (Lange, 1992). And there are lots of other architectures for accomplishing this. The motor system probably functions thus, but there is no reason to think it simulates a serial machine (Viola, Lisberger, and Sejnowski, 1992; Berthier et al, 1992).

Third, should we assume that consciousness involves only one operation at a time? Almost certainly not. Granting that the attentional capacity is much smaller than the extraattentive capacity to represent, why conclude that we can attend to only one thing at a time? Verghese and Pelli (1992) concluded that the capacity of the attentional mechanism is limited to about 44 ± 15 bits per glimpse. They calculated the preattentive capacity to be much greater —about 2106 bits. Their data on the attentional capacity are consistent with paying attention to and being aware of more than one thing at a time. When I look at a bowl of colored M&Ms can I see more than one M&M at once? Probably.

Fourth, is the serial machine simulation necessary to enable recursive properties, such that one can be self-aware (e.g., to think about what one just said to oneself)? Not at all. Recurrent neural nets are powerful enough and complex enough to manage this very nicely. Indeed, recurrence probably is a key feature of various self-monitoring subsystems in the nervous system, including thermoregulation. Is there any rationale for saying that when we are conscious the brain must simulating a serial machine? I see none (PM Churchland, 1995). This does not entail that Dennett must be wrong, but only that we have no reason to think he is on the right track.

Impossible Because the Brain Is Not Smart Enough

Initially, this idea appears to be a modest acknowledgment of our limitations (McGinn, 1990). In fact, it is a powerful prediction based not on solid evidence, but on profound ignorance. For all we can be sure now, the prediction might be correct, but equally, it might very well be false. How feeble is our intelligence? How difficult is the problem? How could we possibly know that solving the problem is beyond our reach, no matter how science and technology develop? Inasmuch as it is not known that the brain is more complicated than it is smart, giving up on the attempt to find out how it works would be disappointing. On the contrary, as long as experiments continue to produce results that contribute to our understanding, why not keep going? (Flanagan, 1992).

THE BINDING PROBLEM

Coined by Christof von der Malsburg, the term binding problem was used first in the context of visual perception. During the last decade, however, its use has greatly expanded to include virtually any integrative task involving perception, memory, and representations generally. Sometimes sensorimotor integration is also considered a species of the binding problem. A highly simplified rendition of the problem can be stated briefly.

How does the brain integrate signals, separated in space and time, such that one experiences a unity? For example, in speech, there is integration across modalities (sight, sound), across time (understanding the sentence, the conversation), as well as within a modality (pitch, loudness, timbre). In vision, information from the two eyes is integrated in such a way that we can see objects in stereoscopic depth. Even though the pathways subserving color processing (parvocellular pathway) appears to be largely segregated from those involved in motion processing (magnocellular pathway), our visual experience is of a unified world; for instance, a blue ball moving diagonally down and a red cylinder moving up. Even though areas of the temporal lobe appear to be specialized for pattern-recognition tasks, whereas regions of the parietal lobe appear specialized for the spatial aspect of visual problem solving, we see a red square in the middle of the screen and a blue triangle lower down. Even though I have no perceptual experience of myself, and even though I fall into deep sleep, I have a representation of a unified self as a repository of memories, experiences, thoughts, and capacities. In addition, as von der Malsburg stressed, the possible combinations of color, shape, movement, location, and the like just within the visual domain is astronomical. Nevertheless, we do not run out of capacity to recognize. Consequently, we cannot expect to find a complete roster of dedicated neurons, each specialized for a particular combination features. Thus, the binding problem.

How does the brain solve its many binding problems? As a first pass, the answers would seem to lie in the brain's exploiting spatial properties of its organization or temporal properties of its organization, or both. The crude idea that the relevant representations are all congregated in a single, small anatomical region seems implausible, for it has been known since the early part of this century that the nervous system does not have such a region where it all comes together. Whatever the neurobiology of the solution, we can expect its anatomy to be distributed.

Still within the spatial dimension, it might be wondered whether registration of topographical maps in sensory structures might provide the answer. Although topographical mapping is not likely to be irrelevant, the secret cannot lie entirely there. Many difficulties cloud the spatial hypothesis, and most of them concern spatial resolution issues. To a first approximation, the more distant a sensory region from the primary region, in vision, for example, the larger the receptive field. The size of the receptive fields in inferotemporal cortex, for example, are on the order to 9 to 15 degrees of visual angle, and hence large enough to encompass a whole bowl full of M&Ms.

How might the brain exploit time to solve the problem? The matter is very puzzling, since different sensory systems have different conduction delays, different neurons have different conduction delays, and any given cortical neuron communicates with only a tiny subset of other cortical neurons. No obvious engineering solution exists, given the anatomy and physiology of the nervous system as we know it. As Carver Mead pointed out, however, and the idea has been echoed by many other electronics engineers, including Acre and Dayar, undoubtedly the answer does depend on exploiting the biophysics to manage time. For time is about the only thing the brain can play with to achieve widespread, complex integration in a fast-moving world. In different but complementary ways, Wolf Singer, Christof von der Malsburg, Francis Crick, Christof Koch, Antonio Damasio, and Rodolfo Llinás are each exploring how timing of neural events, such as synchrony of neuronal firing and entrainment by synchrony, might contribute to the solution(s).

It may be worth pointing out that the answer may not take the form of a mechanism that figures out what items should be bound and performs the binding on them. That idea's metaphorical geneolgy is linked to such activities as binding trout together in a line, or tiling a mosaic likeness of Caesar. A more fruitful approach may emphasize how the very structure of neuronal membrane and neuronal connectivity, given their orchestrated time constants, means that thalamocortical circuits, say, just do yield coherent vectors and trajectories. Such coherence may best be described by parameter spaces, and hence in terms of limits cycles and strange attractors. On this approach, the activity in the relevant well-orchestrated circuits just *is* what we call integration. When consciously experienced, the limit cycle activity just is the quality we refer to with the expression "perceptual unity." Under this characterization, the solution has a rather Kantian flavor, inasmuch as binding is less a process carried out by a dedicated binder than a dynamic property of the organization and structure of the brain itself, or as Kant might have preferred, of the "forms of intuition."

Undoubtedly the micromanagement of the various dynamic properties of neurons is a central and critical job that nervous systems must accomplish. Learning to get the timing right may be *the* central learning problem for brains. A neuron's temporal characteristics in responding to signals, integrating signals, and sending signals is the result of its various structural properties, including the number and arrangement of membrane channels with specific time constants, time constants of gene expression for relevant proteins, time variance of after-hyperpolarization, degree of myelinization, time constants of changes in synaptic reliability, relative position of synapses on dendrites, and soma, spine dynamics, and neuromodulatory time constants. Undoubtedly there are other biophysical variables as well (Llinás, 1988; figure 13.2). Now factor in the specific patterns of recurrent connections—a neuron onto itself as well as back to its input neurons—and it is evident that the dynamic properties of neuronal circuits are complex indeed.

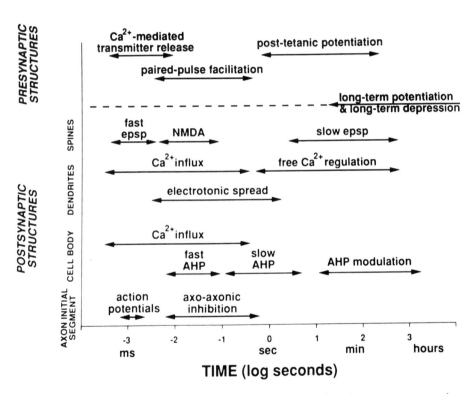

Figure 13.2 Space-time diagram plotting some of the physiological events occurring within neurons. Each process is represented by a horizontal line, arrows indicating the range of time scales over which the process takes place. The vertical scale locates the anatomical structure in which the process takes place. For example, the fast Na^+ spikes initiates in the axon hillock have a time scale of 1 msec. In contrast, Ca^{2+} influx through voltage-sensitive channels known to occur in both the cell bodies and the dendrites of some neurons has a much longer time scale. Some forms of after-hyperpolarization (AHP) following an action potential are activated by Ca^{2+} and have a much longer time course than the action potential itself. Changes in the synaptic efficacy, such as post-tetanic potentiation (PTP) and long term potentiation (LTP) can last for many minutes and hours. NMDA refers to a glutamate receptor that is important in triggering LTP. (From Churchland and Sejnowski, 1992)

CONCLUSION

Scientific discoveries frequently provoke a profound shift in how we think about our universe. In so shifting, they may reconfigure the very questions we ask (PM Churchland, 1995). Thus, after Copernicus, it was no longer worth asking what made the crystal spheres turn daily; after Harvey, it was no longer worth asking how the heart concocted animal spirits; once Newton framed the law of motion, no one cared about an object's natural place or about the properties of impetus; after Lavoisier, the problem of the negative weight of phlogiston could be safely ignored as misbegotten.

Coming to understand mental phenomena in the context of computational-cognitive neuroscience is potentially revolutionary. As we discover the properties of circuits and systems and how they achieve their macroeffects, doubtless some time-honored assumptions about our own nature will be reconfigured. More generally, it is probable that our commonly accepted ideas about reasoning, free will, the self, consciousness, and perception have no more integrity than prescientific ideas about substance, fire, motion, life, space, and time. We still have a long way to go, but the new convergence of research in neuroscience, psychology, and experimental modeling holds out the promise that at least some of the basic principles will be understood.

NOTES

1. Portions of this section are based on material drawn from my 1990 paper, Is neuroscience relevant to philosophy? *Can J Philos* 16:323–341.

2. Portions of the next three sections are based on my presidential address to the American Philosophical Association (PS Churchland 1994).

3. Paul Churchland made this discovery in our kitchen about eight years ago. It seemed to us a bang-up case of someone not really understanding the scientific explanation. Instead of thinking the thermodynamic theory through, Betty Crocker clumsily grafts it onto on old conception as though the old conception required no modification. Someone who thought electricity was caused by moving electrons would tell a comparable Betty Crocker story: voltage forces the electrons to move through the wire, and as they do so, they cause static electricity to build up, and a sparks then jump from electron to electron, on down the wire.

REFERENCES

Beer RD. (1995a). A dynamical systems perspective on agent-environment interaction. *Artif Intell* 72:173–215.

Beer RD. (1995b). On the dynamics of small continuous-time recurrent neural networks. *Adapt Behav* 3:471–511.

Beer RD, Gallagher JC. (1992). Evolving dynamical neural networks for adaptive behavior. *Adapt Behav* 1:91–122.

Bennett BM, Hoffman DD, Prakash C. (1989). *Observer mechanics*. Academic Press, San Diego.

Berthier NE, Singh SP, Barto AG, Houk JC. (1992). A cortico-cerebellar model that learns to generate distributed motor commands to control a kinematic arm. In: *Neural information processing systems 4*. JE Moody, SJ Hanson, RP Lippmann, eds. Morgan-Kaufman, San Mateo, CA, 611–618.

Bickle J. (1992). Revisionary physicalism. *Biol Philos* 7:411–430.

Block N. (1993). Consciousness ignored? Review of D.C. Dennett's *Consciousness explained*. *J Philos* 90(4):83–91.

Chalmers DJ. (1995). The puzzle of conscious experience. *Sci Am* 273:80–86.

Churchland PM. (1988). *Matter and consciousness*, 2nd ed. MIT Press, Cambridge.

Churchland PM. (1993). Evaluating our self conception. *Mind Language* 8:211–222.

Churchland PM. (1994). Betty Crocker's theory of the mind: A review of *The rediscovery of the mind*, by John Searle. *London Review of Books*, May.

Churchland PM. (1995). *The Engine of Reason, the Seat of the Soul*. MIT Press, Cambridge.

Churchland PM, Churchland PS. (1990). Intertheoretic reduction: A neuroscientist's field guide. *Semin Neurosci* 4:249–256.

Churchland PS. (1986). *Neurophilosophy*. MIT Press, Cambridge.

Churchland PS. (1987). Replies to comments. Symposium on Patricia Smith Churchland's *Neurophilosophy*. *Inquiry* 29:241–272.

Churchland PS. (1990). Is neuroscience relevant to philosophy? *Can J Philos* 16:323–341.

Churchland PS. (1994). Can neurobiology teach us anything about consciousness? Presidential address to the American Philosophical Association, Pacific division. In: *Proceedings and addresses of the American Philosophical Association*. Lancaster Press, Lancaster, PA, 23–40.

Churchland PS, Sejnowski TJ. (1989). Brain and cognition. In: *Foundations of cognitive science*. M Posner, ed. MIT Press, Cambridge, 245–300.

Churchland PS, Sejnowski TJ. (1992). *The computational brain*. MIT Press, Cambridge.

Churchland PS, Ramachandran VS. (1993). Filling-in: Why Dennett is wrong. In: *Dennett and his critics*. B Dahlbom, ed. Blackwells, Oxford, pp. 28–52.

Dennett DC. (1991). *Consciousness explained*. Little, Brown, Boston.

Elman JL. (1991). Distributed representations, simple recurrent networks, and grammatical structure. *Machine Leaning* 7:195–225.

Feyerabend PK. (1981). *Philosophical papers*, Vols. 1 and 2. Cambridge University Press, Cambridge.

Finlay BL, Darlington RB. (1995). Linked regularities in the development and evolution of the brain. *Science* 268:1578–1584.

Flanagan O. (1992). *Consciousness reconsidered*. MIT Press, Cambridge.

Flanagan O. (1996). Prospects for a unified theory of consciousness, or, what dreams are made of. In: *Scientific approaches to the question of consciousness: 25th Carnegie symposium on cognition*. J Cohen, J Schooler, eds. L. Erlbaum, Hillsdale, NJ.

Fodor J. (1990). *A theory of content and other essays*. MIT Press, Cambridge, MA.

Giles CL, Miller CB, Chen D, Sun GZ, Chen HH, Lee YC. (1992). Extracting and learning and unknown grammar with recurrent neural nets. In: *Neural information processing systems 4*. JE Moody, SJ Hanson, RP Lippmann, eds. Morgan-Kaufman, San Mateo, CA: 317–324.

Grush R, Churchland PS. (1995). Gaps in Penrose's toilings. *J Consciousness Stud.* 2:10–29.

Hildreth E, Koch C. (1987).

Jain AN. (1992). Generalizing performance in PARSEC—A structured connectionist parsing architecture. In: *Neural information processing systems 4.* JE Moody, SJ Hanson, RP Lippmann, eds. Morgan-Kaufman, San Mateo, CA, 209–216.

Kaas JH, Merzenich MM, Killackey HP. (1983). The reorganization of somatosensory cortex following peripheral nerve damage in adult and developing mammals. *Annu Rev Neurosci* 6:325–356.

Lakoff G. (1987). *Women, fire, and dangerous things.* Chicago University Press, Chicago.

Lange TE. (1992). Dynamically adaptive winner-take-all networks. In: *Neural information processing systems 4.* JE Moody, SJ Hanson, RP Lippmann, eds. Morgan-Kaufman, San Mateo, CA, 341–348.

Llinás RR. (1988). The intrinsic physiological properties of mammalian neurons: Insights into central nervous system function. *Science* 242:1654–1664.

McGinn C. (1990). *The problem of consciousness.* Blackwells, Oxford.

Mozer MC. (1992). Induction of multiscale temporal structure. In: *Neural information processing systems 4.* JE Moody, SJ Hanson, RP Lippmann, eds. Morgan-Kaufman, San Mateo, CA, 275–282.

Mozer MC, Bachrach J. (1991). SLUG: A connectionist architecture for inferring the structure of fine-estate environments. *Machine Learning* 7:139–160.

Penrose R. (1989). *The emperor's new mind.* Oxford University Press, Oxford.

Penrose, R. (1994). *The shadows of the mind.* Oxford University Press, Oxford.

Pinkas G. (1992). Constructing proofs in symmetric networks. In: *neural information processing systems 4.* JE Moody, SJ Hanson, RP Lippmann, eds. Morgan-Kaufman, San Mateo, CA, 217–224.

Pollack JB. (1991). The induction of dynamical recognizers. *Machine Learning* 7:227–252.

Quine WVO. (1961). *Word and object.* MIT Press, Cambridge.

Ramachandran VS. (1993). Behavioral and MEG correlates of neural plasticity in the adult human brain. *Proc Natl Acad Sci* 90:10413–10420.

Roche E. (1981). Prototype classification and logical classification: The two systems. In: *New trends in cognitive representation: Challenges to Piaget's theory,* E Scholnik, ed. Laurence Erlbaum Associates, Hillsdale, NJ. pp 73–86.

Schaffner KF. (1993). Theory structure, reduction, and disciplinary integration in biology. *Biol Philos* 8:319–348.

Searle JR. (1992). *The rediscovery of the mind.* MIT Press, Cambridge.

Singh SP. (1992). The efficient learning of multiple task sequences. In: *Neural information processing systems 4.* JE Moody, SJ Hanson, RP Lippmann, eds. Morgan-Kaufman, San Mateo, CA, 251–258.

Sumida RA, Dyer MG. (1992). Propagation filters in PDS networks for sequencing and ambiguity resolution. In: *Neural information processing systems 4.* JE Moody, SJ Hanson, RP Lippmann, eds. Morgan-Kaufman, San Mateo, CA, 233–240.

Sutton, JP, Mamelak AN, Hobson JA. (1992). Network model of state-dependent sequencing. In: *Neural information processing systems 4.* JE Moody, SJ Hanson, RP Lippmann, eds. Morgan-Kaufman, San Mateo, CA, 283–290.

Taylor C. (1985). *Philosophy and the human sciences: Philosophical Papers*, vol. 2. Cambridge University Press, Cambridge.

Vergehsi P, Pelli DG. (1992). The information capacity of visual attention. *Vision Res* 32:983–995.

Viola PA, Lisberger SG, Sejnowski TJ. (1992). Recurrent eye tracking network using a distributed representation of image motion. In: *Neural information processing systems 4*. JE Moody, SJ Hanson, RP Lippmann, eds. Morgan-Kaufman, San Mateo, CA, 380–387.

Wright R. (1995). It's all in our heads. Review of *The engine of reason, the seat of the soul by P. M. Churchland. New York Times Book Review*, July 9, p. 1.

Contributors

Albert S. Bregman
Department of Psychology
McGill University
Montreal, Quebec, Canada

Patricia S. Churchland
Department of Philosophy
University California at San Diego
La Jolla, California

Martha Constantine-Paton
Department of Biology
Yale University
New Haven, Connecticut

Antonio R. Damasio
Department of Neurology
Division of Behavioral Neurology
and Cognition
University of Iowa College of
Medicine
Iowa City, Iowa

Howard Eichenbaum
Center for Behavioral Neuroscience
State University of New York at
Stony Brook
Stony Brook, New York

Rodolfo R. Llinás
New York University Medical
Center
Department of Physiology and
Neuroscience
New York, New York

Nikos K. Logothetis
Division of Neuroscience
Baylor College of Medicine
Houston, Texas

Stephen McAdams
Laboratoire de Psychologic
Expérimentale (CNRS)
Université René Descartes and
IRCAM
Paris, France

Michael M. Merzenich
W. M. Keck Center for Integrative
Neuroscience
Coleman Laboratory
University of California at San
Francisco
San Francisco, California

Vilayanur S. Ramachandran
Brain and Perception Laboratory
Center for Research on Brain and
Cognition
La Jolla, California

John A. Simmons
Department of Neuroscience
Brown University
Providence, RI

Wolfe Singer
Max-Planck Institute for Brain
Research
Frankfurt, Germany

Christoph von der Malsburg
Institute for Neuroinformatics
Ruhr-University, Bochum, Germany
and Department of Computer Science and
Section for Neurobiology
University of Southern California
Los Angeles, California

Contributors

Index

Binding window
  clutter interference and, 235, 242
  size of, 225–226, 227, 242
    perception of details and, 248
    width of discharge and, 222
Blindsight, 29
Botte, M. C., 272
Brain function
  noninvasive study technologies, 7
  reality emulation, 3
Brain, human. *See also* Image making
  dynamic, interactive view of, 37
  evolutionary changes in, ix, 284
  integration of signals, 297
Bregman, A. S., 252, 254–255
Bunsey, M., 195, 198

Ca fluxes
  NMDA-mediated, 90
  synaptic efficacy and, 84, 88–89
  in synaptic plasticity, 83, 90
Callostomy patients, harmonic perception in,
    262–263
Caloric-induced nystagmus, 49
Caloric-induced reversible hyperamnesia,
    anosognosia and, 51
Catastrophic reaction, 38, 44
Central nervous system. *See also* Plasticity
  as a closed system, 4
  competitive synaptogenic mechanism, 87
  neural activity and synaptic plasticity, 83
Chalmers, David, 289
Churchland, Paul, 295
Classic neural networks. *See also* Neural
    networks
  absence of flexible, dynamic binding
    mechanism in, 135–136
  as cognitive architecture, 132–134
    problems with, 134
  as dynamic link architecture, 136–137
  neural signal organization, 141
Closed-system intrinsic hypothesis, 4–5
CNS. *See* Central nervous system
Cognition
  biologically based theory, 54
  integration of sensory events in, 14
  as an intrinsic CNS property, 6–7
  as an a priori brain property, 5
  unity of, 5
Cognitive architecture, 131–132. *See also*
    Dynamic link architecture
  classic neural networks as, 132–134
Cognitive binding. *See also* Binding problem;
    Cortical binding hypothesis

coherent 40-Hz oscillations in, 9–12
  through cooperative neuronal interactions,
    104–105
Cognitive psychology
  goals of auditory, 251
  multidimensional scaling techniques,
    264–266
Cohen, N. J., 186
Coherence. *See* Neuronal-coherence
    oscillation, cognition and; Temporal
    coherence
Coincidence-detecting neurons
  countervailing intrinsic latency differences
    in, 223
  delay-coincidence mechanisms, 227–
    228
  for determining echo delay, 230, 232
  to evaluate signal correlations, 142
  time-compensated convergence of inputs
    to, 224
Coincident input selection, 73
Compositional property, 203–204
  audition as, 207–210
  predictive power, 206–207
  in speech and sentence perception,
    210–211
  underlying causal factors, 216
Coincident input coselection, 68
Consciousness
  Edelman proposal for primary, 26
  electromagnetism and, 290
  language as condition of, 294–296
  neural mechanisms, 19, 24
  as a neurobiological phenomenon, 290
  physicists' views of, 289–290
  single brain region view of, 22
  virtual machine theory of, 294
    objections to, 295–296
Consciousness Explained (Dennett), 295
Context-dependent analysis, 1
Convergence zones, 21, 25
Cortex
  piriform, in olfaction, 177, 178
  temporal dispersion of visual responses
    across, 227
Cortical binding hypothesis, 12–14
Cortical mapping
  input gating effects, 71
  short- and long-term dynamics, 62–63
Cortical response specificity, 68, 72
Cortico-cortical connections
  abnormalities in, 117
  rearrangement of with strabismus, 114
  in response synchronization, 107, 113

Glutamate receptors, developmental changes in, 90–94. *See also* N-Methyl-D-aspartate receptor
Glutamatergic synaptic transmission, 86–90
Goldstein, K., 38
Grandmother cell argument, 2, 65
GRBFs. *See* Generalized radial basis functions

Haberly, L. B., 178
Harmonic progression
  right hemispheric lateralization of expectancies, 264
  in tonal music, 261
Heat phenomena, 293
Hebb, D. O., 87, 105, 133
Hemineglect syndrome, 40, 45, 56n
Hemispheric specialization, 41–43
  anosognosia and, 42–43
  coping strategies, 42–43
  humor and, 53
  mirror-symmetrical points, 43
  with multiple personalities, 44
Hippocampus. *See also* Theta rhythm
  binding problem, 192–198
  in establishment of relational representation, 192–198
  long-term potentiation and patterned stimulation, 183
  olfactory processing, 180–192
    effect of damage on, 185–192
  in paired associate learning, 192–198
  role in declarative memory, 187
  synaptic plasticity in, 183
Homunculus, 22
Humor
  biological theories of, 52–54
  as a defense mechanism, 53–54

Image making
  breakup by temporal dissociation of neural responses, 220
  definition of image, 19
  early sensory cortices, 19–21, 25
  topographically organized representations, 20
Imaging techniques, 54
Inertia, vision vs. audition, 213
Inferotemporal cortex
  in object recognition, 160–162
  shape selectivity, 161
  view selectivity for three-dimensional objects, 162–163, 164
Intralaminar thalamic complex, 6–7

Jackendoff, R., 268–275
Jacob, Francois, 284
Jordan, D., 257

Kagan, Jerome, 22
Kant, I., 4, 53
Kinsbourne, M., 43
Koch, C., 12, 14, 125
Krumhansl, C. L., 260, 261, 262

Language
  as condition of human consciousness, 294–296
  self and, 22, 26
Lashley, K., 64–65
Latency dispersion
  physiologically generated, 230, 232
  testing in sensory systems, 225, 226
Lateral geniculate nucleus (LGN), 87
Laughter, biological theories of, 52–54
Lerdahl, F., 268–275
LFP. *See* Local field potential responses (LFP)
LGN. *See* Lateral geniculate nucleus (LGN)
Light energy in vision, 212
Llinás, R., 21
Local field potential responses (LFP), 108
Long-term depression (LTD), patterns of stimulation producing, 88
Long-term memory
  mechanisms of organization, 133
  organization mechanism, 132
  synaptic strengths, 133
Long-term potentiation (LTP), 88
  hippocampal, 183
  NMDA receptor function and, 91
LTD. *See* Long-term depression (LTD)
LTP. *See* Long-term potentiation (LTP)

Magnetic resonance imaging (MRI), 7, 283
Magnetoencephalography (MEG), 7–8, 283
  coherent 40-Hz oscillations, 9–12
Matter and Consciousness (Churchland), 290
Mead, Carver, 298
MEG. *See* Magnetoencephalography (MEG)
Memory. *See also* Long-term memory; Odor memory; Short-term memory
  declarative, 186
    role of hippocampus in, 187
  hippocampal-dependent vs. -independent, 186–187
  procedural, 185–186
Metaself, 25
Metric hierarchy in music, 271–272

conditioning-stimulus-specific changes, 74
within cortical nets, 69–70
cortical representational, 61
features of, 67–73
functional activity and, 76
implications for system organization and
    coordination, 74–75
of olfactory bulb, 179
refined, 145
in somatosensory cortex, 8
Polymodal integration, timing for, 21
Positron emission tomography (PET), 7, 283
Premotor template, 3, 5–6
Prosopagnosia, 29
Pseudo-mirror symmetry, 156–158
viewpoint-invariant cells and, 165, 169
Psychology
auditory, 251, 264–266
behavioral studies in, 282
neuroscience and, 291–292
reductionist research strategy, 285
revisionary prediction, 286

Radial basis functions, 149
Rapid synaptic modification hypothesis,
    140–141, 142
Rapid-eye-movement (REM), 51
RBFs. *See* Radial basis functions
Reaction formation, 48
Recognition of visual objects. *See* Object
    recognition
Reductionism, 284–287
objections to research strategy
    absurdity of goals, 287–290
    consciousness as virtual machine
        argument, 294–296
    epithet category error, 288–289
    identifying consciousness with brain
        activities, 292–294
    limitations of intelligence argument, 297
    multiple realizability argument, 290–292
Reflections, vision vs. audition, 212–213
Relational coding, 66–67
Repressed memories in dreams and
    wakefulness, 52
Response synchronization
adaptive synapses, 107
attentional mechanisms and, 119–121
contribution of cortico-cortical connections
    to, 107, 113
in creation of discrete entities, 228
dependence on stimulus configuration,
    109–113

distributed grouping operations, 121–125
experimental testing of predictions, 106–
    109
interhemispheric, 113–114
as a mechanism for response selection,
    105–106
nature and specificity of connections,
    113–114
oscillatory activity and, 117–119
to patterns with temporal structure, 120
perceptual disturbances and impaired,
    114–117
reduction by pharmacological inactivation
    of motion-sensitive cells, 123
self-organizing process, 107
zero-phase lag, 118–119
Rosenblatt, Frank, 134
Rules of simplicity, vision vs. audition,
    211–213

SC. *See* Superior colliculus, synaptogenic
    changes in
Scene representation
definition of scene, 143
dynamic link architecture, 142–149
reconstructing objects from, 220–228
Scene segmentation in dynamic link
    architecture, 143
Schilder, P., 48
Schopenhauer, A., 53
Schriner, Christoph, 73
Scientific explanation, 204
Searle, John, 292, 294
Self
cognitive-neural, 23
definition, 21–22
historical development of, 24
nonhomuncular, 23–24
spatial homunculus solution, 22
subjectivity and, 21–26
third party disposition, 25
universal emergence of, 22
Self-deception, biological theory of, 40–42
Sensory segmentation
binding problem, 102
coherent 40-Hz oscillations in, 9–12
Dalmation dog example, 125
to manage attention, 120
Sensory systems, constructive capability of,
    216
Sentence perception, composition in, 211
Sequential similarity in auditory perception,
    214

Serafine, M. L., 274
Shape selectivity
    inferotemporal cortex in, 161
    transformations in, 205–206
Shepard, R. N., 257
Short-term memory
    data structure, 134
    mechanisms of organization, 133
    neural firing rates, 133
Signal correlations
    in binding, 297
    connectivity patterns, 142
    between descriptors and referents, 143
    in dynamic link architecture, 137–139,
        141–142
    in neural dynamics, 141–142
Somatoparaphrenia, 30
Sound structures, cultural differences, 252
Speech perception
    amplitude of single syllables, 210–211
    composition in, 210–211
    pattern of stress, 210
    signal integration, 297
Stent, G. S., 87–88
Stoeckig, K., 262
Strabismus, rearrangement of cortico-cortical
        connections in, 114
Stroke
    anosognosia with, 37–40
    laterality defects in depression with, 43
Subjectivity
    body signaling and, 24
    mechanisms of emergence, 24–26
    and self, 21–26
Summation of amplitudes, 212
Superior colliculus, synaptogenic changes in,
        93–94
Superposition problem, 105
Surface ambiguity in visual and auditory
        perception, 211–213
Synaptic activity
    adaptive, 107
    in neuromuscular junction, 84–85
    neurophysiological postulate of learning,
        87–88
Synaptic plasticity
    AChR in controlling, 84–86
    adult and developmental forms of, 83
    Ca fluxes and changes in postsynaptic, 90
    developmentally regulated activity-
        dependent, 94
    glutamatergic synaptic transmission and,
        86–90

hippocampal, 183
    in long-term memory, 133
    loss of CNS potential for, 83
    selective presentation for protection of,
        94–95
Synaptogenesis, 83
Synchronization of neuronal response. *See*
    Response synchronization
Syncopation, 272
Syndactyly, surgical correction of, 8
Synfire chains, 142

Temporal binding, 137
    clutter interference as, 241, 247–248
    in echolocation, 240–248
    hierarchy, 138
Temporal coherence
    40-Hz oscillations, 9–12
    detecting, 225–226
    across sets of neurons, 219–220
    in thalamocortical circuits, 298
    transient or oscillatory responses in,
        225–226
Temporal feature-binding hypothesis,
        221–223
    auditory examples, 227–228
    response timing, 228
    testing, 223–228
Tetrodotoxin (TTX), eye-specific dominance
        effects, 87
Thalamocortical system
    cognitive role, 6
    coherence in, 298
    neuronal oscillations, 9
    in olfaction, 177–179
    oscillation near 40 Hz, 14
    time coherence, 8–9
Theta rhythm
    discriminative behaviors, 181, 183
    in nonprimate mammalian limbic system,
        181
    sniff cycles and, 181
Timbre hierarchies, 264–266
Tonal music
    generative theory of, 268–276
    harmonic progression in, 261
    pitch relation systems, 256–257, 259–
        260
Topographical mapping
    of images, 20
    in olfaction, 176–177
    spatial resolution issues, 298
Transparency, vision vs. audition, 212

Trivers, R., 40–41
TTX, eye-specific dominance effects, 87

Unconscious mind, 29

View selectivity
  developmental stages, 166, 169
  to novel objects, 166, 170
  for three-dimensional objects, 162–163,
    164
Virtual machine theory of consciousness, 294
  objections to, 295–296
Virtual reality
  amputation of phantom limb using, 31–33
  relief of phantom limb pain relief with, 34
Virtual serial machine, 26
  anosognosia and, 45–46
Vision. *See also* Object recognition
  vs. audition, 211–213
  connectivity patterns, 121
  identifying neurons with abnormal
    receptive field properties, 115
  vs. olfactory processing, 178
  opaqueness and transparency in, 212
  signal integration, 297
  simplicity rules, 211–213
  surface ambiguity in, 211–213
  use of transformations in, 205–207
Visual awareness, Crick's hypothesis, 26

Zatorre, R. J., 264